DR. HEINERMAN'S

ANTI-AGING
REMEDIES

JOHN HEINERMAN, Ph.D.

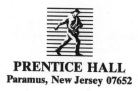

PRENTICE HALL
Paramus, New Jersey 07652

Library of Congress Cataloging-in-Publication Data

Heinerman, John.
    [Encyclopedia of anti-aging remedies]
    Dr. Heinerman's encyclopedia of anti-aging remedies
      p. cm.
    Includes index.
    ISBN 0-13-234212-X (pbk.)
    1. Longevity–Encyclopedias. 2. Aging–Encyclopedias. I. Title
    [RA776.75.H45 1997]
    612.6'8'03–dc21   97-29899
                                                    CIP

The information presented in this book is designed to help you make informed decisions about your health. It is not intended as a substitute for medical care nor a manual for self-treatment. If you feel that you have a medical problem, seek professional medical advice promptly.

Printed in the United States of America

10 9 8 7 6 5 4 3 2

ISBN 0-13-234212-X (p)

ATTENTION: CORPORATIONS AND SCHOOLS

Prentice Hall books are available at quantity discounts with bulk purchase for educational, business, or sales promotional use. For information, please write to: Prentice Hall Career & Personal Development Special Sales, 240 Frisch Court, Paramus, NJ 07652. Please supply: title of book, ISBN number, quantity, how the book will be used, date needed.

PRENTICE HALL
Career & Personal Development
Paramus, NJ 07652
A Simon & Schuster Company

On the World Wide Web at http://www.phdirect.com

Prentice Hall International (UK) Limited, *London*
Prentice Hall of Australia Pty. Limited, *Sydney*
Prentice Hall Canada, Inc., *Toronto*
Prentice Hall Hispanoamericana, S.A., *Mexico*
Prentice Hall of India Private Limited, *New Delhi*
Prentice Hall of Japan, Inc., *Tokyo*
Simon & Schuster Asia Pte. Ltd., *Singapore*
Editora Prentice Hall do Brasil, Ltda., *Rio de Janeiro*

In admiration of

Wilford Woodruff, Lorenzo Snow, George Q. Cannon,
and Joseph F. Smith

*"I notice that when you retire, you keel over. Therefore,
I have no intention of [ever] retiring."*

—Alistair Cooke,
age 88, former host of PBS "Masterpiece
Theater" (as quoted by him on the ABC
Evening News for Friday, March 22, 1996).

Other Books by the Author

Heinerman's Encyclopedia of Juices, Teas, and Tonics
Heinerman's New Encyclopedia of Fruits and Vegetables
Heinerman's Encyclopedia of Healing Herbs and Spices
Heinerman's Encyclopedia of Nuts, Berries, and Seeds
Heinerman's Encyclopedia of Healing Juices

Contents

Foreword

Foreword

🌺 TEN IDEALS TOWARD A MORE YOUTHFUL LIFESTYLE
BY JACOB HEINERMAN, AGE 83

When my son John invited me to write the Foreword to his book on anti-aging, it took me a little by surprise. I wasn't quite prepared for his request, but agreed to do it anyway. I asked him what he would like to see included. He told me, "Why don't you just write down the ten most important things that have kept you young in mind and heart and relatively youthful in your body?"

So I took a few days to give all of this some serious thought, and finally came up with some items that I believe have helped to keep me young in spite of my advanced years. Obviously, no one can expect to remain young forever without old age eventually catching up sooner or later. But, at least, in my case, I've been able to *substantially slow down* the time that the process usually takes.

And it is this *slowing down*, I honestly think, that one can reasonably hope for and expect from reading my son's book, as well as following some of the simple suggestions I've listed here that have worked well for me in my own life.

I. *Be cheerful.* Let your heart be filled with sunshine. It is better than any tonic!

II. *Love people.* Forget yourself and help someone each and every day.

III. *Find peace.* Work in your flower or vegetable garden. There is much contentment to be found in working in the bosom of

Mother Earth—her soil—where life and love are always found.

IV. *Eat live food.* By consuming as much live, raw foods as possible, you will be renewing your physical body each and every day.

V. *Live a simple life.* It will keep the nervous system functioning smoothly.

VI. *Pursue pet therapy.* Keep some animals on the premises. It doesn't matter whether it is a dog, cat, parakeet, turtle, goldfish, or even a pot-bellied pig, so long as you can love and communicate with them.

VII. *Live outdoors.* Do as much living outside the walls of your home as you can. Take a walk in the evenings. If feasible, have a patio and spend time there every night in good weather. You will find it most relaxing.

VIII. *Meditate often.* Silence puts us in tune with the Infinite.

IX. *Exercise daily.* Regular physical workouts of some kind, that are simple and easy to do, will tone up your whole body. By exercising often, your system will feel recharged.

X. *Feel good about yourself.* By thinking good thoughts, feeling good emotions, and doing good deeds, you will radiate a peaceful and calm influence that will benefit others as well as yourself.

Oh, and one more thing. I have discovered in my own life that whenever I'm thinking about others more than myself, I feel a lot more invigorated. On the other hand, selfishness represents contracted feelings and narrow-mindedness. It also makes a person older. But caring for others makes you feel young all over again.

Jacob Heinerman, Age 83
Father of the author

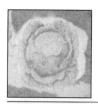

Age Spots

"HOW ONE PORTRAIT ARTIST PREVENTED AGE PIGMENTS IN HIS SKIN TISSUE"

🌿 PORTRAITS OF THE WEALTHY

I met David Kane shortly after he had celebrated his 101st birthday in his Miami Beach, Florida apartment. The place looked like an art gallery with paintings everywhere—they hung on the walls or else rested on shelves and a portion of his wood floor. He was then working on several paintings at once.

"Don't you ever get confused as to which scene belongs on which canvas?" I asked curiously.

"No, not at all," this robust centenarian informed me. "I somehow manage to keep everything in perspective and place things where they rightfully belong."

1

He then told me about some of the portraits he had painted years ago for some of New York's most famous financiers. "I painted some of the Rockefellers, a couple of the Vanderbilts, and yes, the old man J. P. Morgan himself. But in my earlier years back then, there was so damned much prejudice against us Jews, that I decided to play it safe and signed my portraits simply as 'D. E. Kane' so no one would suspect what religion I really was from. Clever devil, wasn't I?"

ASTONISHINGLY GOOD HEALTH

I was amazed to find that Mr. Kane did *not* wear *any* hearing aids or reading glasses, didn't use a cane or shuffle, and walked in large strides with ramrod straightness. He told me he never drank or smoked and only ate light meals with very little meat. "I only eat animal flesh," he said, "during the winter time. And then it is sparingly and, of course, always kosher."

I also noticed a complete absence of the ugly brown age spots on the backs of both hands, that are so common with older people. He noticed my glance down in that direction and answered me before the question was put forth. "I think I can attribute my lack of them to a couple of things. First of all, I've tried to stay away from fried food. I think that hurts the liver and produces a reaction in the pigments of the skin sooner or later. Another thing I've done for many decades is take some dandelion root or peach leaves. I know for a fact, that they've helped keep my liver always in great shape."

In the beginning he took them as teas. He made the dandelion by simmering 2 tablespoons of chopped root in $1^1/_2$ pints of boiling water for 10 minutes, and then steeping the mixture for another 10 minutes, before straining and drinking 1 to 2 cups each day. He followed the same pattern for the peach leaves, except they wouldn't be simmered, only steeped for 20 minutes and taken in the same amount. But in the last couple of decades he switched to take gelatin capsules of both herbs, claiming it was more convenient than always making the teas. He took two capsules of each every day with a meal. He said the morning was the best time to do this.

"Another thing I've done over the years is to rub some gel from one of my aloe vera plants over my skin a couple of times a week," he related. "I also try to avoid over-exposure to the sun and will sometimes wear light cotton work gloves and a long-sleeved shirt and hat to protect my hands, arms, and head from getting burned."

I cordially thanked him for his time and information. Here was one man who seemed to have beaten old age pretty well and still lived long enough to tell others about how he had done it.

Alleviating Allergies/Asthma/Bronchitis

"WHAT THE REAL BETTY CROCKER DOES TO PREVENT RESPIRATORY DISORDERS"

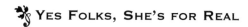 YES FOLKS, SHE'S FOR REAL

Way back in 1921 some executives at General Mills decided to create a fictional character to appear on boxes of some of their products. She was a white woman, somewhere between 40 and 55 years of age, who looked like the All-American mom. It has been said that for those of us who happen to be Caucasian, "there was a little bit of everybody's mother in Betty Crocker," the quintessential American housewife and homebody.

As the years passed, however, there were slightly different versions of her to reflect the ever-changing American society. In 1995 General Mills decided to do an eighth version of this great American advertising icon. Word was sent out through the media of a contest the company was running in which 75 lucky women would be selected to help create an entirely new image.

Among the many thousands who entered was a retired home-maker from the "old money" Holladay district of South Salt Lake right here in my own state of Utah. Actually, she was nom-inated by a niece and sister-in-law residing in Michigan and only found out about it later on when an official from General Mills called to confirm that she was one of the fortunate few to make the final cut of 75 women. A professional photographer took her portrait and it was sent back to the huge food conglomerate.

"Sometime Friday morning, January 12, 1996, I received a call notifying me that I had been one of the lucky winners of the contest," an obviously pleased Mrs. Crocker told me in an interview on Wednesday, March 20th of that Spring. "I was both ecstatic, overwhelmed, and confused all at once. It wasn't until I learned *who* had nominated me that everything became clear."

She also remembered that the person calling her with the good news, made a "big deal out of my name, the fact that I was a *real life* Betty Crocker, and would be turning 75 this same year that General Mills was celebrating their own Betty's 75th birthday." But the coincidences don't just end there. "I've always loved to cook and read every recipe book I can get my hands on. I've been happily married to David Crocker for over 50 years now and am the mother of four boys and the grandmother to four wonderful grandchildren. Except for a brief stint at General Motors as a comptometer operator—that was something like a glorified slide rule before we had pocket calculators—when David and I first got married, I've always been a stay-at-home wife and mother. I've enjoyed raising our kids, cooking for my family, and cleaning the house."

Here, she took a momentary pause of reflection, then added, "Not all the time, mind you, but long enough to have been content with staying at home and letting my husband go out and work to support our family. To keep busy, I've worked in our garden and small orchard for many years, and have bottled thousands of glass quart jars of fruits and vegetables and jams and jellies. When I wasn't doing this, I kept myself busy knitting. I learned the craft as a girl of 16 from a Miss Benson in Michigan, who was somewhere in her late 60s or early 70s. She taught me well and some of my knitted items—a three-colored sweater, for instance—have taken first place at the Utah State Fair."

The *real* Betty Crocker was born Betty Specht, but "never dreamed of becoming such a celebrity when I married David [Crocker]. It's been a fun experience, though, I'll have to admit. Something to share with my family, friends, and neighbors and those we know at Christ Methodist Church [which] we attend regularly."

🦎 WHAT UTAH'S VERSION DOES FOR MAINTAINING GOOD RESPIRATORY HEALTH

"I think part of the reason we're not bothered with respiratory disorders," Mrs. Crocker pointed out during the interview, "is that we tend to laugh a lot. I honestly believe that laughing is good exercise for the lungs, besides making you feel better emotionally." Taking that much air in and letting it out again during a good laugh, she figured, "has to somehow help make them stronger."

Betty also thought that walking has a lot to do with how weak or strong your respiratory system is. "My husband and I are walkers from the word go. We *love* to walk and do it every chance we get." She said they both average between 1 and 2 miles a day in a grassy area near their home lined with trails that are suitable for doing this.

But what I found intriguing were the *forms* of walking employed. "We usually start out with aggressive strides for the first mile or so," she continued, "before slowing down to a more subdued stroll. After some of this, we might then pick up the pace again for a little bit, before finishing off with some more leisure walking."

This back-and-forth pace change from strong to mild walking, done two or three times in a single session, gives the lungs a metabolic workout at varied speeds. "It's comparable to other forms of physical activity," one fitness expert told me. "You always follow up an aggressive period [of exercise] with a short 'cool down' that relaxes the muscles. This way you won't wear the muscles out." The same principle applies with the respiratory system.

Betty Crocker found there is "a real pleasure that comes with walking outdoors." She believed it allows us to experience the beauty and diversity of our surroundings and somehow helps us establish contact not only with our environment but with ourselves and each other. "I think we're more neighborly because we always walk," she added. There is a small but growing body of scientific literature to back her up on this point. The data suggest that combined spiritual and physical benefits are easier to achieve with outdoor, rather than indoor, exercise. Little wonder then that outdoor walking has now become the fastest growing fitness activity in America.

ADDITIONAL EVIDENCE THAT WALKING KEEPS YOU YOUNG

In science or medicine it's always nice to have more than one source of information to draw from. "The more, the merrier," as the old adage goes. From my voluminous files on anti-aging, which span *several* full filing cabinet drawers, I pulled interviews I conducted with two very old people back in 1985. The first one was an international telephone call made to John Evans of Swansea, Wales, who then had just turned 108 (he finally passed away in his 112th year). At the time he was living with his 74-year-old son and his wife. The second interview was in person with Maudie Ryder, who celebrated her 106th Christmas with her daughter Hallalene Ryder in Holladay, a somewhat wealthy suburb of Salt Lake City.

Mr. Evans gave his rules for a long life: don't smoke, drink or swear, but always treat yourself to honey, an onion, and a song every day. Ms. Ryder attributed her long life to many things, including clean living and a clean mind. "I used to say I didn't know how to find fault in people," she told me.

But the chief common denominator shared between them was *walking.* Each one managed to average at least a mile a day. But, unlike the Crockers, they were more into the strolling phase on account of their extremely advanced years. Furthermore, they were big fans of colored vegetables and some berries, both obviously rich in the wonderful antioxidant proanthocyanidins. And neither one of them ever had a history of allergies, asthma, or bronchitis. "Isn't it just wonderful to be able to breathe without any impediments?" the chipper Mr. Evans queried me in his heavily accented English. Then, he added as an afterthought to something mentioned earlier: "I think there should be no cursing and swearing in one's life; it disturbs the nerves, you know." The ever-smiling Ms. Ryder thought that the reason some of her great-grandchildren were now troubled with allergies and asthma was because "they don't eat right, don't eat enough vegetables and, for sure, don't walk enough either."

It's from the simple evidence of good folks like these that we've learned what it takes to *both* prevent as well as treat allergies, asthma, and bronchitis.

ONE.   Walk daily for at least an hour.

TWO.   Work outside as much as possible.

THREE.   Eat a variety of *colored* fruits and vegetables.

FOUR.   Don't allow yourself to get excited.

FIVE.   Don't consume sugary junk foods or beverages. (This last one is my own contribution.)

(For more information on walking see OBESITY.)

But this isn't the only form of outdoor physical exercise that has kept Betty and David free of respiratory problems. They work a lot together—weather permitting, of course—in their garden and small orchard. "We grow all kinds of vegetables," she said, "and have apple, apricot, and peach trees, along with two hazelnut and some raspberry bushes out back. We are eating a lot of natural, unsprayed fruits and vegetables for at least half of the year right out of our backyard. I sincerely believe that this has something to do with our good health."

And she's right. Antioxidant vitamins have become a big thing of late in the world of consumer health. The "Big Three," as I call them, are vitamins A, C, and E or spelled out as A-C-E for easier remembering. The Crockers get plenty of beta-carotene (a form of vitamin A) from their apricots and peaches, as well as from dark leafy greens such as spinach and root vegetables like carrots which they plant and harvest every year. Their vitamin C comes from other garden produce like bell peppers, broccoli, cabbage, kale, tomatoes, and turnip greens. And they pretty much get all the vitamin E their bodies need from "tons of hazelnuts that our bushes give us."

Although Betty and her husband aren't as nutritionally well-informed as a number of others might be, they certainly seem to have found an antidote to aging without conscientiously seeking for one. When oxygen is metabolized or burned by the human body, cells form byproducts known as free radicals. Free radicals travel through the cell, disrupting the structure of other molecules and resulting in cellular damage. Such damage is believed to contribute to aging and a wide variety of health problems.

But the fact that the Crockers eat a lot of fruits and vegetables, even though they consume meat once a day, and that Betty cooks or bakes instead of frying or deep-frying, helps hold their free radical levels to a bare minimum.

ACHOO! RELIEF FOR CAT ALLERGIES

It has been estimated on good authority that 4 in 10 senior citizens over the age of 65 in America own a cat; the majority of such pet owners happen to be women. Roughly 37% of cat owners are allergic to their pets, but still refuse to give them up. They are willing to endure symptoms such as sneezing, wheezing, runny nose, shortness of breath, tightness in the chest, and skin rash or hives before they will surrender old Fur Face.

Here are several reasons why cat allergen is especially bad for those who are hypersensitive to it. The primary offender in cats is a protein called *Felis domesticus allergen 1*, or better remembered in its shortened form Fel d 1. It is found in the saliva and skin of all cats. This allergen is continually shed as tiny airborne particles only one-tenth the size of a bit of dust.

Contrary to popular belief, cat hair itself is *not* allergenic. On the other hand, some Fel d 1 is transferred to the hair as the cat grooms itself. Any hair floating in the air can irritate the respiratory tract of persons afflicted with asthma, bronchitis, or emphysema. Also, other substances like pollen, dust, and mites that can cling to cat hair might contribute to a person's allergy.

A major obstacle to helping cat owners who are allergic to Fel d 1 is that the particles are so tiny that they hang suspended in the air, where they are easily inhaled. Another is that they are sticky and adhere to all porous surfaces, notably to rugs, upholstery, draperies, and bedding but also to walls and ceilings, particularly those that are rough and textured.

Another thing many cat lovers may not realize is that Fel d 1 is feather light and can linger in a house or an apartment for up to half a year after the pet itself has been removed. A final factor is that all cats produce this allergen, but in varying amounts. The situation becomes even more complicated by the fact that every allergic person reacts differently to Fel d 1.

Here are some wonderful tips that should help to successfully *minimize* but not totally eliminate the unfavorable reactions to cat allergen. First of all, try spraying your cat once a week with a solution of *weak* peppermint tea. I think you will be amazed at just how much this helps. To make a weak tea, add 1 teaspoon of peppermint leaves to one pint of boiling water, cover with lid and set aside to steep for 25 minutes. Strain, put into an empty spray bottle and spray over the cat's entire body. It will require some assistance from another person, wearing leather gloves, to hold the animal down while this is being done. It is also a good idea to hold the container nozzle about two inches away from the cat's hair while doing this. It doesn't need to be rubbed in by hand, but should be left alone to dry so as not to cause serious matting problems with long-haired cats.

Having the cat regularly groomed by someone other than the allergy sufferer helps. Regular brushing and combing to remove hair and dander should be done outdoors or in an area where the air is vented to the outdoors so a buildup of allergen won't be produced indoors.

One of the most sensible strategies is for cat lovers to keep their pets *out* of their bedrooms at all times. This will at least give them one place in the house or apartment that is in an allergen-free zone and will afford them wonderful physiological and psychological relief for part of every 24-hour period. But as logical as this sounds, it is going to meet strong resistance from a large number of pet lovers, who can't bear the thought of being without their beloved pusses for more than just a few minutes at a time.

Go easy on the vacuuming, since the exhaust of most machines stirs up particles of cat allergen like you wouldn't believe. I recommend getting a Vita-Vac from the Vita-Mix Corporation (1-800-VITAMIX) for this cleaning chore. Ever since the Anthropological Research Center (the organization that I've been the founding director of for 19 years) got its Vita-Vac a few years ago, our staff has been able to breathe much easier; this takes on even greater significance when you consider the fact that I've kept a pet cat named Jake in the facility for the last 5 or 6 years since he was a kitten. Vita-Vac works better than any other cleaning machine we've ever tried for keeping animal dander to an absolute minimum when used regularly on carpet floors and fabric-covered furniture. (See Product Appendix under Vita-Mix Corp. for further information.)

Also, you should think about using a damp mop wherever possible, especially in the bedroom, instead of the vacuum. Don't think this is a strange suggestion, because damp mopping bedroom carpet helps more than you may realize.

Since cat allergen sticks to porous materials, it would be a good idea, if one can afford it, to eliminate as much fabric material as possible. This includes upholstered furniture, wall-to-wall carpeting, shag and deep pile rugs, down comforters and pillows, draperies, and tapestry wall hangings. Substitute them instead with leather, cane, wood, chrome and glass, plastic slipcovers, washable scatter rugs, and blinds for windows. Enclose mattresses in vinyl and launder bed linens frequently. Replace foam or feather-filled pillows with hypoallergenic ones, wood blankets, afghans, and quilts with synthetic blankets, and put stuffed animal collections inside a glass case for display.

Place a free-standing air cleaner with a high-efficiency particulate HEPA filter in your bedroom. This type of filter can remove 97% of Fel d 1 and other allergens from the air. Also eliminate sources for other allergens in your home or apartment. Use cleansers that kill mold around sinks, showers, drain boards, air conditioners, and humidifiers. Limit plants to only one part of the house or apartment. Control cockroaches as best you can.

Certain herb capsules (burdock, garlic, nettle), herbal teas (coltsfoot, comfrey, horehound, mullein), and herbal sprays and drops (chamomile, myrrh, parsley, watercress) are usually very helpful in alleviating many of the symptoms of cat allergen. About 6 capsules or 2 cups of tea, or 15 to 25 drops of fluid extract (used for sprays and drops) each day is recommended.

Finally, some dietary changes are necessary if an allergic cat lover hopes to feel better. Meat intake should be restricted to once a week. All milk and dairy products should be virtually omitted from the diet. And above all else, *no sugary foods* should be consumed *at all!* Just following this last piece of advice will reduce cat allergen symptoms by as much as 40%.

🦠 A PARTICULAR CLASS OF ANTIOXIDANTS THAT CAN PREVENT RESPIRATORY PROBLEMS

One of the most potent antioxidants is a class of nutrients called flavonols. They are found in fruits and vegetables and other plants and are responsible for the bright colored pigments in them. Flavonols influence the nutritional value of a plant and possess unusual health-giving properties. One particular group of these flavonols, called proanthocyanidins (which refers to their active components), is water soluble and highly bioavailable. They are safe, powerful, and effective for many problems.

Proanthocyandins are more potent than either vitamins C or E. Like vitamin C, proanthocyanidins bind to collagen and elastin fibers, but are even more effective than vitamin C. Vitamin C leaves the body fast, while proanthocyanidins remain in the system for several days after.

Russian scientists have been looking at this highly interesting group of compounds for some time now. The science journal *Terapevticheskii Arkhiv* (66(3):32-34, 1994) pointed out that asthma and bronchitis patients tend to have high oxidative stress levels and are seriously lacking in sufficient antioxidant defenses. But when these same patients were given daily supplements of proanthocyanidins, their respiratory problems immediately cleared up. Other journals have noted that consumption of antioxidant-rich foods helps to prevent as well as treat allergies and lung disease.

So, when you're thinking about what kinds of food to eat that may be high in proanthocyanidins, remember that *color is everything* when it comes to this. Green, red, and yellow bell peppers, purple eggplant, red cabbage, orange carrots, pink grapefruit, yellow squash and melons, crimson tomatoes, and golden peaches are just a few of the items offered by nature that contain whopping amounts of these proanthocyanidins. *Bon appetit!*

Alzheimer's Disease Assistance

"NUTRIENTS FOR THE BRAIN THAT PREVENT NEURON DEGENERATION"

❧ WHAT IS IT?

A famous German neurologist by the name of Alois Alzheimer (1864-1915) was the first one to investigate and report the condition eventually named after him. Originally it was known simply as dementia and recognized by these various symptoms:

- Increasing forgetfulness and short-term memory losses.
- Difficulty making decisions.
- Impaired judgment.
- An inability to make math calculations or handle money.
- Decreased knowledge of current events.
- Anxiety, withdrawal, and depression as awareness of deficits becomes frightening and embarrassing.
- Language difficulties.
- Loss of the ability to write or understand written words.
- Complete loss of ability to speak.
- Delusions, hallucinations, paranoia, or irrational accusations of family members.
- Agitation and combativeness.

- Unusual quiet and serenity at times.
- Wandering and frequently getting lost.
- Urinary and fecal incontinence.
- Inappropriate social behavior; an indifference to others; failure to recognize friends and family.
- Inability to dress, eat, shave, bathe, or use a toilet without some assistance.
- Walking difficulty, leading to falls and bedsores.

All or many of these manifestations indicate gradual to severe degeneration of crucial neurons in that part of the brain which handles cognitive functioning. Most patients die within five to ten years of contracting Alzheimer's disease.

97-YEAR-OLD PROFESSOR'S SECRETS FOR RAZOR-SHARP MEMORY

I go to New York City at least twice a year on book business. Some of it has to do with my publisher, Prentice Hall, being located across the river in Englewood Cliffs, New Jersey. And other parts of it have to do with fulfilling the buying urge in me as a book collector; hence, I visit several antiquarian book shops within Manhattan hoping to find a few more treasures to add to an already enormous library (over 13,000 volumes as of 1996).

It was on one of these trips not too long ago that I met up with Abraham Goldstein. Abe, as he's fondly known by his colleagues at Baruch College in Manhattan (part of the City University of New York system), is still an adjunct professor of law, in spite of his age. He's been teaching there every single year since 1929–66 years in all. Abe, by the way, was 94 when we visited together (he turned 97 in 1996).

Abe started work with a private law firm in New York in 1926 and it remained his full-time profession until 1975. But early on, in 1929, he took on the second job of being a part-time, two-class-a-week instructor at Baruch, then known in those days as City College's School of Business and Civic Administration. He got hired at the college when he handled a legal matter for the dean, who was quite impressed and offered him a faculty appointment.

I asked this Energizer Bunny of education, who just seems to keep going and going, what he attributed his excellent memory to.

"First of all, I'm not married," he joked. "I believe that married men lose their minds a lot sooner than those of us who remain bachelors.

"The second thing is retaining a good sense of humor. As you can see, I haven't lost mine by any means. Seriously though, I think that a judicious sprinkling of levity every day in your general conversation helps the mind to retain its elasticity. By that I mean, its flexibility. I think that those who take life or themselves too seriously are in danger of ossifying their brains to the point where it won't work as well once they become older.

"The third thing is to try and maintain a general routine as much as possible. I'm a creature of habit, at least when it comes to my workday lunch. Typically I make a peanut butter and jelly sandwich at home.

"The next thing is to be concise and deliberate in every undertaking. I teach a business contracts law class to 35 students. I always deliver my lectures in a very orderly fashion. I believe that there is a procedure for everything in life, and once we find out what it is for something then we should faithfully adhere to it. This helps the mind to become better trained in following a set course, without having to expend a lot of extra energy trying to make order out of confusion."

Goldstein told me he was in pretty good health in spite of some minor hearing problems. He was thin with a full head of white hair and immaculately dressed; the day I met him he had on beige pants, a blue shirt and striped-tie-tucked-inside-the-belt type of an outfit.

"If you don't remember everything I just told you," he chided me, "then please don't forget that humor is probably one of the most important things towards retaining a sharp memory in the later years of your life." He then concluded our amiable visit with a cute little story of his own.

"This reminds me of the time the Lord was speaking with Saint Peter. He told Peter, 'Maybe you should go down to Earth to see what's going on.' So Peter goes down, surveys things a bit and comes back to make his report. He informs the Lord that 10% of the people are doing real good in their daily lives, but that the other 90% are not. So Peter suggests to the Lord that he write a letter to that 10% who are trying to live honorable lives. And so the Lord takes him up on his suggestion and does so."

Pausing for a moment to catch his breath, Professor Goldstein eyes me with a glint and asks somewhat mischievously, "Do *you* know what the Lord wrote in that letter?"

I shrugged honestly and answered with a straight face, "No, I don't."

Whereupon, the good prof asks in mock surprise: "*What*, you didn't get a letter?"

🐉 NUTRIENTS FOR THE BRAIN

The brain requires constant nourishment in order to function properly. As we get older, these needs dramatically increase. Brain foods can be obtained two ways: through eating them or else taking a wide variety of supplements.

The safest way to proceed in obtaining optimal brain nutrition is outlined in some simple steps below:

1. Eat a balanced diet, low in fat and high in carbohydrates, but definitely with protein foods added.

2. Take a daily supplement of the RDA for vitamins and minerals.

3. Take a broad-spectrum antioxidant once a day.

4. Eat foods high in antioxidants.

5. Avoid smoking, drinking, over-consuming caffeinated beverages and eating too many simple sugars.

6. Talk to a doctor or nutritionist about brain booster preparations to make sure they are safe and to clarify any pre-existing conditions—such as hypertension or gout—which could cause problems down the road.

A brief discussion of some of the foregoing suggestions may provide additional details for those willing to give their brains better nourishment.

A great deal has been written about antioxidants and the important roles they play in removing free radicals from the system. Think of free radicals as molecular sharks zipping around in the cellular sea of your body, nibbling here and there. After so much biochemical nibbling, things stop working in a normal fashion. For the brain, memory impairment soon becomes evident.

The three best supplements in the health food marketplace that I know of for zapping these free radicals in the brain are Kyolic garlic from Wakunaga, Mighty Greens from Pines International, and Gingko Biloba Plus from Wakunaga. I advise taking two capsules of each of the fine Wakunaga products once a day on an empty stomach. Mix one level tablespoonful of the Mighty Greens powder with 8 ounces of water. Stir thoroughly and drink it while swallowing the capsules. Mighty Greens is composed of wheat grass, barley grass, beet juice, rhubarb juice, peppermint, and over 20 other herbs. It is the single best chlorophyll product in the entire health food industry. And all three items come from companies you can trust and rely on for safe, wholesome and *honest* products. They are available from most health food stores. (Consult the Product Appendix for additional information on where to obtain them, if necessary.)

B-complex vitamins directly affect brain function in a variety of different ways. Therefore, it behooves the reader to take a daily supplement of this on a regular basis. A high potency B-complex (two tablets daily) will improve the memory very quickly. Don't worry if your urine becomes a little more yellow—this is just a natural consequence of taking B vitamins.

Vitamin C is important to brain function. I recommend a daily supplementation of at least 1,000 milligrams. Taking a vitamin C that is obtained from calcium ascorbate and ascorbyl palmitate is the best. Unfortunately, most of the vitamin C products sold in health food stores aren't up to much. Especially those sold by KAL, Thompson, and Twin Labs. Avoid them wherever possible and look for other brands instead. Pines International will soon be marketing a Super C under a separate Native American Nutrition label. It is one you can safely take and not have to worry about any hidden additives being slipped in without your knowledge. (See Product Appendix for more information.)

The best source of vitamin E is from wheat germ oil. Vitamin E makes a marvelous antioxidant and clears the brain and body of harmful debris. It keeps cell membranes from being damaged by free radicals. You can obtain vitamin E from soybeans, eggs, nuts, seeds, and whole grains. But you won't find the best wheat germ oil or vitamin E oil, for that matter, in a health food store. Rather, you'll find it at your local veterinary supply house or livestock center. The best in the business is Rex's Wheat Germ Oil. It has a dark amber color to it and a strong, nutty taste. It comes in a metal quart can. On the back side it tells you how much to give to various livestock animals.

But for over 30 years my family, friends, and I have been relying on this particular product for all of our own vitamin E needs. We simply don't trust anything else to put into our bodies but this. Unless you're a veterinarian, getting this stuff is mighty difficult. Therefore, as a public service to readers, our research center here in Salt Lake City makes it available for purchase. (To obtain some for yourself contact: Anthropological Research Center, P. O. Box 11471, Salt Lake City, UT 84147.) Because of its potency, you only need to take a teaspoon every morning. A quart can should last you several months.

Choline and lecithin are two other nutrients necessary for normal brain functions. Daily supplementation will expand them and increase the memory. Through the diet, choline can be taken in by eating cheese, fish, liver, egg yolks (in moderation, of course), seed oils, peanuts, peas, beans, brewer's yeast, green leafy vegetables, cauliflower, and cabbage. In supplements, choline can be found in Pines Mighty Greens drink and Wakunaga's Kyo-Ginseng (see Product Appendix on these). One tablespoon in 8 ounces of water for the first and 4 capsules daily for the second, are sufficient.

Lecithin, as long as it includes phosphatidyl choline, is a good brain booster. Lecithin can be used in liquid or granule forms; take one teaspoon every morning with breakfast.

Brain performance depends a lot on the actions of certain minerals such as potassium, sodium, magnesium, and calcium. If any of these aren't present in adequate amounts, the mind will soon suffer from problems such as depression, irritability, memory loss, and insomnia. It has been estimated by some health experts that close to 40% of all Americans may have a deficiency in one or more of these minerals. Food sources for all of them range from dairy products, sardines and salmon to dark leafy greens, nuts, and seeds.

One supplement, though, which is quite rich in all four of these minerals, plus many other valuable trace elements needed for boosting brain activity, is the Mighty Greens plant mixture drink from Pines International (see Product Appendix). Put one level tablespoonful in an 8-ounce glass of water, stir, drink, and let your brain enjoy its marvelous energizing effects.

Don't forget about fats and oils either. Some fat is needed to make glial cells, which speed messages across the brain, and an adequate amount is required for all proper brain and body functioning. You should obtain most of your fat through a normal, healthy diet. But supplementation is necessary to get two very important kinds of fat: essential fatty acids called linoleic acid (omega 6) and alpha-linolenic acid (omega 3). You can get the first by taking one tablespoon of evening primrose oil every day; you obtain the second by eating salmon, trout, mackerel, tuna, and sardines—*lots* of sardines, I might add!

A number of Americans are starting to try new ways to enhance their mental powers with so-called "smart drugs" and "power drinks." Two of the best herbal products in the health food industry for making you smarter are Kyo-Ginseng (four capsules daily) and Ginkgo Biloba Plus (two capsules daily) from Wakunaga of America (see Product Appendix). And a terrific "smart drink" can be made using the Mighty Greens from Pines International (see Product Appendix).

A Smart Drink

1. Gently crush into powder with a rolling pin, hammer, or similar heavy object, one tablet each of these vitamins: glutamine, folic acid, vitamin B-6, and vitamin C. Do this on a piece of wax paper or clean linen cloth, then shake into a small bowl and set aside.

2. Empty two gelatin capsules of each of these powders: Kyo-Ginseng and Ginkgo Biloba Plus from Wakunaga of America. Include them in the bowl with the other powders.

3. Mix 1 1/2 tablespoons of Mighty Greens from Pines in 8 ounces of spring water. Stir thoroughly. Then add the other powders and stir again. Or else put everything into a Vita-Mix container and blend for 1 minute on medium speed. Drink in the morning before breakfast.

SOME THINGS TO DO TO FIGHT BRAIN FATIGUE

When you get up in the morning, be sure to have a high-protein breakfast before leaving your dwelling. Protein helps the brain make the neurotransmitters dopamine and norepinephrine, both of which maintain alertness and the ability to think clearly. This will also build up the brain's supply of the alertness chemical tryosine, and shore up its glucose stores.

A light lunch is recommended. I've discovered from my own occasional sad experiences that the brain and body will slump in the afternoon if called upon to digest too much at once. Also, it might not be a bad idea to include some form of protein again at noontime. Munching on nuts and seeds helps fulfill this.

You shouldn't be eating big meals at night if you want to sleep well. And you should especially avoid high protein meals such as a succulent steak or prime rib dinner. Tryptophan (found in carbohydrates) is used by the brain to make serotonin (a calming chemical). But it competes with the tyrosine in protein to cross the blood-brain barrier, with tyrosine usually winning. So to sleep well at night diet mostly on carbohydrate-rich foods, unless subject to blood sugar disorders like hypoglycemia or diabetes. Then a combination of some protein and carbohydrates becomes essential to physical well-being.

Above all else, *DO NOT SKIP MEALS*. Better to eat a little but often, than a big meal and infrequently. And stay away from fried and deep-fried foods as much as possible. They're murder on your liver and wreck your brain, heart, and kidneys for sure! (See also MEMORY LOSS and SENILITY)

Arteriosclerosis/Atherosclerosis

(see Coronary Artery Disease)

Arthritis Rebound

"FORMER BRITISH PRIME MINISTER'S SECRETS FOR AGILITY AT AGE 71"

THE 'IRON LADY' COMES TO UTAH

The first convert immigrants from the British Isles to Utah had to trudge through a rugged ring of mountains in order to get there. But on Friday, March 1, 1996, former Prime Minister Margaret Thatcher soared over them in a private jet belonging to a wealthy Utah industrialist.

"My views were undoubtedly much better than your pioneers had," she quipped. Thatcher praised Utah's beauty and heritage during brief remarks at a newly completed International Arrival Terminal at the Salt Lake International Airport. Her arrival marked the commencement of a month-long United

Kingdom-Utah Festival 1996. Thatcher and Salt Lake City Mayor Deedee Corradini each stressed the link between Utah and the UK.

Thatcher's plane arrived more than an hour late. Fire engines sprayed arches of water over the jet after it landed. Bagpipes and drummers preceded her into the terminal, and balloons fell from the ceiling when Corradini announced the beginning of the festival. Utah's Governor Mike Leavitt had invited Thatcher to Utah back in 1994. Merrick Baker-Bates, the British consul general in Los Angeles, encouraged Thatcher to visit Utah. Mormon Church President Gordon B. Hinckley (age 86), who served a church mission to England as a young man back in the mid-1930s, also was instrumental in persuading the "Iron Lady" to come to the Beehive State. The event took 18 months to pull off.

Security was extremely tight for this diminutive woman and her husband, Sir Denis Thatcher, whom she married in 1951 and had twin children by. Virtually none of the public ever got close enough to even shake her hand. I was one of the lucky ones, however, to "sneak" in an interview with her, however brief it was.

🌿 MRS. THATCHER'S SECRETS FOR STAYING AGILE

She turned her attention in my direction and smiled. We exchanged the usual formal greetings and I immediately got down to the business of why I was there. I realized that I only had about a minute and a half, and I wanted to make every moment count so as to get my money's worth.

I asked her, "Have you ever been troubled with arthritis in your life?" She replied in her typical forthright manner, "No, I haven't been. Neither has Denis" (meaning her husband, of course). She explained that "both of us are quite agile, you see, for our ages."

"To what do you attribute this agility?" I promptly inquired. She laid out several things in logical order that they adhere to faithfully, which she felt "keeps us nimble as deer."

The first of these, not surprisingly, was tea. Being very British as both of them are, one wouldn't expect anything less. "We take tea around 2 o'clock past every noontime," she said. "And we always take it without sugar, but do like a wee bit of cream in it."

Plenty of scientific evidence backs up Mrs. Thatcher's beverage habit. Tea contains one very important mineral, namely fluoride—lots of it, as a matter of fact. Green tea (which the Thatchers prefer) has twice as much per cup as does black tea; an added bonus is that it also has far *less* caffeine than the other. Now fluoride is essential for the preservation of minerals in the bones such as calcium, magnesium, potassium, and phosphorus. When enough fluoride is present in the bones, these other minerals won't leach out as easily, thereby making for stronger bones and healthier joints. Green tea also yields a lot of antioxidants per cup. These are compounds which check the erratic behavior of free radicals within the system. Free radicals are scavenger molecules that can wreak biological havoc to the body if left unchecked. They are virtually responsible for everything that goes with old age. But antioxidants act as policemen and chemically "arrest" their crazy activities so they do far less harm.

The Thatchers prefer using spring water for tea infusion, believing it is healthier and safer. Their house servants back in England prepare their daily cups of tea in a very simple fashion. The servants put the equivalent of two glasses (or about 16 fluid ounces) of boiling spring water in a beautifully decorated porcelain china teapot and add 3 level tablespoons of loose, cut, dried, tea leaves. These are stirred around with a silver spoon and the top put on the teapot. After the leaves have infused for about five minutes, the servants then pour out some tea into two cups for the former prime minister and her husband.

The next thing from Mrs. Thatcher's lips took me somewhat by surprise. She thought that the time she and her husband spent in their backyard garden, planting flowers and "smelling the blooms quite often" (as she put it), contributed to their great agility. She had no medical explanation for her theory, only that when she *didn't* spend time "with my blooms, then do I feel a bit stiff sometimes."

Later it dawned on me that what the Thatchers unintentionally practice while working in their flower garden is a form of aromatherapy. This system of natural medicine draws on the healing powers of the plant world. But instead of using the entire plant or part of it, aromatherapy employs just the essential oils of plants. These potent, aromatic substances are housed in tiny glands on the outside or deep inside the roots, wood, leaves, flowers, or fruit of plants. Aromatherapy is a dynamic, concentrated representation of the healing properties of the plant, and is believed by some to contain its life force. Hence, great care must be taken to extract the oil in its purest state.

In aromatherapy, inhalation, application, and baths are the principal methods used to encourage essential oils to enter the body. Essential oils are highly volatile, evaporating quite readily on exposure to air, and when inhaled, may enter the system through the nostrils. When diluted and applied externally, essential oil molecules may permeate the skin. Bath treatments enable the user to both inhale and absorb the oils.

Aromatherapy is covered more in depth in one of my other books, *Heinerman's Encyclopedia of Healing Herbs and Spices* (Englewood Cliffs, NJ: Prentice Hall, 1996). There are several other good books on the subject, too. One of the simplest is *Aromatherapy for Common Ailments* by Shirley Price (New York: Simon & Schuster, 1991). I took the foregoing brief description of aromatherapy from the opening paragraphs of the book's first chapter. And towards the very end of the book, the author mentions that "aromatherapy can help to relax muscles and relieve pain" in arthritic conditions, "but it cannot renew worn cartilage nor can it always help to relieve pain in the bone."

The best way to utilize some of the oils recommended in aromatherapy is with the cabbage leaf compress. Peel several of the large, outer leaves off of a head of green cabbage. Cut out their midrib veins so they lay out flat. Then put each one on an ironing board and with a steam iron, gently iron each of them.

Prior to doing this, however, prepare the following formula in advance. In two tablespoons of olive or sesame seed oil, combine the following herbal essential oils (purchased from any health food store): rosemary (4 drops), lavender (2 drops), and ginger

(3 drops). Stir or shake the contents well. Then pour some of the oil mixture on to the *ironed* side of each cabbage leaf and evenly spread around with the fingertips. Then place the leaf over that arthritic body part desired with the ironed side *towards* the skin and hold in place with some adhesive tape. Place a dry hand towel over the leaf in order to retain the heat as long as possible. In 15 minutes, untape each leaf, iron again, apply some more oil, and repeat the process over again. Do this for an hour 3 or 4 times daily, using fresh leaves during each course of treatment. Remember to work quickly doing all of this to prevent much loss of heat.

Realizing that my interview time was diminishing, I hurriedly asked the former prime minister if there was anything in their dietary habits that they did differently from everyone else. "We don't eat fried foods," she stated matter-of-factly. Limited research has shown that this may contribute to both kinds of arthritis (rheumatoid and osteo-) in some way.

I discerned by her countenance that she was already getting somewhat weary of being verbally hammered with my questions. So I wrapped this very brief interview up by asking if there was anything else they did to stay so fit and limber? "We do a lot of walking, and when gardening, a fair amount of stooping and bending," she replied with a straight face. 'That tends to keep us agile, don't you agree?" I nodded and graciously thanked her for her time as the elevator doors opened just then. She smiled the consummate smile indicative of most politicians and her small party quickly exited.

❧ HOW ONE MAN OBTAINED FREEDOM FROM PAIN

Isaac Haynes is a retired 67-year-old African-American minister residing in Harlem, New York. He served in the pulpit faithfully for many years, but decided to bow out of the ministry at age 63 due to a worsening condition of rheumatoid arthritis. "It got so bad in my fingers that I couldn't even turn the pages of my scriptures or hymnal," he wrote in a letter to me.

So, the good reverend went on a "health quest" to search for those things which might improve his painful condition. "I wanted to try those things that were more natural for my body," he stated, "instead of relying on synthetic drugs that I didn't think were too good for my body." He visited several health food stores in Manhattan, including one of the Vitamin Shoppe outlets located at 120 West 57th Street.

Quoting again from the narrative in his letter, he continued as follows: "I told the clerk who waited on me what my problem was. She told me that by law she couldn't do any actual prescribing as such. But she did direct me to several different books which recommended some things for arthritis.

"I made a list of the best things I thought might help my problem and purchased them from the lady. I started taking them according to instructions given in the books or else those appearing on the product labels themselves. I started noticing a difference right away, and within ten days I could move my fingers and wrists again without any pain."

Here is the list of what Reverend Haynes used and the quantities he took them in. His self-created supplement program lasted for a total of three months. He reported no recurring problems of swelling or excruciating pain after that. (Consult the Product Appendix for more information on where to obtain some of the items mentioned here.)

EVENING PRIMROSE OIL.	4 capsules with breakfast.
FLAXSEED OIL.	1 teaspoon every day with food.
COENZYME Q-10.	90 mg. once a day with food.
KYOLIC GARLIC.	6 capsules daily of Kyolic Super Formula 106.
WHEAT GRASS.	10 tablets of Pines Wheat Grass daily with food.
ALFALFA.	6 tablets twice daily with food.
TEA TREE OIL.	Rub 3-5 drops on swollen joints twice daily.
B-COMPLEX.	3 tablets of high-potency once daily.
MAGNESIUM-CALCIUM.	4 tablets of Arth-X Plus from Trace Minerals Research.
VITAMIN C.	1,000 mg. twice daily with food.
BIOFLAVONOIDS.	50 mg. each of rutin and hesperidin daily.

ARTHRITIS AND BEES

This next therapy may, at first glance, appear to be somewhat unorthodox, if not downright radical. But rest assured that in the mid-to-late 1970s it was one of the most popular folk treatments in the country for rheumatoid arthritis. Tens of thousands of people flocked to a variety of beekeepers around the country for their daily bee stings, which not only greatly relieved their arthritic suffering, but in many instances, actually seemed to cure their problems.

A freelance writer by the name of Patrick Frazier wrote one of the earliest and most insightful, evenhanded articles on the subject for the May 19, 1974 edition of *The Washington Post.* Appropriately entitled, "Arthritis and Bees: Venom Research Overcoming Old Prejudices," he outlined for readers the benefits which many arthritic-prone beekeepers had obtained for themselves when periodically stung by some of their bees. Those who were stung noticed that almost immediately afterwards their arthritic swelling went down and their joint pain greatly subsided. He mentioned one Vermont beekeeper in particular who seemed to have found permanent relief from his own arthritis with this highly controversial therapy.

The man's name was Charles Marz, who in May 1934, at the age of 29, still suffered acute arthritic pains in his knees from an attack of rheumatic fever the previous winter. For him just to stand and walk made him appear as an elderly person three or four times his age. But it was spring and he had to get out and work in his apiary as usual.

Charles knew about the old wives' tale of bee stings being used as a remedy for arthritis, but like most others believed it was a bunch of nonsense. However, figuring he had nothing to lose he decided to experiment for himself to see if such a thing really worked or not. He caught two of his own honeybees and made them sting the inside of his knees where the pain was the most severe. Two welts raised from the stings but nothing else happened. He soon forgot about it and continued working with his hives the rest of the day.

By the next morning, however, he realized something wonderful had happened overnight. As he eased himself out of bed, it dawned on him that the arthritic pain in both of his knees was *completely gone*. His first reaction was, "My God, am I imagining "that I had arthritis yesterday, or is it my imagination that I haven't got it today?" "To this day [May 1974] I cannot believe what happened," he told reporter Frazier. And that was the start of Marz' life-long interest in bee venom therapy for one of mankind's most crippling diseases.

Over the next five decades, Charles became an active proponent of this therapy for the treatment of arthritis. He worked closely with a few open-minded medical doctors, such as rheumatologists, in helping to treat thousands of patients suffering from excruciating joint pain. He usually worked through their clinics to do this, but wasn't adverse about helping those who came to seek out his services at his large bee farm (Champlain Valley Apiaries) in Middlebury, VT.

AN INTRODUCTION TO BEE VENOM THERAPY (BVT) FOR ARTHRITIS

I was fortunate enough in the latter part of 1970s to become personally acquainted with Charles Marz. At that time he was entering his early 70s. I watched in amazement as he treated different individuals with *live* honeybee venom and see individuals get up and move around without *any* pain whatsoever in just a matter of a few hours. I interviewed him at length, took copious notes of everything I saw and heard, and filed it away for future reference.

Mr. Marz eventually passed on, but the extensive materials I had gleaned in my brief association with him remained intact. Eventually, I found a use for it in this book. The following data came from Mr. Marz *first-hand* and is given in his own words. Now, just because this information is presented here, in no way suggests or encourages readers to attempt this therapy for themselves. Bear in mind that it is still medically controversial, and that nothing so radical should ever be attempted *without* strict medical supervision. Marz believed in working closely with doctors; the same pattern should continue for those who may wish to explore this matter further for themselves. But, neither myself nor my publisher recommend bee venom therapy as a substitute for more conventional arthritis treatments. The material given here is for informational purposes *only* and *not*—I repeat *not*—intended for actual self treatment of arthritis.

And now Charles Marz in his own words: "If one considers seriously trying bee venom therapy (BVT), a source of bees is necessary. There is no better source than [from] local beekeepers. They can be very helpful with instructions on how to handle the bees. The simplest method to carry bees is in a glass jar, with holes in the metal cover for air. In the jar some honey must be supplied for food and a piece of cardboard inside the jar for the bees to cling to. A half pint jar will hold 50 or more bees for about a week. When more are needed, it is only necessary to clean the jar, put in more fresh honey and cardboard and take it to the beekeeper to be replenished.

"When picking up bees to use, they must be picked up by the head or thorax (where wings and legs are attached) and crushed with the tweezers. The sting is at the tail end of the bees and it is only necessary to touch the skin with it. The sting will immediately stick to the skin and come out of the bee and remain in the skin. The sting gland of the honey bee is a very complex mechanism. The two shafts of the sting are barbed and slide alongside of each other and are activated by a bunch of muscles. This will cause the sting to bury itself into the skin even after it leaves the body of the bee and at the same time, pump the venom into the wound. The longer the sting is left in the skin, the more venom will be introduced, up to about 5 minutes or so that the muscles are active.

THE 'ACUPUNCTURE METHOD' OF ADMINISTERING BEE STINGS

"The next step after one has the bees available and knows how to handle them [just ask a beekeeper for this information], is where and how much bee venom to use. As a rule, the patient needs someone to help them apply the stings. It is difficult to do alone especially in the spine area. Also, the person assisting can help determine where the stings should be applied. The most effective areas seem to be the 'trigger points' [in Oriental medicine, they would be the acupuncture or acupressure points]. These can be found by pressing different places in the area where the arthritis is located. When a 'trigger point' is pressed, it will produce a very sharp pain and the patient will jump. These are the areas where the stings should then be applied and can be marked with a ball point pen." (He noted here that in some respects this does closely correspond with the acupuncture points of Chinese medicine.)

"Before stings are applied, it is well to first apply ice or a frozen 'Scotch ice can' to make the skin cold. This will greatly reduce the pain produced by the sting when it is first applied. Before any therapy is started, the person must first be tested for any possible allergic reaction. This is done by applying a sting and then removing it instantly, after being assured that there is *no* history of allergy. Wait for 15 minutes or a half hour and if there is no allergic reaction in this time, there is no allergic problem. In half an hour another sting can be applied and this also removed quickly. This is usually enough for the first treatment.

"After then the serious business of therapy can be started. If the arthritis is of an acute type, or short duration, no damage to the joints and only a few local points involved, the treatment is usually only of short duration and only a few stings are necessary. Sometimes a local condition will clear up with only one sting, but normally, the treatment requires a series of treatments. The first day, start out with just the two test stings and continue every day for about a week with two to four stings each day, depending on the severity of the arthritis.

"While bee venom has a systemic as well as a local reaction, the best results are found by treating the 'trigger points' all over the body where the arthritis is involved. Basically, arthritis of the upper part of the body, stems from the lower spine and the upper spine and the lower part of the body from the lower spine. For this reason, it is a good idea to use the spine areas as a base of operations. Treat the spine first. Then work down from the spine towards the extremities; the shoulders, neck, elbows, wrists, hands, and so forth. From the lower spine, work towards the hips, knees and ankles, where 'trigger points' are found.

Treatment Phase and Reactions

"With experience one can soon find out how many stings they can take without too much discomfort. At first, the stings may produce very little pain, but as the treatment is continued, the body will again be more sensitive to pain as the arthritic symptoms leave the areas. This is a good sign that there is improvement in the condition. If the arthritic condition is severe, after the first week of two to four stings each day, treat every other day using more stings as needed. It may be necessary to give 10 to 20 stings with each treatment for bad cases. It must be remembered, in serious cases of joint damage, no type of treatment can make new joints or tissue. In such cases, one can only expect to get relief of pain, and to stop the progress of the disease.

"A full course of treatment generally will last from four to eight weeks, with treatments every other day. The stings should be applied to different areas each time so as not to treat an area that is still swollen.

"Usually when treatments are first started, there is very little or no swelling. Then as the treatment is continued, the areas will begin to swell much more, with redness and itching of the areas treated. Sometimes during this stage, the patient will feel worse, with more pain and pain in areas never before affected. There may even be nausea and a general feeling of discouragement. It is important to remember that this is a good sign that the treatment is working and treatment must be continued in order to be effective. The number of stings can be reduced, if desired. It appears that the cause for this reaction is the purging of toxins from the body by the stimulation of the biotic processes of the system. It follows the classic Hans Selye, M.D. [a renowned epidemiologist, since deceased] syndrome of the stages of reaction and then the stage of resistance. Soon after this, the stings will no longer swell and a person becomes 'immune,' just as a bee-keeper might become immune after working with bees for a long time. When one reaches this 'immune stage,' the first course of treatment can be terminated.

"At this point a person will usually find their condition much improved. No more treatment is necessary for another month or two, and if there is no return of the arthritic symptoms, there is no longer need of any further treatments for a period of perhaps several years or as long as 20 years or more. However, if after a 'rest period' of a month or two, there are still arthritic symptoms, another course of treatments can be followed, starting with one sting and gradually building up as with the first course. However, with subsequent courses, the treatments are usually more effective and with quicker results so that a shorter course of treatments usually suffices. In very bad cases, three or more courses of treatments may be necessary covering a period of two years or more. However, in the usual cases where there is little or no joint damage, a few weeks of treatment will suffice.

❧ ARTHRITIS TYPES THAT RESPOND BEST TO BEE STINGS

"There is often the question for which types of arthritis BVT is effective. It appears to be effective in most all kinds of true arthritis. Gout and other acute forms respond quickly. Spondylitis and rheumatoid arthritis forms where serious joint damage is involved, will find limited results, unless treatment can be started before serious damage develops. It is interesting to relate that with children BVT seems to be of special benefit as they seem to respond quicker than adults.

❧ IS IT SAFE?

"The final thing which seems to worry most people who are thinking about starting something like this is, 'Is BVT safe for us to use?' My answer to that question is an emphatic 'yes!' Conventional drugs such as cortisone, which are routinely used to treat arthritis, can do the body far more harm than a little bee venom could. There are thousands of beekeepers all over the world to demonstrate that this substance has no adverse side effects even when taken over a long period of time. Just look at me as an example of that. I personally have taken a thousand stings or more per year for the past 50 years as have many other beekeepers. Many beekeepers live to be 80 years of age or more. Your chances of dying from a bad reaction to a potent drug are 1,000 times more likely than from a honey bee sting!"

SOME THINGS TO KEEP IN MIND WHEN ATTEMPTING IT

This concludes the information which the late Charles Marz kindly provided me with back in the Spring of 1978. The reader should keep in mind, however, that some individuals are extremely hypersensitive to insect venom. If stung, such persons could suffer anaphylaxis, which certainly is life threatening. *Before BVT is attempted, individuals should check with their allergenists to make sure that they are not hypersensitive to bee venom!* It may also be worthwhile to keep on hand a hypodermic needle filled with adrenalin in the event that anaphylaxis occurs during an administration of BVT. The adrenalin can then be immediately injected intramuscularly and bring the person out of such an acute allergic reaction before it becomes too severe.

AQUATIC EXERCISE

If you have arthritis, a dip in the pool may be just what the doctor ordered. The Arthritis Foundation and National YMCA have developed an aquatics program that can help reduce pain and stiffness, increase the strength of muscles and improve joint flexibility and personal stamina.

There are some basic advantages to water exercise. For one thing, arthritic joints and muscles can be greatly strengthened with low impact exercises in the water due to its buoyancy. And water permits a type of aerobic exercise with wrist or hand weights that would be impossible to do otherwise. Also, warm water tends to relax sore muscles and decreases the pain from arthritis and other conditions.

If you have access to a warm swimming pool and can use it often, here are some simple aquatic exercises you may want to try out. Just be sure to always keep your swollen joints submerged while exercising.

FORWARD ARM RAISE: Lifting up each arm in front of you enables the shoulder joints to be loosened more.

CALF STRETCH: Holding on to the edge of the pool and bending up and down helps to work the muscles in your lower legs.

LEG EXTENSION: While floating in the water, grasp one leg above the knee with both hands and momentarily hold it up while stretching the limb out. Balance yourself with the other leg. Do the same to both legs. This helps tone your upper thighs.

TORSO STRETCH: With the legs spread about two feet apart, bend the upper part of the body sideways, first to the left and then to the right. This works the muscles on both sides of your trunk.

CHEST EXPANSION: With the legs spread one foot apart and both arms elevated above the head, take some slow, deep breaths, holding in the air for several seconds longer before blowing it out with a loud burst of energy. Repeated efforts of such deep breathing increase the lungs' capacity for greater oxygen intake.

TRUNK STRETCH: With the legs spread two feet apart, elevate both arms holding them out directly in front of you until nearly level with your chin. Then swing your upper body and arms sideways, always keeping your feet pointed straight ahead. Do this both ways several times. This exercise works the muscles located on both sides of your torso.

SHOULDER ROTATION: Again, with the feet spread apart as before, raise both arms until square with the shoulders, while at the same time turning both forearms in a downward, perpendicular position. This improves your range of motion.

ARM CROSS: The positioning of both forearms to form an "x" by the abdomen, helps to loosen the shoulders and upper back. The feet, of course, are spread apart as usual.

MARCH: Walking in a military style by swinging both arms and raising each leg high helps you warm up as well as cool down.

Attractive Teeth

"LIGHTS! CAMERA! ACTION!—SMILE AND SAY
'CHEESE' FOR THE PHOTOGRAPHER"

 ## CAN YOU HEAR ME BETTER?

I never know when I might run across a new or different remedy of some kind. Life has taught me to find the unusual in the most unexpected places. Natural remedies for helping you to look better in the later years don't always turn up at health food conventions or herbal conferences. They can sometimes appear out of the blue as the following account will show.

On Friday, April 19, 1996, I decided to take a short five-minute walk from my research center over to the Salt Palace Convention Center, which is one block directly west of the building I'm in. The American Academy of Audiology was in town for its four-day convention. I secured an exhibitor's badge and roamed freely among the aisles of this huge facility.

PEARLY WHITES BUT NOT THE PEARLY GATES

At one particular exhibit I met a 52-year-old lady named Connie. She was attired in, how shall I say, a rather provocative dress. Put another way, it wasn't how much she had on, but how *little* that brought droves of audiologists to this particular booth.

She inquired where my practice was located. I answered that I wasn't an audiologist, but a medical anthropologist who specialized in writing books on folk medicine. She asked what that was and I told her that I did research on the benefits of herbs. Upon hearing that word, she steered the course of our conversation in the following direction.

"Then you might probably be interested in something I use on my teeth," she continued. "I learned this trick from my mom years ago. Both of us are smokers. And in my business, where you are continually meeting the public, having nice, white teeth is part of the attraction I use to help me get people interested in what I sell and to close as many sales as I can."

Connie then explained how her mother started using powdered black walnut hulls a long time ago to get rid of any tobacco, coffee, or food stains that might have accumulated on her teeth. The daughter pointed out that she has followed the same practice herself since then.

"We get our toothbrush wet by running it under the basin tap a little. Then we dip the end of it into a little dish containing black walnut hull powder, which had been obtained by emptying it out of gelatin capsules. After covering the bristles with some of it, we brush our teeth, always making sure to get the front top and bottom teeth really good. Afterwards, we rinse our mouths with cold water."

Connie said that she and her mom do this routine no more than three times a week, "since the herb powder can wear away your enamel if you're not careful about how frequently you use it." She also has found that rubbing a half slice of strawberry across her teeth several times a day helps to keep them pretty. "I also like to rinse with a half cup of cold green tea," she concluded. "It helps to hold the cavities down."

Connie might not become a candidate for the Pearly Gates any time soon considering the sexually tempting image that she wants to portray. But she will certainly continue to be an ageless picture of perfect dental beauty as long as she keeps on using black walnut and strawberries.

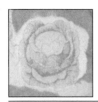

B

Back Pain Removal

🌱 ONE OF SOCIETY'S MAJOR DISABILITIES

Low back pain happens to be one of the major causes of physical disability in our society. Back pain in general, however, has been associated with a number of disorders. These include, but are not limited to the following problems, many of which are rather common:

ANKYLOSING SPONDYLITIS: inflammation of joints between spine and pelvis.

ENDOMETRIOSIS: migration of uterine lining to other sex or abdominal organs.

FIBROIDS (UTERINE): benign growths of the muscular wall of uterus.

36

FIBROMYALGIA: generalized fatigue and pain in muscles, tendons, and ligaments.

Gallbladder disorders, which can include gallstones and liver disturbances.

Herniated disk in the lower spinal back somewhere.

Kidney cancer, kidney cysts, and general kidney infection.

OBESITY: usually ranks as one of the major causes of back pain.

OSTEOARTHRITIS: degeneration of cartilage that lines the joints.

OSTEOMALACIA/RICKETS: softening of bones due to poor calcification.

OSTEOMYELITIS: infection of bone and bone marrow.

OSTEOPOROSIS: loss of bone mass due to calcium depletion.

PAGET'S DISEASE: weakening, thickening and deformity of bones.

PANCREATITIS: inflammation of the pancreas.

PROSTATE CANCER: frequently attributed to self-abuse or excessive sex.

Renal calculi or kidney stones.

SCOLIOSIS: gradual bending of spine to one side or into an S-shape.

Spinal cord trauma due to falls or auto accidents.

Sprains and strains from heavy lifting and improper bending.

CHIROPRACTIC AND MASSAGE TREATMENTS

Open-minded doctors who practice alternative medicine have advocated aggressive nonsurgical treatments as being superior to surgery in dealing with low back pain. One recent study seems to back up their claims. According to a report that appeared in the *Journal of Manipulative and Physiological Therapeutics* (18:335-42, 1995), researchers reviewed 3,531 charts of consecutive patients visiting a teaching chiropractic clinic between 1990 and 1993. Seventy-one of these were from cases of low back pain with radiating leg pain clinically diagnosed as lumbar disk herniation. Better than 40% of these patients were 50 years or older. Of 59 patients who received a course of spinal adjustment, 90% reported significant improvement in their conditions. The report concluded that "chiropractic care may be an effective and safe treatment for low back pain and sciatica."

In selecting a chiropractor to treat your own back pain, make sure that the one you pick is right for you. Ask around to see who the best chiropractor may be. Find out through your local state chiropractic review board, those chiropractors who may have had some additional medical training beyond that offered by most chiropractic colleges, which would better qualify them to treat back injuries through spinal manipulation.

Massage is also a good approach to treating back pain. About 10 to 15 drops of peppermint oil may be applied over that area of the lower back where pain is greatest. The person administering the massage should kneel astride the patient's head and work from the middle of the back in even, downward strokes, pushing forward with the meaty parts of both palms and the fingers spread apart all the way to the tailbone. Both hands are then cupped, turned sideways, and placed at an angle against the skin. With slight pushing exertion they are pulled upwards towards the shoulder blades in a squeegee action similar to that used by window washers. Apply more drops of oil as necessary to keep the skin surface lubricated enough to permit the hands and fingers to easily glide over it with minimal friction. Repeat these back-and-forth motions for up to ten minutes and perform the treatment every six hours, if possible, for maximum relief.

WAYS TO MAKE BACK PAIN LESS AGONIZING

A number of other things can be done to assuage the excruciating stabs of back pain. Doctors routinely tell their patients to take two aspirins. This might sound redundant to some, but many studies show it's still the best course to follow. A natural alternative would be to substitute 4 capsules of white willow bark or two capsules each of capsicum and yarrow. Also, arthritic roll-on creams containing capsaicin, the fiery compound from red pepper, might be helpful, especially if accompanied by some mild massage strokes immediately following application.

According to a 1994 report by the federal government's Agency for Health Care Policy and Research (AHCPR), drugs such as aspirin and ibuprofen might even induce some side effects. This is why using the herbs is much better. The report also concludes, after analyzing the results of nearly 4,000 back pain studies, that most people with acute back pain should do exercises instead of lying down. Aerobic exercises are the best and build up endurance to pain either by walking, using a stationary bike, swimming, or jogging slowly for half an hour every day. Any of these activities should be initiated within two weeks of the pain's onset. There may be a tendency for you to take it easy, but resist this inclination. A Finnish study published in *The New England Journal of Medicine* sometime in 1995 noted that as little as two days of bed rest can actually *slow* recovery from low back pain by deconditioning the muscles. Going about one's normal activities produced the best results. Though beneficial for preventing future attacks, stretching exercises should be deferred until the acute episode subsides.

In 1992, some 653,400 Americans reported work-related back injuries, according to the Bureau of Labor Statistics. Undoubtedly, many more injuries went unreported. A ranking epidemiologist for the National Institute of Occupational Safety and Health observed that nurses and heavy-industry workers rank among the highest in reports of occupational back pain.

Sprains (affecting the muscles) and strains (affecting the ligaments) make up more than 80% of all work-related injuries. Unsafe motions like twisting or bending at the waist are the leading causes of injury. Inflammatory pain may be eased by drinking cups of *warm* tea made from a combination of peppermint leaves (1 tbsp.), fennel seeds (1 tsp.), and valerian root (1 tsp.). Boil $1^1/_2$ pints water and add the seeds and root; cover and simmer on low heat for 7 minutes. Set aside, uncover and add the leaves; stir thoroughly, replace the lid and steep for 25 minutes. Strain one cup, warm again if necessary and drink on an empty stomach.

However, merely *sitting* for long periods of time is usually a major culprit for bringing on back pain. Sitting, particularly slouching, puts continuous pressure on lower back muscles and disks, and looking up and down from computer screens to key-boards can strain the upper back. Vehicular vibrations or poorly designed airline seats contribute additional stress to the backs of those whose work involves driving or flying long distances. To get around this, I sometimes slip a small pillow or cushion behind my back just below my shoulder blades. This enables me to sit upright more comfortably for longer periods of time than I might otherwise be able to do.

There are other things you can do to make sitting easier on your spine. Sit straight and close to your desk and don't hunch forward. The knees should be elevated slightly above your hips, so a footrest under the desk may be needed. Pay attention to heights and angles. Your work surface should be at elbow level and the top of your computer screen at eye level.

I find that getting up at regular intervals and stretching helps immensely. I work long hours in my research center, typing out many different health manuscripts and newsletter articles for my publisher. Every 45 minutes or so I will shift positions, or stand and stretch. I follow a simple exercise routine recommended by the American Academy of Orthopedic Surgeons. I stand with my feet slightly apart and gently bend backwards with my hands on my lower back. Keeping my knees straight, I bend backwards at the waist as far as I can and hold that position for two seconds.

Be sure to always get the proper chair that's right for your body. Don't be misled by products marketed as being "ergonomic." A number of furniture manufacturers use the term to mean different things, including comfortable, easy to use, or efficient. The ideal chair, I've discovered, should support the length and width of your back, and has a flexible backrest, adjustable arm-rests, and a seat height that I can adjust to let my feet rest on the floor. The seat pad should be firm and leave space behind the knees. A five-pronged base with caster that turn easily is the one I most prefer.

Correct footwear is also very important to consider. A person should wear low-heeled shoes to cushion your weight and keep your spine aligned. Prop one foot on a short stool or phone book, and alternate. Sit on a high stool or stand on carpeting when possible. Sometimes I get so tired of sitting that I will actually stand over a desk or table top and read material or write things by hand for awhile. Again, it's variation and gives the body different choices of position.

Yoga Is the Key to Keeping Your Spine Young

If, as the old adage goes, "You are what you eat," then surely "you are as young as your spine is." A spine that is both supple and strong is a great blessing in disguise. From a practical standpoint, maintaining spinal health enables you the freedom to perform with grace and ease the most ordinary of everyday tasks. These range from tying your shoes and vacuuming the carpet to mowing grass or planting flowers in your garden. A healthy spine means better posture, better breathing, increased energy, and improved body health in later years.

The best way to insure that your spine stays young as you get older, is by taking up yoga. This system of simple stretching exercises combined with quiet contemplation offers you a wise repertoire of postures—from beginning to advanced—to keep your spine limber, strong and youthful. A balanced practice includes forward bends, back bends, sideways stretches, and twists. One basic posture that addresses the side-to-side movements of the spine is an easy standing stretch known in yoga tradition as Ardha Chandrasana or the Half Moon Pose.

The pose is relatively simple in terms of its mechanics. At the same time, in addition to working the spine, it can offer you a number of benefits. Raising the arms over your head encourages flexibility of the shoulder joints and tones the muscles of the arms. The lateral stretch tends to strengthen the overall musculature of the torso, including the abdominals. The overall pose greatly benefits the kidneys, liver, spleen, and digestive system.

To properly begin this simple exercise, you must first clear your mind of all anxiety and tension. Do this in a basic standing position with both feet together and arms at your sides. Imagine yourself standing by the seashore, near a lake, or beside a babbling mountain brook. Your stance should feel balanced and relaxed within five minutes.

Now slowly open your eyes and focus your gaze on one point at eye level or slightly above it. Contract your quads, gently firm up the buttocks, and then draw the abdominal area in and up. The shoulders should be down and the chest lifted. Breathe deeply, bringing awareness to your entire body. Commit your whole tabernacle to this posture.

Inhale as you begin to rotate your palms out and bring your arms from your sides to well above your head. Interlace your fingers, pointing upward and crossing one thumb over the other. Take another couple of breaths as you extend through your arms, straightening your elbows as firmly as you can. Be sure to keep the arms in the same place as your body. The throat and neck should remain relaxed.

When you are ready to stretch to the side, breathe in, stretching upward. As you exhale, stretch directly to your right, hips pressed toward the left. Keep the underside of the rib cage in as long as possible. I might suggest that you stand in front of a full-length mirror while doing this. You'll find it to be helpful.

Hold here and breathe. Continue to look at your chosen spot. Keep the legs very firm, with buttocks and abdominals lifted. When you're ready to come up, focus on the left side of the abdominal area and waist and come up on the inhalation. Once you are upright again, pause and exhale.

Now take another deep breath in and, as you move over to the left side, exhale. Again, keep as much length as possible underneath the left side of the rib cage and waist. The bottom elbow will have a tendency to bend or buckle a little. So it may be necessary to work a little harder on the underneath arm until this problem has been corrected. Also, use caution and be sure not to twist the neck or chin. Both the neck and head should move in line with the rest of the spine, following the arc described by your fingertips.

When you're ready, come up to center on the inhalation. Pause and exhale, then stretch up again as you inhale. Open your arms down to your sides as you exhale, completing the pose. Stand for a few well-deserved breaths, keeping your focus on your chosen spot, resting in another yoga position known as the Mountain Pose. Then repeat this exercise one more time.

By now you will be feeling a surge of warm energy flowing throughout your body. Your legs, torso, and arms will be alive with a pleasant tingling sensation. This is due to the increased rush of blood through your system. The Half Moon Pose is wonderful to do at intervals during a series of standing postures. It also serves as a nice counterpose to balancing out both forward and backward bending postures in yoga. It is good in preparation for twists also.

I am grateful to Mara Carrico of San Diego, California, for her kind assistance in providing me with information on this particular stretching exercise. Her book, *Ten-Minute Yoga Work-In* and *Jane Fonda's Yoga Exercise Workout* video (which Ms. Carrico helped to create) are available from The Yoga Institute and Bookshop, 2150 Portsmouth, Houston, Texas 77098.

CAUTION: Always practice yoga with care. If a woman is pregnant or menstruating, she should not engage in yoga exercises. If a person has had previous back surgery, he or she should check with his or her doctor before attempting any kind of stretching exercises. Also, those bothered with hiatal hernias or heart problems should get medical approval before undertaking *any* yoga.

How I Conquered My Own Lower Back Pain

I stand 6 feet 4 inches tall in stocking feet. Sometimes when I'm walking I will forget correct posture and tend to slump a bit. Sitting a lot and typing lengthy books also leads to unintentional slouching. Sometimes reaching up high for a book on a top shelf will, likewise, create problems for me. And, if I'm not careful when bending over to pick up a heavy box, I can also put my back out of place. All of these likely scenarios have happened in times past, resulting in very severe back pain.

One day while watching an experienced animal trainer run some German Shepherd police dogs through a series of maneuvers, the idea struck me to borrow from a couple of the positions he had these obedient canines in. I call them my Hanging Dog and Half-Dog Poses.

The idea with the first is to make an inverted V shape with my body, mimicking the stretch I saw some of these dogs take upon first rising from their sleep. At other times I'll loop a belt around my hips and over a doorknob to help support my body weight. As I hang, the abdomen relaxes. It is this feeling of letting go that brings tremendous relief when you are afflicted with lower back pain.

The props required for this are a nonskid mat and a door with strong doorknobs. Spread out the mat, with the narrow end centered on the edge of the open door. Firmly fasten the belt into a wide loop and place it around both doorknobs. Step inside the loop and stand with your back to the door. Hold the belt and walk forward until it presses against your body, where the thighs meet the torso.

Then bend your knees, lean forward, and put your hands on the floor. Walk your feet back toward the door and walk your hands forward until your body is in the shape of an inverted V. Let the belt hold the weight of your body. Make sure that the belt pulls evenly against both sides of the door. If your hamstrings are too tight to practice comfortably with your hands on the floor, work with your hands on a chair seat.

Your hands should be placed approximately 20 inches apart; the same applies to your feet. Besides, your hands and feet should be a wide distance from each other. Often this pose is practiced with hands and feet too close together. This makes it harder to feel the tonifying stretch that releases the spine and abdomen.

Permit your head to hang down as you allow the belt to hold your weight. Breathe slowly and evenly as your back muscles lengthen. As you exhale, move your stomach into the pelvis so it forms a concave shape. Then relax a bit. You can practice this Hanging Dog Pose for up to 3 minutes. To come out of it, simply bend your knees, walk your hands toward your feet, and stand up *slowly*. Remain still for one minute. Keeping your eyes open, take a few deep breaths before stepping out of the belt loop.

I've found from my own experience that this exercise pose tends to place the long muscles of my lower back in traction.

And with gravity assisting, this simple stretch relieves much of the tension in these long muscles, as well as in other muscles of my lower back. In addition, my Hanging Dog Pose is an inversion, which reverses the normal position that the vertebral structures have in relationship to gravity. This, in turn, relieves the habitual effects of upright posture.

An even simpler version of the first is my Half-Dog Pose. All you need for this is a sturdy table with a single-fold blanket on top of it to support your torso when you bend forward. This pose gently stretches the long muscles of the back by placing the lower back in traction. As your torso rests on the table, gravity's pull on the back muscles is greatly relieved.

To start this, stand in front of the table, with your feet spread hip-wide apart. Now gradually bend forward from where your torso meets your thighs, and rest your torso on the table. Your torso and legs should be at 90° to each other, with your legs straight and feet resting lightly on the floor. If you're not at a 90° angle, come up and stack another blanket (single-fold) over the first blanket. Then move forward again and rest your torso on the blankets. Stretch your arms out in front of you and hold on to the far edge or rest them on the table, or fold your arms and place them on the table. Rest your forehead either on the table or on your folded arms. You can also turn your head to one side as long as you spend an equal amount of time with your head facing the other side, too.

Try to breathe slowly and easily. Let your torso and arms rest completely on the table. Slightly bend your knees and let the weight of your legs drop toward the floor. Allow your back and neck to lengthen on each exhalation. Try stretching in this supported position: Walk backward a few steps or reach forward with your arms. If you feel uneasy about any of this, discontinue for a short time.

You can practice this Supported Half-Dog Pose for up to 3 minutes, if need be. Keeping your knees bent, use your arms to help you come to a standing position. Stand quietly for a few breaths before going about your regular activities again. This pose helps to stretch the muscles along the spinal column, and relieves tightness and stiffness in your lower back.

CAUTION: Remove your socks when doing both poses. If you feel *more* pain when attempting to do this, cease at once and do later when your back is more cooperative. Have someone massage the painful area by hand or with a mechanical vibrator to loosen the muscles up a bit before trying it again.

Those who have acute hypertension or migraine headaches shouldn't attempt doing either of these without consulting a physician first. If dizziness is experienced when coming into or out of either pose, make sure that you aren't holding your breath while moving up and down. **Don't practice** either pose if you are pregnant, have taken medication, or just finished a big meal. It is best to do these exercises on an empty stomach devoid of food or drugs.

Other variations include: simple backbends supported by a long-roll blanket placed directly under the middle of the back; a child's pose in which you kneel and bend over with your chest supported by a couple of folded sleeping bags or quilts or several pillows or sofa cushions; and a basic relaxation pose that calls for a prone position on a carpeted floor flat on your back with the hips elevated and legs draped across a chair (place a single-fold blanket behind the neck and a sandbag directly over your abdomen for greater benefit).

Take care when practicing any of these simple stretching techniques. They're relatively safe provided one doesn't have any of the aforementioned conditions. When coming out of one or several of these poses, do so *gradually*. Then walk around the room for a couple of minutes to try out your relaxed back. You will be pleasantly surprised to see just how quickly much, if not all, of the pain has subsided. And when resuming your normal activities, be careful to not bend and twist at the same time. You may need to do repeated performances of each pose several times a day for up to a week before your back is in great shape again.

But yoga exercises like these are guaranteed to not only free you of back pain, but also to make your spine feel as young as one belonging to a high school or college athlete or cheerleader.

Balancing Blood Sugar Imbalances

"BALTIMORE'S HISTORIC WATERING HOLE YIELDS UP SOME SURPRISING REMEDIES"

🌿 AN ORIGINAL NEIGHBORHOOD KEPT INTACT

As one of the original neighborhoods that merged in the 18th century to form the city of Baltimore, Fells Point exudes a unique and salty warmth—a combination of hospitality and hipness difficult to define. One thing is certain for sure: this waterfront community located southeast of the Inner Harbor knows how to serve up the good times.

Some believe it's the proximity to the sea, or the fact that Fells Point has been quenching the thirst of sailors and seafarers since the early 1700s. With several dozen pubs, taverns, and inns, it is the place to go in Baltimore to unload the urban angst.

But this authentic Federal period village is more than a bar district. With more than 350 structures dating back to the 1760s, Fells Point is one of Baltimore's best-preserved neighborhoods. It was the first district in Maryland to be placed on the National Register of Historic Places. It was once a thriving center for shipbuilding, trade, and other nautical activities, and the still bustling harbor echoes this past.

What is perhaps most enticing about this point is that in spite of its closeness to the touristy and often crowded Inner Harbor and Baltimore Aquarium, it still remains virtually undiscovered by outsiders.

Book business had taken me to that city the week of September 15-18, 1995. I was there to sign several hundred books being given away at the Prentice Hall exhibit at the Natural Products Expo East being held in the huge Baltimore Convention Center. One of the local health food retailers who happened by, informed me about the Robert Long House (built around 1765) and said I might find the adjacent garden interesting, since it was right up my alley anyway.

I found the L-shaped garden to be an exact replica of how a colonial garden was cultivated. There were numerous plants everywhere which once served as food seasonings, scents, fabric dyes, and above all, medicines.

🌿 HANDY REMEDIES FOR BLOOD-SUGAR PROBLEMS

Several other visitors were there to enjoy the lovely sights that this garden offered up. One of them was Elaine Juzak, a practicing herbalist. She was sketching one of the plants on a large white notepad as I strolled by.

My curiosity got the better of me and I paused to inquire of her activity. After some small talk, we made a formal introduction to each other. Upon learning my last name and the type of books I wrote, she warmed up to me even more and mentioned having several of 50-plus books in her small library.

I pointed over to one plant for no apparent reason and casually remarked, "Looks like garden artichoke to me." She agreed with my identification and then related how she recommends this all the time to many of her clients who suffer blood sugar disorders.

"I find globe artichoke to be one of the best *food medicines* around for diabetes or hypoglycemia," she said. "I encourage my customers to eat it all the time. Steaming them is probably the best way to go with them. I also have them make a tea of the flower heads and leaves." To do this, simply add one-half cup of these vegetable parts to 1½ pints boiling water. Cover and simmer for 15 minutes. Then set aside and steep another ten minutes. Strain and drink 3 cups each day, one per meal.

I noticed some dandelion growing haphazardly in a few places. "Probably for medicinal purposes back then," I wondered aloud. Just then one of the caretakers happened by and told us both that such an herb had no place being there.

"Simply ruins the garden," he grumbled. "Detracts from the beauty of everything else. Must get my herbicide and spray it soon to get rid of the noxious thing. Blasted weeds anyway!" He then passed on by us mumbling some more to himself.

Ms. Juzak and I looked at each other in astonishment. We were greatly surprised by the blatant ignorance of people like this. The man had absolutely no idea that he had just been cursing one of the *best* herbs given to us by nature for treating diabetes and hypoglycemia. Both Elaine and I only knew too well the different ways it can be used in either condition.

Diabetes/Hypoglycemia

Dandelion Flower:	Consumed raw in the Spring in salads.
Dandelion Leaves:	Excellent when used fresh in Spring salads. Ideal for juicing in a Vita-Mix blender. Wonderful as a tea when sun-dried.
Dandelion Root:	Terrific medicine in capsule form (3 daily). Makes a dandy tea (2 cups daily with meals). Nice coffee substitute, too.

Together we spied some flax growing off in one corner by itself. "That's good for diabetes," I observed, "when 2 tablespoons of the mature seeds are boiled for 35 minutes in one quart of distilled water, until only half the liquid remains. People who've followed this suggestion have reported back to me that after drinking 1-2 cups a day for 6 weeks, they need to take *less* insulin."

"Ditto, ditto, and ditto," laughed Elaine. "Same thing applies for those with low blood sugar."

Some stinging nettle was spotted not too far from the flax. "Euell Gibbons praised them in his book *Stalking the Healthful Herbs* (New York: David McKay Company, Inc., 1966; p. 15). He suggested that equal parts of them and horseradish leaves be gathered with gloved hands in the early Spring, washed under running water, and be parboiled, with a little lemon juice and apple cider vinegar spritzed over them afterwards to improve their flavor. They're a great tonic food combination for diabetics and hypoglycemics."

"I haven't ever heard horseradish leaves being used for that purpose," Ms. Juzak chimed in. "But I certainly know all about the benefits of nettle for blood sugar disorders. I prescribe it as a tea (2 cups a day) or in capsules (3 twice daily)."

Just then the crotchety caretaker returned with his sprayer. He walked over to the dandelions and gave them several good squirts of powerful herbicides. "There, you rascals," he exclaimed to himself. "Take that and that!" Elaine and I looked at each other and shrugged our shoulders in helpless amazement.

Deciding to have a little fun with the old gent, I loudly remarked, "Oh, sir, there's some more weeds over here." I then pointed out the stinging nettle.

Whereupon, he drew himself up with some indignity. "You apparently don't know much about herbs, do you?" he rejoined. "That's *supposed to be there*. It was a valuable food staple in colonial times. If you read your brochure they give inside the house, then you'd know better, wouldn't you." With that he walked away, satisfied that this presumed upstart had been put in his proper place and fully corrected on his apparent mistake.

Ms. Juzak and I both laughed at the irony of the whole episode. "Takes all kinds to make the world go round, doesn't it?" she asked. I nodded in agreement.

The only thing over which we were divided so far as our expert opinions went, was onion, some of which grew in the garden that afternoon. She stated that boiled onion consumed whole and its cooking water were both very good for blood sugar problems.

I respectfully begged to disagree with her. "Might be for diabetes," I mentioned, "same as garlic, goldenseal, cayenne pepper, and pau d'arco are. But the person with hypoglycemia, who takes any of these internally, will have the devil to pay later on with increased aggravations to his or her problem. The scientific literature and my own experiments bear this out."

She said she had never heard anything like this and wasn't aware of such side-effects from these particular plants for those with low blood sugar. But we shook hands and parted on good terms, nevertheless.

Baldness Beautified

"HOW ONE UTAH MAN KEPT MOST OF HIS HAIR FOR ALMOST A CENTURY"

🌿 Mr. Kitchens' Great Culinary Secret

I met George Washington Kitchens a couple of years ago in my capacity as editor of *Utah Prime Times* (the state's largest seniors newspaper); he was then 98 years of age. At that time he was South Salt Lake's oldest resident. He had resided there for 61 years when I interviewed him.

In young manhood George wheeled cement for the footings of the State Capitol. He was very sports-minded. George boxed with Jack Dempsey, won a golf tournament at Bonneville Golf Course and amazed many of his senior friends when he walked on his hands off the diving board at Saratoga resort at age 71.

George's life spanned the eras from horse-and-buggy to rocket ship. When he was born the United States still flew the Civil War Flag with its 37 stars. He courted his wife in a surrey with a fringe on top and saw a man land on the moon.

Two very remarkable things struck me about this man. One was his happy personality: "I always try and leave people with a smile; it makes them feel a whole lot better." The other was his near full head of hair. "How come you're not bald like every other older fellow?" I asked, knowing full well that in my late forties I had gotten "pretty thin through the middle" on my own scalp.

"It's a trade secret," he teased me with a sly grin. "Been in the family forever, least ways as long as I can remember. My father died with most of his own hair still intact. As did his father before him."

"Oh, then it's a genetic thing?" I replied.

"More like a dietary thing," he quickly responded. "Both of my great-uncles and uncle on my dad's side became bald as billiard balls when they reached 70. And two of my own three sons probably have less hair on their heads by now, than what I have on my chest." Here he paused for a good-natured chuckle.

✤ GREENS, GREENS, AND MORE GREENS

George claimed that the "food secret" to the lack of baldness in himself, his dad, and his granddad was "cooked greens, like the kind they make in the South." George was certainly one to know, since he spent part of his growing up years in Dawson, Georgia. "My mom always fixed us greens every chance she could," he said. "I took a hankering to them myself at an early age and have been eating 'em ever since."

The "cooked greens" to which George referred were mostly collards, turnip greens, beet greens, mustard greens, and spinach. "They're cooked best when flavored with a little lemon juice and fried bacon bits," he observed. When his family relocated to the Mountain West, first in Idaho and then later in Utah, stinging nettle was substituted for collards.

George believed it was the high amount of iron in such cooked leafy greens that "has helped my hair to stay in place and pretty much kept it from all falling out." He said an oldtime barber told him many years ago that a diet high in iron-rich foods was good for keeping a healthy head of hair in place. "I guess his advice seems to have worked for the most part," George reflected as he ran his hand over the top of his head. (George Kitchens died a few years later at the age of 102.)

While it may not always be practical to cook up a bunch of mixed greens and eat them on a regular basis, a person could certainly take them in a different form that's more convenient with the same results. Pines International has a product called Mighty Greens, which consists of over two dozen leafy green herbs and vegetables that are packed with iron and other vital nutrients necessary for a healthy scalp. One tablespoon of this powder mixed in with a glass of juice or water makes a delicious chlorophyll drink.

There should also be added to this about seven drops of ConcenTrace, a natural trace mineral product from Trace Minerals Research of Ogden, Utah. This will supply the body with other important elements that keep hair follicles alive, healthy, and *in place* for many, many years. Both products are available from some health food stores. Or consult the Product Appendix for more information on how to obtain them.

GIVE THE SCALP A GOOD MASSAGE

George also told me that this same oldtime barber suggested giving the scalp a good massage every morning upon arising. He said this could be easily accomplished by sitting on the edge of your bed, bending forward and vigorously rubbing the scalp with the fingertips in all directions for about five minutes.

"This gets the circulation really going in an area of the body, which seldom gets any attention," he noted. "The barber told me that you could tell when the circulation had increased when the top of your head started tingling all over. That's the sign the blood was rushing in and nourishing the hair follicles." George said it could also be done with a hand-held vibrator, if necessary.

I decided to give this thing a try myself some years ago. And while it was a bit too late to rescue my already formed male pattern baldness syndrome, it did manage to *stop further* hair loss. My father Jacob, who was age 83 during the writing of this book, is 85% bald. At least I was able to slow mine down considerably and retain more of my own hair follicles by giving myself regular scalp messages several times a week.

Bladder Strengtheners

"TECHNIQUES FOR CONTROLLING URINE LEAKAGE"

WHAT CAUSES IT?

This medical problem may be characterized as the partial or total inability to control the urge to urinate. It is prevalent in older folks, being twice as frequent in women over the age of 50. While aging does exert some obvious influence, more than likely this problem is produced by some underlying disorder.

There are different kinds of incontinence: stress and urge incontinence are two of the most common. Stress incontinence occurs when some activity—coughing, laughing, or lifting, for

instance-temporarily increases the pressure on the bladder, causing a small amount of urine leakage. Urge incontinence happens
when an unexpected inclination to urinate is followed by an
inability to control the bladder, sometimes releasing copious
amounts of urine.

Incontinence leads to social embarrassment, mental depression, and public isolation. More often than not, it is the major
reason why people are put in nursing homes by their relatives.
Particular treatment measures and the degree of success
achieved with treatment depend on the underlying cause, but in
most instances, incontinence can be at least controlled if not
eliminated.

Several factors are believed to be responsible for this problem. Abnormalities of the detrusor muscle, which contracts to
force urine out of the bladder is one of them. Another is weak-
ness of the muscles of the pelvic floor that support the bladder
and control urine flow in women who've just delivered new-
borns. Then there are age-related changes in the urinary tract,
like bladder shrinkage. Atrophy of the urethra due to decreased
estrogen production in postmenopausal women should probably
be mentioned. Another reason may be the use of the over-the-
counter or prescription medications that include diuretics,
sleeping pills, and tranquilizers. And sometimes a urinary tract
infection may be involved. Occasionally there may be damage to
the nerves that control bladder function, causing either excessive contraction of the bladder or loss of sensation governing the
urge to urinate. An eighth factor can sometimes be surgery or
radiation therapy of the pelvic area. An obstruction of the flow
of urine may be due to an enlarged prostate or urethal stricture.
A final consideration are psychological disorders, especially
depression.

WAYS OF RESOLVING THE MATTER

In a number of cases, older men and women have regained control of their bladders with techniques known as bladder training
(for urge incontinence) and Kegel exercises (for stress inconti-

nence). Bladder training begins by scheduling a bathroom visit every two hours, whether a person needs to go or not. The interval is steadily increased by 30 minutes at a time, toward a goal of four-hour intervals. In most cases the body adapts to this schedule, eliminating incontinence. Kegel exercises involve repetitive contractions of the pelvic-floor muscles to strengthen them and prevent stress incontinence. Ask your urologist for more information on how to do them properly.

One middle-aged woman I know, who only wanted her first name of Ruth used in this book, told me she received considerable help for her problem from biofeedback. This is a technique using electronic equipment that provides visual and auditory feedback to increase patient awareness and control of the bladder muscles. She claimed that the sights and sounds of a waterfall were incentive enough to sharply focus on controlling her bladder. As a result of this strong determination to reverse the course of the falling water, her own incontinence was eventually cured.

A number of botanicals have proven helpful sometimes in treating incontinence. The forms in which they're taken often determine just how effective they may be. The list below gives both pieces of data.

ASPARAGUS:	one cup of the water they are cooked in.
BARBERRY:	one cup of tea or 4 capsules.
BLACK CURRANT:	1/2 cup of the juice.
BUCHU:	one cup of tea or 3 capsules.
CARROT:	one cup of juice.
CELERY:	1/2 cup juice mixed with 1 cup carrot juice.
CHERVIL:	1/2 to 1 cup of tea.
CHICKWEED:	one cup of tea or 2 capsules.
CHICORY:	1/2 cup of juice made from the leaves mixed with 1 cup of carrot juice; 1 cup of tea made from the root.
DANDELION:	1/2 cup of juice made from the tender leaves and combined with 1 cup of tomato juice; 1 cup of tea made from the root; or 3 capsules.

GARDEN VIOLET: 1 cup of tea made from the spring leaves or fall harvested rootstock.

HORSERADISH: $1/4$ teaspoon sauce consumed with $1/2$ slice of bread or 2 capsules.

JUNIPER: 1 cup of tea periodically.

LICORICE: 2 capsules or 1 cup of tea made from the rootbark.

ONION: $1/2$ cup of tea made from the boiled bulb or $1/2$ of the bulb, sliced, lightly sautéed, and eaten.

PARSLEY: $1/4$ cup of juice mixed with 1 cup of carrot juice.

PEACH: one fresh peach peeled and eaten; 1 cup of tea made from the leaves; or 15 drops of the tincture.

RADISH: $1/4$ cup of juice mixed with 1 cup of tomato juice.

WILLOW: 1 cup of tea; 3 capsules; or 15 drops of tincture.

To make tea, boil one pint of water and add 2 teaspoons of any botanicals mentioned in the list. If the plant materials are delicate (flowers and leaves), then stir them with a spoon, cover with a lid, and set aside to steep for 25 minutes. On the other hand, if the parts are of tougher materials (seeds, twigs, bark, and root) then stir, cover with lid and simmer on low heat for 5 minutes, before setting aside to steep 20 minutes. Strain and drink the amount directed twice daily, once in the morning and again in the early evening, always on an empty stomach.

Juices can be made by submitting vegetables to a Vita-Mix whole food machine. Add $1/2$ to 1 cup of ice cubes, secure the lid, and run for two minutes. Use the juice in the manner previously directed.

Herbal antibiotics may sometimes be necessary to treat a bacterial infection that could be associated with urinary incontinence. Some of the better ones include echinacea, goldenseal, myrrh, and wild Oregon grape. They are best taken in capsules (about 2 a day) on account of their bad tastes. Kyolic Garlic from Wakunaga of America is another perfect remedy: take 4 capsules or one tablespoon of the liquid regularly.

If over-the-counter or prescription drugs are believed to be a cause of the incontinence, consult with your doctor. He may either change the prescription or reduce the intake. An operation may be recommend by your urologist to relieve pressure on bladder nerves, reduce blockage of the urethra, or repair damaged muscles or other structures. Personally, if it were me in this same situation, I would refuse surgery and instead rely on herbs and faith-healing to correct the matter.

Adult diapers and pads are easy enough to resort to, but could actually promote complications if they're used for a long time. Therefore, short-term applications are suggested instead. A bedside toilet will help with nighttime urgency. Avoid drinking excess fluids for two to three hours prior to retiring for the night.

Bursitis Rectified

"'SINGIN' IN THE RAIN' ACTOR KEPT LIMBER BY DANCING A LOT"

 HE DANCED HIS WAY INTO OUR HEARTS

On Friday, February 2, 1996, one of Hollywood's most successful and beloved performers died at the age of 83. His name was Gene Kelly. His film and stage career spanned over half a century. His life was the stuff of a Hollywood musical. A would-be baseball player and failed law student, he once made money teaching dance in the basement of his parents' Pennsylvania home. After a few Depression-era amateur contests, he conquered Broadway and then Hollywood, starring in such films as "Singin' in the Rain," "On the Town" and "An American in Paris."

In 1942, Judy Garland was Kelly's first dance partner on the big screen. Later he would be teamed up with Fred Astaire, Rita Hayworth, Frank Sinatra, Leslie Caron, Donald O'Connor, Shirley MacLaine, and many others. But of all his dance partners, none was more memorable than that famous umbrella, which he used in his classic film "Singin' in the Rain." This much beloved 1952 Hollywood spoof with Debbie Reynolds and Donald O'Connor as his co-stars, provided the lasting image of

Kelly's winning screen persona: an affable, optimistic man with a fine Irish grin and soft spot in his heart.

A BAD CASE OF BURSITIS

The daily program, "Entertainment Tonight" devoted several minutes of its Monday evening, February 5th broadcast to Kelly's life and cinematic accomplishments. Several of his former co-stars were interviewed, including Debbie Reynolds and Frank Sinatra. It was revealed in the program that when Kelly was about 26 years of age (roughly 1939), he developed an unexplained case of bursitis in parts of his lower torso. The bursa or small, fluid-filled sacs located at or near the joints in his hips, knees, and heels, became inflamed. This resulted in joint swelling and made every movement quite painful for him.

HOW KELLY FOUND RELIEF

Two things that a doctor recommended for him to use were cold and hot packs. Kelly applied ice packs over these areas a couple of times every day, then switched to heat packs for awhile after that. This stimulated blood flow to these areas and helped to ease the pain there.

But the thing that seemed to work the most was when he started dancing. Not the perfect ballroom dancing of a Fred Astaire or the sophisticated toe tapping of an Eleanor Powell. But more of a loose-limbed jig of a sailor on leave, that was reminiscent of some of the old dancers from the South who did vaudeville frequently in those years. It seemed like every part of his body moved whenever he danced: his arms swung out wide, his legs and feet moved in every direction, his head kept turning; in fact, his entire torso was in constant motion.

Eventually this painful bursitis cleared up of its own accord. Undoubtedly, what happened was that this type of energetic dancing, involving different parts of the body, greatly enhanced blood flow throughout his entire system. This helped to reduce his swollen joint bursas and make the pain disappear.

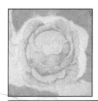

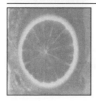

Circulatory Disorders Diminished

"'WRONG-WAY CORRIGAN' HAD IT RIGHT WHEN IT
CAME TO HIS OWN HEALTH"

❧ CALIFORNIA BY WAY OF IRELAND

Douglas Corrigan, a brash, errant aviator, captured the imagination of a Depression-weary public in 1938 when he took off from Brooklyn on a nonstop solo flight to Los Angeles and instead landed his improbable aircraft in Dublin, Ireland, a day later. The few people who were at Floyd Bennett Field that early July 17, 1938 morning at 5:15 A.M. were baffled when the 31-year-old aviator turned into a cloud bank and disappeared to the east.

According to his flight plan, he should have been heading west. But his friends and the world learned something quite different when his jerry-built, overloaded second-hand airplane touched down at Dublin's Baldonnel Airport some 28 hours and 13 minutes later. Corrigan had no real sense of which direction he was headed in. This honest mistake, however, helped him to fly straight into the hearts of the American people.

"I'm Doug Corrigan," he told a group of startled Irish airport personnel who eagerly gathered around him moments after he landed. "Just got in from New York. Where am I now, Los Angeles County? I intended to fly to California."

He had his plane crated up, loaded aboard a cargo vessel bound for America, and sailed back to his native land. The ship Manhattan cruised into New York Harbor on August 4th, where he received a tumultuous greeting. There was an even bigger welcome the very next day when an estimated 1 million New Yorkers lined lower Broadway for a ticker-tape parade that eclipsed the one given for Charles A. Lindbergh after his solo flight to Paris in 1927.

 ## AN AMERICAN HERO IS BORN

The man's 3,150-mile flight was an instant sensation, pushing depressing economic news and grim international reports aside on the front pages of American newspapers and dominating the radio airwaves for days across the entire nation. Although six renowned pilots, among them Amelia Earhart and Wylie Post, had made solo flights across the Atlantic since Lindbergh had blazed the trail in the "Spirit of St. Louis" in 1927, none struck such a chord with the American public as this fellow did.

Part of this was because 'Wrong-Way' Corrigan was seen as an engaging and impish young pilot who had boldly thumbed his nose at authority. Another part was due to the fact that he had made the flight in a pile of junk instead of a state-of-the-art plane with cutting-edge instruments. Fact of the matter is, his rickety plane was so precariously patched together that it was variously dubbed an airborne crate and a flying bucket of bolts.

When I visited Mr. Corrigan at his home in Orange, California, sometime in 1990, he was then 83 years old. He related to me how he put the plane together. "I bought it as a wreck for $310 in 1935. I managed to hop from cow pasture to cow pasture all the way back to California from New York. I ripped out the original 90-horsepower engine and replaced it with a 165-horsepower model that I cobbled together from two old Wright engines. I also decided to install five extra fuel tanks, but they totally blocked my forward view. I don't mind telling you that other parts of the aircraft, including my cabin door, were held together with nothing but *baling wire!*"

Within months of his infamous error he had completed a triumphant American tour, endorsed wrong-way products like a watch that ran backward, and signed lucrative contracts for an autobiography and a movie, "The Flying Irishman," in which he played himself.

🎋 RIGHT SOLUTIONS FOR WRONG HEALTH PROBLEMS

It was 'Wrong-Way's' sister, Evelyn of Santa Ynez, California, who introduced her brother to the 'Right-Way' diet. And also the same person who put us in contact with each other. The event happened this way: A dignified woman of older years came by an exhibit at one of the annual National Health Federation conventions in the Pasadena Convention Center in the early part of 1989, where I was busy selling and autographing some of my health books.

When it came to writing something appropriate on the inside flyleaf of her copy of *Heinerman's Encyclopedia of Fruits, Vegetables and Herbs* (Englewood Cliffs, NJ: Prentice Hall, 1988), I asked for her name, and she replied, "My first name's Evelyn, but I don't care to give out my married name to strangers. Why don't you just put, "To 'Wrong-Way' Corrigan's kid sister from the author." I complied with her wishes and we shortly chatted some more thereafter.

Evelyn stated that her brother started developing circulatory problems at the beginning of the early 1980s. He experienced vein congestion due to years of poor eating habits and lack of adequate exercise. His feet swelled and a few skin ulcers showed up on the back part of the lower legs. Symptoms were also manifested, she said, in some engorged veins which stood out like "giant loops of blue spaghetti." In addition to these things, Corrigan frequently complained of leg weariness, painful arches, and occasional calf cramps.

Getting him to where he would even listen to her was a challenge in and of itself. His attitude in the beginning was typical of that of so many Americans: he viewed alternative health measures outside the purview of orthodox medicine as "a bunch of nonsense." She had to work with her brother and "sell" him on the idea of doing something about his problems *naturally* instead of surgically and with drug therapy.

An older doctor who had been practicing for many years recommended that Evelyn have him wear a pair of support hose. He suggested an old reliable brand by the name of "Teds," which would allow Corrigan to fit them to his own measurements. His sister purchased a pair at an orthopedic shop, but it is also available at any hospital supply center.

A chiropractor showed her a simple exercise for him to do. Corrigan would remove his shoes, lie down on his back, and stretch his feet way up in the air, bracing his hips with both hands by planting his elbows on the carpet surface on which he was then lying. He made sure to keep his feet and calf muscles loose, while he jiggled each foot for about a minute. He also purchased a mini-trampoline at her insistence and lightly bounced up and down on that every morning and evening for 10 minutes. He also began taking short walks upon arising and before retiring, which helped to get the blood moving through his veins again. Eventually he invested in a hand-held vibrator which he used periodically on the backs of his thighs, calves, and ankles to relieve some of the cramping.

An in-house herbalist at a health food store advised Corrigan's sister to have him take some kind of chlorophyll every day. Unfortunately, an inferior brand was recommended, which, though poor in quality, nevertheless managed to improve his sluggish circulation somewhat. Had it been me counseling Evelyn, I would have mentioned the Mighty Greens drink blend and Beet Root Juice Powder without hesitation. Knowing that they are outstanding products from personal use myself, I would have informed her to have the brother mix one tablespoon of the Mighty Greens and one teaspoon of the beet powder together in an 8-ounce glass of water and then drink it on an empty stomach or with a meal.

Furthermore, I would have strongly advised her to have him take 3 capsules of Kyolic EPA from Wakunaga of America, in order to ward off TIAs—transient (brief) ischemic (lack of blood supply) attacks—that are advance warnings a stroke is likely. (See Product Appendix under Pines and Wakunaga for more details.)

The same herbalist also suggested capsules of ginger root (2 a day) and cayenne pepper (1-2), which she bought for him, but doubted he took as regularly as he should have. However, on most of the other things, 'Wrong-Way' seemed favorably inclined to follow her advice. Eventually his problems cleared up enough to give him reasonable freedom from the pain and discomfort that he had been suffering before.

I was informed by members of the family that Corrigan died in late 1995 while in his 88th year of life.

Comebacks from Cancer

"THE BEST ALTERNATIVE TREATMENT PROGRAM DEVELOPED BY AN 84-YEAR-OLD WOMAN"

 ### SHE CURED HERSELF OF COLON CANCER AT 50

The following information originally appeared in a longer form in my 49th book, *Heinerman's Encyclopedia of Juices, Teas and Tonics* (Englewood Cliffs, NJ: Prentice Hall, 1996). But because of its significance to life extension and the process of wellness in general, I feel duty-bound to include some of it here.

The world lost one of its greatest advocates of healthy eating and natural living. Her name was Ann Wigmore and she died from smoke inhalation in her Boston apartment on Thursday, February 17, 1994. She was 84 at the time of her unhappy demise. Ms. Wigmore had been in the process of making some chamomile tea to help her sleep better, when the hot plate she was using for this purpose suddenly caught on fire.

I knew this grand dame of healthy living for more than a decade. We often met at various alternative medical conventions where both of us were on the same program, but usually speaking at different times. We often spent quality time together comparing notes on different health-related matters. But it is probably fair to say that I learned more from listening to her than what I was probably able to teach her.

"Doctor Ann," as she was lovingly called by those who knew her well, never had any formal medical training. And she had little patience with scientists, believing them to be "dimwitted fools." Which probably explains why I purposely kept my Ph.D. in medical anthropology in my back pocket and out of sight, once I learned her true feelings about college-educated people with degrees behind their names.

It was at the Health Horizons Expo held in Pittsburgh the weekend of November 4-6, 1983 at the old Soldiers & Sailors Memorial Hall on 5th Avenue and Bigelow, where she and I spent 3 to 4 hours discussing a wide range of health matters. It was probably one of the most meaningful interviews I've ever conducted in my life. Much of the information given here is from that interview and appears for *the very first time* in print. Ironically enough, none of the holistic health journalists who had written up on her through the years had ever probed as far into her personal life as I had. And she told me that by saying, matter-of-factly, "You're the first one I've ever let go this deep into my private affairs."

Anne Wigmore was born on March 4, 1909 on a farm in Cropos, Lithuania. She emigrated to America when she was sixteen years of age. "I knew nothing about the laws of good health in those days," she sheepishly admitted. "My eating habits were very indiscriminate. And I paid the price for it—by the time I was 50, my hair had turned completely white, and I suffered from arthritis, asthma, colon cancer, and migraine headaches. To have seen me then, you would have said 'there is one sick, old lady.' I was that far from the grave (holding a thumb and fore-finger an inch apart)."

Desperate for help, Ann didn't know exactly where to turn. "At first I consulted with all the doctors, but soon found them to be a bunch of damned old fools who knew nothing and just kept people like myself in a constant state of sickness and pretty well doped up with drugs so we wouldn't feel so much of the pain."

Being of a religious turn—"I was born Catholic but switched to Methodist and Congregational"—she attended the Unity School of Christianity in Missouri. "This wasn't your typical the-ological school," she reminded me. "I received my ministerial license from them, but got my doctor of divinity from the College of Metaphysics." So, in the belief that the Universe had something more to offer her than did the "stupid philosophies of ignorant quacks" (meaning medical doctors), she turned to "the powers that be in the Great Beyond" (as she so eloquently phrased it). "I got the beginnings of my knowledge from the galaxy," she laughed. "Now how's that for believability?"

The "cosmic influences" from space (as she styled it), "told me that if I wanted to live, then I needed to stop eating 'dead food' and start eating 'living food.' It was plainly shown to me that 'liv-ing foods' had enzymes and vitamins in them. And that *ferment-ed* foods were really good for the body because they were 'predi-gested,' that is to say partially digested. And, therefore, could be more easily assimilated into the system with a minimum amount of digestive effort. '*These* are the foods,' I was told in plain English, 'that will destroy the cancers and other diseases in you and restore your body to good health again.' So, I became con-vinced then and there, to overhaul my life, get rid of all my old, bad habits and begin anew with the things I'd been told to do."

WIGMORE'S "ANSWER TO CANCER" PROGRAM: A SUMMARY

"Dr. Ann's" natural approach to cancer involves a number of dif-ferent elements. Some have to do with diet and herbs, while others focus more on lifestyle and psychological changes. They are each presented in detail under separate sub-headings, but are briefly summarized here.

The first step involves preparing a simple, fermented drink from wheat berries, which Ms. Wigmore referred to as Rejuvelac. The second calls for some rather creative and novel ways of using nuts and seeds. All three foods, she noted, provide a sick body with "predigested protein" to help it rebuild itself. The power of *fresh* juices came in third, but, in a sense, formed the nucleus of her outstanding nutrition program. For this reason there is more information on juicing, than on any of the other steps involved.

The last two items she continually emphasized were a determined desire to get well and living in harmony with the environment around you. "I can't make people get well," she was always fond of saying. "I can only give them the *inspiration* for doing so. It is left for them to decide whether or not they really *want* to recover." And once recovery is evident, it is the duty of every former cancer patient to live in such an ordered way that everything between the body, mind, and sprit is in near perfect balance.

REJUVELAC, THE "MIRACLE FOOD" FOR GETTING WELL

The first thing Ann started making was a simple, predigested food which she appropriately called Rejuvelac. She washed some whole grains of wheat enough times in a glass jar until the water ran clear. "I prefer organically grown wheat and the soft kind if it's available; but you can substitute the hard wheat, if necessary," she told me in our interview some years ago.

She then soaked one cup of wheat berries in three cups of water for 48 hours. The first soaking took her the longest time to ferment and would produce a mild-tastirng Rejuvelac. "It's a good thing to have around the kitchen several stoneware crocks for fermenting and storing the finished drink," she added. She poured the first batch into an empty crock and used it as needed. The second batch was made by using the same seed from the first batch. Without rinsing the seeds, she added more water to the crock and permitted it to soak for just 24 hours. This batch, she assured me, wouldn't take nearly as long to ferment as it had already commenced fermenting.

Rejuvelac took the place of water and Ann started drinking it "by the quartfuls." "This fermented wheat berry beverage of mine," she noted, "was the foundation on which I built everything else years later." Every sick person who walked into her ornate brick mansion, called The Hippocrates Health Institute, at the corner of Commonwealth Avenue and Exeter Street in Boston, and paid the standard $1,250 for a two-week stay, received ample quantities of Rejuvelac. "It doesn't cure anything," she cautioned, "but only *builds the foundation* for the cure to rest on."

 ## "PREDIGESTED PROTEIN" FROM SEEDS & NUTS

I can still remember that memorable visit we had with each other way back in 1983. Even after all these years, the humor, good-naturedness, and considerable health wisdom still shine through in that woman. In my heart I still feel an admiration for someone who fairly sparkled with humanity and compassion.

In that old Soldiers & Sailors Memorial hall in downtown Pittsburgh, she continued spelling out for my benefit the details of her fascinating "Answer to Cancer" recovery program.

"The body always needs some form of protein," she said, "even when it's ailing and dying. I quickly discovered this with my own colon cancer—here I was wasting away into oblivion, but couldn't eat any of the standard sources of protein, such as meat, milk, eggs, and butter. My body kept rejecting them."

So Ann ingeniously figured out her own "predigested protein," as she aptly named. "*Everything* I consume is 'predigested!'" she stated with obvious enthusiasm. In other words, what she was telling me was that EVERY FOOD she consumed and gave her many hundreds of patients to consume had in some way been FERMENTED! Her special "seed yogurt" became the *second* mainstay of her recovery program.

She experimented with different nuts and seeds to find out what each one tasted like. "Almonds are relatively sweet, sesame has a sharp taste, and sunflower seeds give a blander flavor," she observed. "Cashews are quite rich, but peanuts are difficult to digest. All the seeds become sweeter once they're sprouted."

To make her "seed yogurt," fill a two-quart glass Mason jar three-fourths full with seeds of your choice; they can be separate or mixed together. Figure on using one cup each of dehulled sunflower seeds and sesame seeds. Pour over them $2^1/_2$ cups of Rejuvelac. Soak for $5^1/_2$ hours and sprout 13 hours. Blend with some more Rejuvelac (another $2^1/_2$ cups) to make a fine thick cream. Pour this into a sprout bag made of muslin material and hang over a bowl to drip during the fermentation process.

"I always like to cut up some bell peppers, celery, and onions," she continued, "and mix them in with the seeds and liquid. When I add them I generally use a larger bowl to let everything ferment in. I keep it at room temperature the whole time it's fermenting. I cover the bowl, but never tightly. I let things sit for about 5 hours. Then I pour off the whey into another container. The seed yogurt can be refrigerated for several days. It has many uses. At the 'Mansion' [Hippocrates Health Institute], we often add it to salads to make interesting creamy concoctions. I will even add a little bit sometimes to my green drinks, to give them more 'perk and spunk!' We use it just as we would yogurt, over fruit salads, as an in between snack mixed with some Rejuvelac, and so forth.

"When I started putting this 'predigested protein' into my body, wonderful things began happening. My body experienced more energy, I gained weight, and my colon cancer started *diminishing*! No person with cancer should ever be without my Rejuvelac and this 'seed yogurt.'"

🦎 JUICES ARE THE "POWER OF LIFE"

The late Paul Bragg had a very simple dietary philosophy that he lived by for most of his adult life: "Juices are the real *power of life*, and the more you consume them the longer you'll live!" He certainly was a living testament of this, dying in a drowning accident off Waikiki Beach, Hawaii, in December, 1976, just shy of his 97th birthday!

"Dr. Ann" also subscribed to the same ideology. "I could easily live to be 95 if I wanted to," I recall her telling me. At the time of our interview she described herself as "a feisty 75-year-old" who was "a ball of energy." Dr. Bernard Jensen, a noted nutritionist, health practitioner, author, and speaker, still held to this "juicing theory" in the 89th year of his own existence.

Every single one of these people was what might be called an "apostle of good health and rightful living." Each one came from a troubled background filled with sickness, pain, and utter despair early in their lives. But the one thing they shared in common together was that *fresh juices* helped them to fully recuperate and get their lives and health back in working order again.

Ann told me that after World War I, there was "total devastation" of the area in which she and her family lived. So her grandmother Maria Warnisky went out with her and gathered "ordinary meadow grasses, like clover, lambsquarter, and timothy, and brought them home for us to eat," Ms. Wigmore recalled. "I never knew that such nourishing and simple meals could be made from *common weeds*. That experience helped to convince me later on in life that *grasses are essential* to making *worthwhile juices*! You just can't do without them. Practically no leafy vegetable can hold a candle to them in terms of the wonderful vitamin, mineral, and enzyme nourishment they provide."

Ann ranked the following plants as critical to cancer recovery and invariably included most if not all of them in her juices.

ALFALFA, because it is the "King of Mineral Content."

BEET, because its dark red pigment enriches the blood.

CARROT, because it is high in antioxidant vitamin A components.

DANDELION, because it does the liver a world of good.

LAMBSQUARTER, because "wilderness nutrition" is at work here.

WATERCRESS, because of the valuable sulphur—a virtually unknown nutrient.

These six herbs, she felt, constituted "the perfect juice" for cancer prevention and treatment. While battling her own colon cancer, she not only drank two glasses of this mixture a day, but gave herself enemas with some of it, too.

 ## Ann Wigmore's Juicing Secrets

I've modified some of "Dr. Ann's" recipe instructions to make it easier for readers to create it themselves. I also changed the name to reflect a broader, more positive use for this dynamic juice formula beyond its somewhat self-limiting and negative association with cancer. In fact, there are a number of other health benefits to it, some of which are cited near the end of this section.

 ## The Urge to Get Well

The late Ms. Wigmore believed that discipline was critical to recovery. "While I may believe in compromising under certain circumstances," she once told me, "I've never done so when it comes to sick patients. Life has taught me that you can *never* compromise with illness. You must give a person sick with cancer or any other illness for that matter, what he or she *needs*, and not what the individual may want. I don't pussyfoot around. Time is always of the essence when you have a serious life-threatening disease on your hands. It is urgent that the person gets back to health again as soon as possible.

"Four things I've found to be very helpful to me in treating sick patients. First of all, there must be a *desire* to heal and want to get well. Without it, neither the therapist in charge nor his patient under his immediate care, will ever be successful in getting results that last. And once you and your patient have that desire, then both must *act upon it* while interest is still high and hope very strong. Also each one must *believe in it* or have faith that once the desire is acted upon, it will eventually come to pass. The last thing is to always have *patience*. This is probably the one quality that so many therapists and patients lack. Nature works very slow and the recovery process takes time, sometimes longer than we think."

Juice Powerhouse

¹/₂ cup alfalfa sprouts

2 tablespoons Pines organic beet root juice powder (see Product Appendix for more information)

1¹/₂ cups carrots, cut in 1-inch pieces

¹/₂ cup young dandelion greens

¹/₂ cup lambsquarter

¹/₂ cup watercress

2 cups water

2 cups ice cubes

1. Put the first three ingredients into a Vita-Mix container or equivalent food blender. Add 1 cup water and 1 cup ice cubes. Secure the two-part lid and run the machine for 1¹/₂ minutes.

2. Empty the contents into a large punch bowl or pot and set aside temporarily.

3. Put the container back on the machine (no need to rinse it out first).

4. Next add the remaining three ingredients and the other cups of water and ice cubes. Secure the lid and mix again for the same amount of time.

5. Empty these contents into the large bowl or pot and stir thoroughly with a wooden spoon.

6. Ladle equal amounts into two empty glass quart jars. Seal with lids and refrigerate. Drink one 6 fluid ounce glass four times daily.

7. If some of it is intended to be used for an enema, make sure a little more water is added to dilute down a bit, if necessary. Also, set it out several hours in advance so it reaches room temperature before injecting into the rectum.

WALKING IN HARMONY WITH NATURE

Living in balance with your surrounding environment will keep you well in body, mind, and soul. One of Ann's statements culled out from my lengthy interview with her back in the early winter of 1983 in Pittsburgh, still stands out as being noteworthy and begs to be cited here.

"Sex is like food," she said. "If the person is upset, he or she will indulge in it or food or drink. That individual is always looking for a way out of the problem. But when the person is healthy and happy and productive, then he or she simply does not need the overindulgence in anything, not in food, drink, or sex.

"If you teach an alcoholic restraint, he'll go off the sauce for a period, but then go right back on it again because the original cause for his drinking in the first place, hasn't yet been removed. Or an overweight person, who is always stuffing his or her face with food. That person is doing so because there is a great deal of pain and sorrow there. But when someone is healthy, happy, and productive, then his or her expression comes from another direction. That's the way Nature works. Everything must sooner or later link up with Nature, because Nature always moves forward, is always evolving and growing.

"If we get linked up with Nature, then we automatically do what Nature does. I believe God and Nature are one and the same. And as we are one with Nature, so are we with God, too. But when we are not one with Nature, then we become abnormal in our behavior and habits. This lets disease in. Remember, though, that *nothing in Nature is ever abnormal!*"

The last time I briefly saw Ann Wigmore shortly before her accidental death, she was then 83 and still displayed her same physical exuberance, ruddy complexion, and dark hair that I remembered from a decade ago in Pittsburgh. "I haven't lost any of my spunk yet," she joked, obviously still showing a keen sense of humor, too.

Coronary Artery Disease Antidotes

"CELEBRATED SENIOR DIES AT AGE 137 WITH VIRTUALLY NO ATHEROSCLEROSIS"

❧ LEADING CAUSE OF DEATHS IN AMERICA

It is a well known and established medical fact that the leading cause of death in the United States is coronary artery disease. It is especially fatal to those 50 years of age and above. With every five years of life above middle age, old people with imprudent diets are 5 times at risk of contracting this disease. Thus, someone 65 years of age would be 15 times more likely to get it than someone only 50 years old.

The problem usually begins with a buildup of plaques in the arterial walls, which is called atherosclerosis. These plaques or atheromas (as they're also called) consist mostly of cholesterol-rich fatty deposits, collagen, other proteins, and excess smooth muscle cells. The process usually takes a lifetime to develop. Gradual thickening and narrowing of the arterial walls of the heart impede the flow of blood. Over the course of time these greatly narrowed arteries are unable to meet the increased oxygen requirements of the heart. Essentially this is what coronary artery disease is all about.

❧ AMERICA'S OLDEST SENIOR CITIZEN

I was in Florida in 1976 lecturing for an herb company. I happened to hear about Charlie Smith and had some of those who sponsored me there drive me on over to the Bartow Convalescent Center in the city of Bartow. Then-administrator Ruth Aiple let me spend a couple of enjoyable hours visiting with this very remarkable gentleman.

Charlie was of medium height, slight build, bald as a billiard ball, with gentle eyes and soft voice to match, and a hound dog expression to his face. At that time he had just barely celebrated his 134th birthday. The Polk County school board had awarded him an honorary high school diploma. Along with that the ceremony also included a presentation of a Winnie-the-Pooh bear from newsmen eager to interview and photograph him and a congratulatory telegram from then-President Gerald Ford. Charlie showed me these things with obvious delight, but remained modest as to his own importance. He said he hated being in the limelight so much.

🌿 CAME OVER ON A SLAVE SHIP AS A BOY

Charlie was never certain about his birthdate and there were always questions about his true age. He was 133 years old when discovered picking oranges in a citrus grove in central Florida. Social Security officials told the convalescent center's administrator that they had managed to confirm his age when they found reliable documents in nearby New Orleans and matching papers in faraway Texas confirming his sale into slavery in 1842.

For all of his ancientness, Charlie still had a pretty good memory, especially of his early childhood. He related in almost a whisper sometimes what it had been like as a child living in his native Liberia. He spoke fondly of those early childhood years when he romped and played on the beaches and swam naked in the ocean with his little friends. And then described in more melancholy tones of the time when "the big ship came and took me away from all I knew and brought me here to this strange land."

🌿 "I EAT WHAT I WANT"

I inquired into the man's diet, hoping to find a clue or two there with regard to his remarkable longevity. "I eat what I want to," he softly spoke. "I never worried about anything so's long as it don't wiggle or squirm on my plate. But I do like garlic and onions. Have munched on many of them in my time. Eat them like apples and keeps the people away from me." Here he paused long enough to slowly flash another warm and winning, toothless smile.

"I drink what I please, but don't touch much liquor. Bad stuff for you if you get too much in you. Makes people do crazy things." Charlie admitted that in the last few years he had even given up drinking any more alcohol, but still relished "a good, strong black cup of coffee" and now seemed to prefer soda pop to water. We parted soon thereafter, but I kept in touch periodically with some of the staff at the nursing home as to his progress and condition.

In my last communication with the administrator, Ms. Aiple, she told me that "he had been slipping away gradually. It wasn't anything that we didn't expect, of course." But she reassured me that in the end, "Mr. Smith had a quiet, peaceful, and comfortable demise. He passed on in his sleep without pain. Everyone who came into the room was amazed to see a faint smile traced across his dark face. He died with the dignity befitting a man of his stature. He was a noble soul to the very end. And such a sweet one, too." (The actual time of expiration was October 5, 1979 at 6:30 P.M.)

AMAZINGLY GOOD HEALTH OF THE HEART AUTOPSY REPORT SHOWS

Charlie's remains were conveyed from the Bartow Convalescent Center to Lakeland General Hospital in nearby Lakeland, Florida. Charlie's 70-year-old, sole surviving son Chester Smith signed an autopsy permit, which was then witnessed and signed by two Registered Nurses working at the hospital, Sue Best and Marilyn J. Ness.

Doctors were anxious to learn more about Charlie's overall health. They hoped by performing an autopsy to learn some internal secrets, which might have contributed to his incredible longevity. In this thing they were not to be disappointed at all. The pathological team was headed by Robert K. Ramsey, M.D., with five other surgeons assisting: Francis D. Drake, M.D., James L. Holimon, M.D., D. Richard Jones, M.D., Wilton M. Reavis, Jr., M.D., and Luther A. Youngs III, M.D.

I am deeply indebted to Dr. Ramsey most of all for furnishing me with a complete copy of the "Autopsy Protocol," which he sent to me over 15 years ago from his office at the Lakeland Regional Medical Center where he then practiced. This report remained in my files until the writing of this book took place in the first quarter of 1996. It is herewith produced, in part, for the very first time.

Readers will note that I have greatly simplified those excerpted portions pertinent to the state of Mr. Smith's heart. I have taken the liberty to do this on account of the very technical medical terminology employed by Dr. Ramsey and the others when they completed their report. The language I've used is in layman's terms and, therefore, quite easy to understand.

While Charlie's "cause of death" was listed as "chronic renal failure, chronic congestive heart failure, and bronchopneumonia," due to the natural causes of old age, yet his heart overall was remarkably quite sound, considering his extreme age. The "Gross Description" of the HEART on page 3 of the autopsy report revealed the following things:

Right and left ventricles were of normal thickness.

The aortic valve had very slight atherosclerosis.

Both coronary arteries manifested negligible atherosclerosis and medial calcification.

These more remote coronary arteries also exhibited "only mild atherosclerosis."

Furthermore, the autopsy report declared that the descedent's aorta had "only mild atherosclerosis" and that the renal arteries in both kidneys had "minimal atherosclerosis." Even the cerebral arteries in the brain indicated very "mild atherosclerosis present." In other words, for a man so old, this Charlie Smith's body showed virtually no atherosclerosis to speak of. Or, to put it in Dr. Ramsey's own words when he and I chatted briefly by telephone: "Of all the autopsies I ever did on elderly cadavers, his was the most *unremarkable* when it came to looking for evidence of atherosclerosis in all the usual places that we routinely look. This guy's heart was in the best condition of any I'd ever seen, because it had *so little* evidence of atherosclerosis."

❧ WHAT WERE CHARLIE SMITH'S HEALTH SECRETS?

Based on the information gathered from a personal interview with Charlie when he was still alive, a brief summary can be made of those few important factors that kept this man's heart, like the Energizer Battery bunny of television ad fame, "going and going and going" forever it seemed.

FIRST HEALTH CLUE: He ate lots of garlic and onions most of his life. Scientific research has shown that those people who regularly incorporate one or the other or both in their diets often, usually have the *least* amount of coronary artery disease. Supplementing your daily diet with 1 teaspoon of liquid Kyolic Garlic or 3 capsules of Kyolic EPA (see Product Appendix) will help you to maintain a healthy heart longer.

SECOND HEALTH CLUE: Charlie *occasionally* sipped some liquor, preferring rum and brandy whenever he could obtain some. Recent medical evidence from France, that has been widely reported in the media, has shown that even one *small* glass of red wine each day with a meal will help to prevent hardening of the arteries.

THIRD HEALTH CLUE: Mr. Smith was very, very active for most of his life, except the last few years when he was confined to a nursing home because of his enfeebled condition. He worked for many years as a slave, doing a lot of hard labor that involved considerable bending, lifting, and carrying of heavy loads upon his back. Later, when he obtained his freedom and eventually got around to marrying, he still worked long hours at different jobs. Most were menial tasks of labor that ranged from janitorial work to citrus picking. And when he wasn't doing this, he was *always walking.* All of this activity was usually unhurried and measured as a rule. Charlie never rushed in anything. He told me, "I believe in taking my time. No sense in hurrying when I'll get there soon enough as is."

By incorporating these same three health principles in your own life, you will greatly *decrease* your chances of ever contracting coronary artery disease. And, who knows—you might even wind up living almost as long as Charlie did!

AN ASTONISHING SURPRISE

Charlie Smith's autopsy report concluded with one piece of astounding information. Doctors discovered tiny fragments of a fine metallic substance in the pelvic region near the sacrum (the triangular bone just below the lumbar vertebrae). They belonged to bigger portions of what eventually turned out to be an *old bullet* from the Civil War period. Charlie had apparently been wounded as a young man sometime during this conflict, but had been unable to have the bullet removed. His body eventually took care of the matter by encasing it in a tough protein cocoon where the bullet remained for the rest of his life. Which just goes to show how capable the body is of taking care of itself, often without a physician's assistance!

Creativity for Coping

"SOME POSITIVE WAYS TO CHALLENGE HOPELESSNESS AND DESPAIR"

INPUT FROM THE EXPERTS

In preparation for this particular section of my book, I spent some time interviewing by telephone several mental health professionals and theologians in Florida and Arizona, where the greatest number of America's seniors like to congregate. These individuals have worked with many of the elderly who have given some consideration to ending their lives in one way or another. From them I've culled the best strategies for coping with the pain, despair, frustration, loneliness and depression, which inevitably leads to thoughts of suicide. I am grateful for their assistance, but have honored their requests for anonymity so that they may continue serving their elderly clients in the same efficient manner without the stains of any breach of confidence on their good names.

Life-Saving Technique #1: Admit Problems

Without a doubt acknowledging feelings of hopelessness and desperation is to the person's greatest advantage. Most seniors won't admit they are having emotional troubles. But my informed experts told me that acknowledging such feelings of depression is the first real step toward recovery. Suicidal-prone oldsters grew up in an era when acknowledging emotional problems or going to a psychiatrist or psychologist was tantamount to admitting you were crazy, which is far from the truth. In fact, just the opposite is true: facing up to one's emotional problems shows not only courage but also demonstrates a serious willingness to continue living.

Life-Saving Technique #2: Be Active

The leading reason for emotional problems and suicide among seniors is isolation and loneliness. Staying active and interacting with people is the way to avoid it. Miner Cobb, 67, of Leesburg, Florida, and his pal, Emil Faltin, 77, of nearby Eustis came to a National Health Federation convention that I was speaking at in Orlando in the late Fall of 1993. My subject at the time happened to be on "Depression in Seniors." They shared with me their own secret way of coping with it: "We don't have it [depression] because we talk it out at the Lake Square Mall, where we meet just about every day for doughnuts and coffee." As editor of *Utah Prime Times* (a seniors newspaper) I interviewed a number of older people at the Orem Friendship Center on Tuesday, December 12, 1995 for an article I was doing on the place. There I met Thelma Carter, age 71, and her friend, Elsie Aston, age 68. Both were then in the middle of a major quilting project. "It helps us to pass the time," they said. "Keeps us busy and out of mischief. Better still, keeps our minds off our problems. We don't think as much on them when we're occupied with something like this."

Life-Saving Technique #3: See a Doctor

Always be sure to treat depression for what it really is: *a very serious and life-threatening disease*. Just as you might visit a physician for a mysterious mole on the skin or unexplained abdominal pain, one should never hesitate to call a psychologist or psychiatrist. They are specially trained to assist in such matters. Remember, there is *no shame* attached to such visits. And no, a person is *not* crazy by going for professional counseling. In fact, just the opposite is true. You are quite *sensible* in seeing them before it is too late.

Life-Saving Technique #4: Talk It Out

San Francisco offers one of the most unique and innovative services to its senior citizens of any place in the country that I know of. It is a 24-hour suicide hot line that helps the elderly stay in touch with life. Started back in 1989 and officially certified in 1991, the Center for Elderly Suicide Prevention & Grief Related Services has handled an estimated 119,647 calls, according to staff member Perrie Ancheta, age 27. This averages out to about 1,424 calls per month or some 17,092 calls annually, he said in our phone conversation of Monday evening, January 29, 1996.

"Most of our calls at the hot line number (415)-752-3778," he noted, "are handled by psychology interns, who volunteer their time to man the phone banks when people call in. We train them on how to answer the 'Friendship Line' in a cheery, positive way, to make our callers feel at ease. Our 45 volunteers are here to listen, offer words of encouragement, and, more importantly, help the emotionally desperate feel better about themselves.

"We have a number of 'regulars,' who just check in with us from time to time. We also call out to a sizeable number of clients to see how they are faring. Some are wheelchair-bound or in a frail physical condition and cannot get out as they would like to. Still others, while physically able to move about, may be feeling down because of impoverished circumstances. We've noticed over the years, that as the state of our nation's economy has declined, there has also been a corresponding increase in the number of calls we get from many seniors, who are fearful over financial matters.

"We've found that the *best help* by far, that we've been able to offer all of those who contact us is to let them talk and then let them know that the persons listening on the other end here, really do *care* about them. I think that if more of my [younger] generation would just take the time to listen to more of the older generation, then there would not be so many emotional problems with our elderly citizens like there has been. *Talking* about it and *getting it out* of the system is wonderful therapy, you know. I'm so glad we can offer this service to our city's elderly residents; I wish other cities would try to introduce a similar service for their own seniors. It would be one of the best things they ever did for their citizens."

Life-Saving Technique #5: Pray a Lot

There is something sublime in the power of prayer that defies description. An unspeakable majesty of strength enters into the soul of the one who prays often. There is an invigorating awakening that takes place and diverts burdens of the mind and heart to the soul instead. With each offered prayer comes a spiritual renewal that essentially absorbs whatever problems are laid upon the soul.

The act of prayer is as basic to man and woman as is eating, sleeping, bathing, dressing, eliminating, working, and playing. It is, in fact, the very exercise that makes the human conscience more strong with each passing prayer.

James Montgomery (1771-1854) understood well the power embodied within prayer itself. This son of a Scottish minister was an ardent champion of reformer principles that the British government found offensive and subsequently imprisoned him for on two different occasions. While thus incarcerated in a dark dungeon, he penned the following hymn under inspiration (one of more than 400 published in his lifetime). From it he and countless others have drawn considerable hope and strength.

"PRAYER IS THE SOUL'S SINCERE DESIRE"

Prayer is the soul's sincere desire,
Uttered or unexpressed;
The motion of a hidden fire
That trembles in the breast.

Prayer is the burden of a sigh,
The falling of a tear,
The upward glancing of an eye,
When none but God is near.

Prayer is the simplest form of speech
That infant lips can try;
Prayer, the sublimest strains that reach
The Majesty on high.

Prayer is the believer's vital breath,
The believer's native air;
His watchword at the gates of death;
He enters heav'n with prayer.

Prayer is the contrite sinner's voice,
Returning from his ways,
While angels in their songs rejoice,
And cry, Behold he prays.

There should never be a set form of prayer (except in special religious rituals). Rather the things to be said should be freely expressed from the depths of the soul as one is moved upon by inward emotion as much as by inspiration from Above.

Of all the live-saving techniques that I can think of, this one of prayer is the most important of all. It is like mouth-to-mouth resuscitation for the ebbing of life. It is, in fact, the great soul of God Himself reaching out to touch the human soul when an individual gasps for help and receives the best kind of first-aid treatment possible, exclusively intended for just such spiritual emergencies.

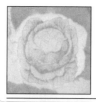

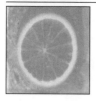

Dynamic Digestion

"GOOD EMOTIONAL HEALTH THE REAL KEY TO
IMPROVED FOOD ABSORPTION"

🌿 THE BODY'S "SECOND BRAIN"

You may think that what I'm about to tell you is pretty far-fetched. But before there is a rush to judgment, please read on and become just as amazed as I was when I first came across the information about to be presented here. It will probably change forever the way you view eating and, hopefully, lead to as much attention being given to *how* you feel as well as *what* you eat when hunger occurs.

On Tuesday, January 23, 1996, while scanning the pages of the Health section of *The New York Times*, I came across the following very remarkable item. Recently, medical researchers have determined that each of our bodies has a "second brain" of sorts. It is located in the gut and contains neurons, neurotransmitters, and proteins.

Dr. Michael Gershon of Columbia-Presbyterian Medical Center in Bronx, New York, believed that this second brain could help to explain the reason for conditions such as ulcers, chronic abdominal pain, gastrointestinal disorders like colitis, and the "butterflies" many of us get from time to time in our stomach when we become nervous for some reason.

Your Stomach's "Brain"

The gut's brain is known as the enteric nervous system, and may be found in the tissues that line the digestive organs. The gut contains 100 million neurons as well as nearly every major substance found in the brain itself. Dr. Gershon pointed out that this second brain or nervous system has major neurotransmitters such as serotonin and dopamine; brain proteins known as neuropeptides; even major immune system cells; enkephalins, a set of natural opiates; and benzodiazepines, a set of psychoactive chemicals that act like Valium and Xanax. The gut's brain can operate largely independently of the central nervous system. But it does seem to interact very closely with the body's other brain through a connection by the vagus nerve (one of the body's major nerves).

Herbs for Creating Good-Eating Emotions

There are several wonderful herbs for putting the body in the right kind of mood that is conducive to good digestion. They are German chamomile and several members of the mint family: catnip, peppermint, and spearmint. Hyssop, lavender, and rose petals also help. All of these herbs work best in a *warm tea* form.

Boil one pint of spring or distilled water. Turn off the heat and add 1 1/2 tablespoons flowers or leaves of any of the botanicals mentioned. Stir, cover with a lid, and set aside to steep for about

12 minutes. Strain, add a little pure maple syrup if desired, and slowly sip ten or fifteen minutes *before* a meal is to be consumed. This will give the tea time to penetrate the enteric nervous system and remove any agitation that may be felt there. Whatever food is then consumed will have a much better chance of being fully digested under more relaxed conditions.

COLOSTRUM AS A DIGESTIVE ENHANCER

Colostrum is the milk-like fluid produced by all female mammals in the first 24 to 36 hours directly after giving birth. It lasts until the onset of lactation, which occurs within 36 to 72 hours post-partum. Chemically, colostrum is a highly complex substance rich in protein, antibodies, and growth factors. It has less than 6% lactose and contains none of the allergy-inducing proteins traditionally associated with milk itself.

Back in the late 1980s, colostrum was big news; numerous magazine articles and print ads touted it as an effective muscle-building substance for athletes. More recently, though, it has been noted for its effect on reducing diarrhea, particularly in AIDS patients.

Research has shown that the main biological benefits of colostrum supplementation is increased gut efficiency—attributable to the immunological factors in colostrum controlling subclinical and clinical gut infection. Also, the growth factors in colostrum are able to keep the intestinal mucosa sealed and healthy. This, in turn, enhances uptake of important nutrients, which explains its benefits for diarrhea.

Due to its ability to heal both clinical and subclinical intestinal infections, colostrum is believed to benefit athletes in training by enhancing the efficiency of amino acid and carbohydrate fuel uptake in the intestine. Colostrum has certain important growth factors, chief among which is insulin-like growth factor 1 or IGF-1. They tend to "seal" the gut from ulceration, which would reduce uptake efficiency if left unchecked. Thus, transport of both carbohydrates and amino acids, the building blocks of protein, are enhanced, and more nutrients are made available faster for the working athlete's muscle cells.

But many Americans, who aren't necessarily athletes by any means, are suspected of suffering from some small amount of "gut seepage." Doctors refer to this condition as "leaky gut syndrome." In extreme cases, people suffer from clinical disorders that cause ulcerations—some due to actions by microorganisms and leading to diarrhea—and in all cases result in inefficient uptake of nutrients. In fact, chronic subclinical bouts with such microorganisms account for the vast majority of all gut inefficiencies, reducing absorption of food energy to only 80% with the rest being passed through the colon.

A reasonably healthy person suffering such a gut inefficiency would definitely notice small perturbations in any physical activity, resulting in a drop in energy levels. But if some colostrum were able to seal that leakage of 15% and the individual experiences a 100% food energy burst for the first time in a long time, then he or she would definitely notice it. This might be of significance to anyone suffering from irritable bowel syndrome and incomplete digestion due to protein supplementation.

The United States Department of Agriculture has certified a number of milking facilities around the country for the production of colostrum for human consumption. They have specialized arrangements for obtaining post-partum cows and milking them during the first 24-36 hours, with the understanding that this is when colostrum contains the highest concentrations of growth and immune factors. Organically produced colostrum is generally the best-quality colostrum available because it is free of pesticides, herbicides, anabolic hormones such as rBST (cow growth hormone shots), steroids, or clenbuterol. Also, the animals from which it is taken have not been given teat antibiotic injections.

You may find quality colostrum in most health food stores or nutrition centers. One reliable brand is Lambda Biolife Colostrum. But consumers should beware of any brands being offered too cheaply, because it usually means that manufacturers have cut their colostrum with cheese whey protein. A reliable company will generally offer independent certification of its colostrum.

❧ THE IMPORTANCE OF SLIPPERY ELM

A word needs to be said here about powdered slippery elm bark. The inner bark has been used for a couple of centuries by Native American tribes and early pioneer settlers in the Central and Eastern United States. It is available by mail order (Southern Utah Herb Co., P.O. Box 160, Tropic, UT 84776) or from most herb shops or health food stores.

Slippery elm clears up leaky gut syndrome by healing any ulceration of the mucosal lining in the stomach. It is recommended that three capsules of slippery elm bark be taken daily with a meal for five to ten weeks to completely stop any small amount of such gut seepage.

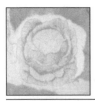

E

Emotional Trauma

"NATURAL HERBAL SEDATIVES FOR UPSETTING
EXPERIENCES"

PSYCHIC TRAUMA DEFINED

In life all of us have experienced, at one time or another, situations that have proven to be extremely aggravating or vexing to say the least. They can range all the way from an unexpected tax audit from the Internal Revenue Service to the sudden death of a loved one. Or they can span the gamut from news that one of your teenage drivers just wrecked the family car to an announcement that you no longer have a job due to company down-sizing and layoffs.

No matter what such occurrences may be, they are usually extreme in nature, quite sudden in their happening, and almost always produce an emotional shock of some kind upon the nervous system. This is basically what psychiatrists and psychologists have characterized as psychic trauma.

🌿 HERBS TO ALLEVIATE TRAUMA

There are some botanicals which might be useful in alleviating the mental and emotional distresses accompanying psychic trauma. Some work better in one form, while others work better in another way. The table below lists the best form for taking each one.

ASAFOETIDA	Taken as a tincture: $1/2$ to 1 teaspoon.
CATNIP	Taken as a warm tea: 1 cup.
CHAMOMILE	Taken as a warm tea: 1 cup.
PEPPERMINT	Taken as a warm tea: 1 cup. Taken as an essential oil: 3 drops in 6 oz. warm water.
SPEARMINT	Taken as a warm tea: 2 cups.
VALERIAN	Taken in capsules: 4 daily. Taken in tincture: 15 drops beneath the tongue.
WORMWOOD	Taken as a tincture: 15 drops beneath the tongue.
ZEODARY	Taken as a warm tea: 1 cup.

In the event you cannot find these herbs, you may write to:

OLD AMISH HERBS
4141 Iris St. North
St. Petersburg, FL 33703.

Estrogen Replacement Therapy

"BOTANICAL SUBSTITUTES TO HELP A WOMAN FEEL
BETTER IN MID-LIFE"

❧ THE AVAILABLE ESTROGENS

Christiane Northrup, M.D., is a physician practicing alternative women's medicine in New England (principally in Yarmouth, Maine). In her book *Women's Bodies, Women's Wisdom* (New York: Bantam Books, 1994; p. 470), she discussed the basics of estrogen. There are three types: estrone (E1), estradiol (E2), and estriol (E3). The middle one, estradiol, is the kind produced within the ovary. The first one, however, is formed from a conversion of the second type. The last, estriol, is also made within the ovary but in much smaller quantities than the other two are. Estriol levels tend to be rather high, though, during pregnancy when it's produced in generous amounts.

Dr. Northrup stated that "the type of estrogens used in conventional Estrogen Replacement Therapy" (or ERT) "are estrone and estradiol." But, she cautioned, they have also been implicated in breast cancer. "Estriol, on the other hand, [is] a somewhat weaker estrogen [and] must be given in higher doses to achieve the same effect." She speculated that because of its low potency, it could "well have a protective effect against breast cancer" in general.

❧ PHYTOESTROGENS: ARE THEY GOOD SUBSTITUTES FOR ERT?

On a preceding page in her book, Dr. Northrup mentioned that plant-derived sources of estrogen, called phytoestrogens, might be helpful as *mild* therapy in the treatment of hot flashes and other menopausal symptoms. She cited one particular study in passing which showed that Japanese women subsisting on large amounts of soybean products like tofu, miso, and the beans themselves, actually experienced less menopausal and premenstrual syndrome symptoms than their European and American female counterparts who didn't eat any of these things.

She also pointed out that some nuts (cashews, almonds, and peanuts), fruits (apple), and grains (corn, oats, and wheat) "contain significant amounts of phytoestrogens." But she reminded her readers not to expect the same results that can be gained from regular ERT, since such phytoestrogens are rather weak to begin with.

🦎 WHAT ALFALFA AND RED CLOVER CAN DO FOR OLDER WOMEN

Almost a quarter-of-a-century ago, a Dr. Sheldon H. Cherry of Mount Sinai Medical School wrote a best-selling health book entitled, *The Menopause Myth* (New York: Ballantine Books, 1975) in which he emphatically declared that "the indiscriminate use of estrogen therapy by all women of climacteric age . . . is not warranted; indeed, it may well be dangerous [too]."

Furthermore, Dr. Cherry threw cold water on the idea that ERT could ever reverse the aging process. "Estrogen doesn't help wrinkles, doesn't keep women young, and doesn't prevent aging [either]." Women are "plain stupid" he insisted, if they expect miraculous youth from Estrogen Replacement Therapy.

Certainly, this doctor's "bedside manners" left something to be desired in some of his female readers whom he undoubtedly offended with his straight-talking style. But with what is *now* known concerning ERT, no intelligent woman would ever want to put ERT into her own body and run the risk of getting cancer and dying a very painful death.

Because of the obvious hazards with ERT—more notably breast and uterine cancers, heart attacks, blood clots, and strokes—many health-minded women are now seeking safer and more natural alternatives to estrogenic agents such as estrone and estradiol, which form the core of ERT. I have recommended several grasses quite common to agriculture for grazing and animal feed purposes; they are alfalfa and red clover. The first contains compounds such as coumestrol, genistein, biochanin A, and daidzein, all of which have manifested noticeable estrogenic activities in ruminants. The second herb, red clover, contains some isoflavones (coumarin, medicagol, and coumestrol) which have displayed definite estrogenic properties in ruminants like cows, sheep, deer, giraffes, and camels.

But, unlike other herbalists who've recommended these same herbs somewhat indiscriminately to women having difficulty going through their menopausal years, I've gone one step further and *added* a couple of botanical nervines to this therapy. Dr. Cherry correctly noted in his book that the psychological symptoms usually connected to menopause—anxiety, depression, and irritability—are really extensions of a previously existing *mental* or *nervous* disorder, and can't be helped or solved by an estrogen pill.

So, while I can't necessarily guarantee my female audience gaining back any of their lost youth, I can provide some *real* solutions to their menopausal miseries that will bring them out of the Dark Ages of suffering and into the dawn of feeling a whole lot better and being happier with themselves. This much I *can* promise you: if you're a woman getting close to or already into the menopause phase of your life and stay on my simple Herbal Estrogen Replacement Therapy or HERT *faithfully* for as long as it takes, you will be amazed at just how easy you'll breeze through it!

🌿 A NATURAL PROGRAM THAT REALLY WORKS

My HERT is quite simple to follow. Here's how it goes:

1. All four herbs are taken as *teas*.

2. The herbal estrogens are alternated with the nervines.

3. Somewhere around 8:00 A.M., you should drink *two* cups of *warm* alfalfa tea. Around 10:00 A.M. you should drink *one* cup of *cool* peppermint tea. Close to 2 P.M. you should drink *two* cups of *warm* red clover tea in succession. And about 6:00 P.M. you should

first savor (by smelling the aroma) and then *slowly sip* two cups of German chamomile tea.

4. Near your bedtime, drink one cup of *hot* peppermint tea to help you enjoy a relaxing sleep.

It is important for readers to understand that these herbs will *not* work as expected in any form other than the teas. So forget taking capsules, tablets, or tincture drops of the same; you're just wasting time, money, and valuable resources doing this.

Making the teas is elementary, but for those who've strayed afar from their pioneer folk medicine heritages of the distant past, here's a brief refresher course for you to follow.

Making an Herbal Tea

A. Boil one pint of spring water.

B. Add *two* tablespoons of any of these herbs.

C. Stir quickly with a spoon, set aside, and cover with a lid.

D. Steep for 10 minutes if the tea is to be *hot*, 15 minutes if taken *warm*, and about 25 minutes if taken *cool*.

E. Pour liquid contents through a fine wire-mesh strainer and drink.

F. Repeat as often as needed in the manner previously prescribed.

G. Refrigerate excess tea; strain when necessary and reheat on stove or in a microwave oven.

Again, I must remind my readers that this simple HERT isn't promising them the sun, moon, and stars of youthfulness. To do so would be hyping things a great deal, not to mention being somewhat irresponsible. But by faithfully adhering to it for months at a time, it will certainly smooth out the rough bumps in the long road of menopause and make a woman's journey through this life phase very pleasant and enjoyable to say the least.

SOME OTHER ESTROGENIC HERBS

Alfalfa and red clover are by no means the only herbs containing residual amounts of estrogenic compounds. There are a number of others that do too, but certainly in far less quantities than the former pair. A few of the more prominent herbs falling into this category would be licorice, wild Mexican yam, sarsaparilla, black cohosh, elder, and unicorn root.

These can be taken in capsule or tablet form if one so chooses, but don't expect as much from them as you could from the alfalfa-peppermint and red clover-chamomile duos. However, these other botanicals, when used regularly, might help decrease a woman's dosage of Premarin. This is an estrogen cream made from a pregnant mare's urine (hence the name). An ad for Premarin that appeared in a number of widely circulated women's magazines in 1993-94, showed a beautiful middle-aged lady with a beguiling smile on her countenance as a man was in the act of tenderly kissing her neck. The caption below read as follows: "You think it's good medicine. [But] she thinks it's wonderful!"

In her book on women's health, Dr. Northrup wisely counseled women to stop believing the "estrogen companies and gynecologists [who] plant . . . seeds of fear . . . as soon as . . . menopause [happens]." A woman's body will *not* fall apart and *won't* waste away without hormonal medication, she reassured. And if you follow my previously outlined HERT you, as a woman approaching menopause, should never feel depressed, fatigued, incontinent, forgetful, or senile. In that sense, it might be said these herbs will keep the symptoms of aging away somewhat.

Exercise Rejuvenation

"PHYSICAL ACTIVITY OF SOME KIND IS THE KEY TO FEELING YOUNGER"

Those exercises which can keep you young and forever rejuvenate your body cells should always be simple and easy to do. Furthermore, they should involve things that are quite handy around the house and not entail the purchase of expensive equipment. Such physical movements should also strengthen parts of the body like the brain or bones that ordinarily don't figure much in exercise regimens. And finally, exercises to help turn back the hands on your body's time clock, should incorporate the *spiritual* dimension in some way. After all, what good is a fit and trim physical being, if the spiritual one inside still remains a lazy and slouchy couch potato from a moral perspective?

❧ 'THE TERMINATOR' PUSHES THE ONE-MINUTE NAVAJO WORKOUT

In the summer of 1993, Nina Begay of Window Rock, Arizona, told me that between May 18th and 20th of that same year, Hollywood strongman and tough-guy actor Arnold Schwarzenegger was a special guest at the tribal fairgrounds in that city. Known especially for his lead role in the science-fiction/action thriller, "The Terminator" (in which he played the role of a destructive human-like robot), Schwarzenegger introduced the huge crowd to a very simple exercise to help young and old get rid of their abdominal "love handles."

Standing next to the somewhat paunchy tribal president Peterson Zah, the very muscular chairman of the President's

Council on Physical Fitness and Sports, had everyone stand on their feet and follow his lead. He raised his right arm high overhead while at the same time bending his upper body to the left as far as possible. "Remember to keep both feet together and to hold your left arm beside you," he reminded them. "And be sure not to overstrain yourself either." He encouraged them to *gently* stretch their torsos as much to the left as possible in a *rocking* rhythm, but without hurting themselves.

Then everyone followed his example and switched by bringing down their right arms and lifting up their left ones instead. "That's it—just keep stretching in slow motion," he said, holding his own left arm at an angle over his head. "You look like ballet dancers down there," he joked, and everyone laughed back.

"Listen to me," he continued. "All you need to do is just practice this stretching exercise for 30 seconds on each side. It takes no more than a minute at the most. You should try doing this a couple of times a day, at least once in the morning and again before you go to bed." He said that those who stayed with this would discover their love handles disappearing in a matter of just a few weeks.

Nina wrote in her letter that her father, brother, and boy friend, all of whom had been paunchy and sporting side rolls of fat above their hips, decided to take the big man's offer up and try it for themselves. In less than three weeks, she noted, "their love handles have disappeared and their stomach muscles are much tighter."

"RUNNING CURED MY CANCER"

In the early part of 1992, I met Bill Shrader of Albany, New York, at a holistic health convention in New York City. He was then in his 76th year of life and "feeling just great." He told me a highly interesting story worth repeating here.

"In 1956 I developed my first cancerous growth and stupidly allowed the doctors to give me 30 radiation treatments," he began. "I believe that's what put the cancer in my system a second time. Well, the doctors told me it would come back, but I wasn't paying any attention to them. Well, sure enough when I turned 70, the damned thing returned with an even greater vengeance."

He first noticed something was wrong when "I started putting some spray paint on my car and the next day I had a sore throat." After lasting for three days, he looked into the bathroom mirror and opened his mouth. There on his tongue was a growth of some kind. A biopsy later revealed terminal oral cancer.

"The doctors expected me to only last a year at the most," he said with a chuckle. Bill Shrader has laughed a lot since then, especially when he considered what might have been. "Can you believe that they wanted to cut a third of my tongue away and cut all through here," he said pointing at his shoulder. "Why I would have lost the use of this arm and it would have taken me six months to learn to talk again. I told them all in no uncertain terms 'to go straight to hell' and walked out of the hospital mad as a wet hen."

He went to the library and started studying up on cancer. He devised his own treatment, which included many sulphur containing fruits and vegetables: figs, dried apricots, cabbage, kale, kohlrabi, Brussels sprouts, cauliflower, broccoli, garlic, and onion.

But his *main* prescription was *running*—"lots of it," he added. "The thing I started noticing with my exercises is that whenever I ran five to 10 miles at a stretch, all of my oral tumors practically went away. My theory was that it was kicking up my immune system."

Shrader's running began in high school in Norwalk, Connecticut, where he became the record-setting captain of his high school track team. He went on to Harvard University and graduated with the class of 1937. He retreated to rural upstate New York just west of Albany, opened an export-import business, and raised a family of 12 kids. His wife died in 1986.

Bill's own brother died from cancer not long after returning from active duty in World War II. "When he came back, he was a total nervous wreck," Shrader continued. "Cigarette after cigarette. Three packs a day. I believe that's what did the poor guy in."

Shrader was quick to point out that the kind of intensive running he regularly does may not be for everyone. I asked him if simple jogging might be enough to help someone get rid of cancer if that person wasn't up to running many miles every day. "I don't know," he said with a moment's pause of reflection. "But I'll tell you this. I think that when a person can compete against himself some way in the fight against cancer, your body has a much better chance of rallying. Of course, you have to be eating right to begin with and consume enough foods that will give you the great amount of energy required for such intensive exercise as this. But I think cancer tumors don't like the body to be put through such vigorous activity. In my case, it seems that my constant running upset their balance and they simply disappeared."

Shrader claimed that "even in old age, being a marathon runner has its obvious benefits, if you can leave your cancer in the dust for good."

Exercise Can Be a Religious Experience

Mainstream Christianity and Judaism consider the soul, the spiritual self in each of one of us, as being essentially distinct and separate from our bodies. As a result, Americans are unlikely to ever associate spiritual discipline with something like exercise. So, whenever an exercise-altered mental state is achieved, people are more apt to think of the experience as simply a good feeling or a pleasant way to escape from the stresses and problems vexing them in ordinary life.

But somehow managing to incorporate aspects of the spiritual dimension in with intense physical activity of some kind, will enable the participant to more fully utilize the powers of the mind while the body is being put through a good workout. The limited number of studies that have been done on yoga exercise, for instance, have shown that when meditation is linked with breathing and stretching exercises, the brain and nervous system receive enhanced benefits above and beyond what advantages the muscles of the body may gain.

One of the best ways in getting there is to create for yourself an exercise environment that is conducive to peace. This would suggest that loud noise, frenetic dance music, jarring jumps and teeth-gritting pumps all be eliminated. In their place would come more serene activities done in slow-motion fashion in an atmosphere of soft lighting, acoustic music, natural light, and earth-tone colors.

In such a renovated setting as this can the mind and nerves become more relaxed, while the body itself is being put through measured paces of physical activity. A lot more is being strengthened here than just muscles, bones, heart, and lungs. Two forms of exercise work in parallel but different ways to help you feel better: tranquillity rules the brain and central nervous system, while physical motion governs some of the major organs, the skeletal frame and muscle tissue. In this way exercise can become more meaningful to you by acquiring certain spiritual overtones. The end result is always a much *more complete* and satisfying feeling than if you just did exercise alone.

🌿 THE PLACEBO SIDE

This little ditty appeared sometime ago in *The Wall Street Journal* (Thursday, January 31, 1988, D-31):

> *My health, these days is fine*
> *And I'm no longer irked—*
> *Having finally found*
> *A placebo that worked.*
>
> *—Joshua Adams*

It probably best illustrates the mysterious power connected with an empty agent, be it a simple sugar pill, a syringe filled with salt water or a method of activity without specific purpose to it.

The basic human emotions of faith, hope, and trust are all vital components in making a seemingly worthless placebo work. The placebo effect has been known at different times to heal wounds, alter body chemistry, and even change the course of the most relentless diseases.

Doctors who've studied the placebo effect for years, have usually focused on presumed "miracle pills" or sham surgeries that were made to appear to relieve pain. But very little, if anything, has been done in regard to exercise as a potential placebo for some medical problems.

The second entry in this section examined one cancer patient's personal experience with running to cure him of his disease. While there were some very real benefits to this form of exercise, there was obviously a placebo effect in place somewhere too. Now the benefits to physical health which can come from exercise are generally well known. Activities like jogging and aerobics are commonly believed to enhance our psychological well-being.

But exactly just how does physical activity of any kind improve our mental outlook? Surprisingly, until now, no one had really looked to find a definite answer to this question. But some scientists are bold enough to venture a guess that the placebo effect may be at play here. They claim that exercise may improve our psychological health simply because we *think* it will. Just as taking the well known sugar pill in medicine may help some people to feel better, so might some forms of exercise help to improve our mindset.

In order to fully test this idea out, five Canadian researchers randomly assigned 48 volunteers (24 men, 24 women) to one of two exercise groups. The same exercise leaders guided both groups through a 10-week fitness program involving a variety of activities (jogging, aerobic dancing, swimming, and soccer). Only those in the experimental group, however, were told that the training program would improve *both* their physical and psychological health. Those in the control group were told only that they would benefit physically.

At the end of 10 weeks, according to the journal *Psychosomatic Medicine* (Vol. 55, No. 2, March/April 1993), the physical fitness of both groups had improved about the same. But the psychological well-being of the experimental group had also improved significantly. They specifically reported a *substantial* increase in their own personal confidence levels.

❧ HAVE YOU BEEN DOING THE OTHER KIND OF EXERCISE?

Nearly everyone who is into exercise and fitness to some degree, is aware of aerobic activity. At its most basic level, you put one foot in front of the other and work up a good sweat while going at it. While making you huff and puff it also strengthens your heart and the rest of your cardiovascular system, thus reducing your chances of ever contracting heart disease.

But not so well known is another form of exercise known as isotonics; it also goes by the names of strength training, weight training, or resistance training. Isotonics is crucial to being in the best of health because it is especially designed to build muscle mass. The more muscle you have, the stronger you are, so that you can carry heavy loads or perform other physically difficult tasks without becoming short-winded. By the second week of isotonics a person feels stronger. By the end of 3 months individual strength capacity has been doubled or tripled.

And by increasing your own muscle mass, you're also resetting your internal "fat thermostat" a few degrees higher. This means that your body's metabolic rate has substantially increased and is now capable of burning off those "extra" calories you may have been worrying about.

Another benefit to greater muscle mass is that it decreases the risk of you ever getting diabetes. The more muscle your body takes on, the less insulin is needed to get sugar or glucose out of your circulating blood plasma.

Isotonics also is very promising in terms of protecting you against heart disease, but does it in a different way than aerobic activity would. When a person is engaged in strength training of any kind, his or her "good" HDL-cholesterol is elevated and the "bad" LDL-cholesterol significantly lowered.

Bone density is, likewise, increased through isotonic procedures. This form of exercise helps to protect against the fractures often associated with brittle bones in old age. There is now even some evidence to show that isotonics could assist in mitigating the effects of rheumatoid arthritis. (Please consult these several other entries located elsewhere in the text for additional information: ARTHRITIS REBOUND, FRAILNESS PREVENTION, HEALTHY BONES, and OPTIMISM FOR OSTEOPOROSIS.)

Doing isotonics isn't all that difficult. The most elementary step is to learn to push against the weight of your own body without any equipment. One movement that's good for this is the pushup. Every time you lift your body off the floor (and thereby overcome the resistance of its weight), you are, in reality, strengthening the muscles in your arms, chest, shoulders, and back. If a woman is pregnant, however, or a person has had recent abdominal or back surgery, a physician should be consulted before attempting this.

For the next several isotonic maneuvers I'm going to recommend, you don't need any type of special exercise equipment. In fact, everything you'll need, believe it or not, will come directly from your local *supermarket*. Sounds a bit weird doesn't it, telling you to look for the best devices to train with from the grocery store instead of an athletic equipment place? But as you read on, you'll be delighted to learn that what may, at first glance, seem ridiculous actually has a lot of common sense to it.

I put my own office staff of female secretaries on the regimen one afternoon on Wednesday, May 8th, 1996 just to see how effective my recommendations would be. Now the ladies who perform contract labor for me on a full- or part-time basis, ranged in age from 26 to 67. On that particular busy day, there happened to have been four of them present during the half-hour exercise session that I ran them through.

For arm curls, they sat on stools or the edge of office chairs (the non-swivel kind) and holding *cans of food* of varying weights, slowly bent their elbows and "curled" these weights to shoulder level. After which they slowly returned them to the starting position and resumed the same movement again for several minutes. Below is a simple table of the can weights which each age group felt the most comfortable in using.

ARM/BICEPS CURL

Canned Food Item	Weight	Age Bracket
Campbell's Family-Size Vegetable Soup	26$^{1}/_{2}$ oz.	20-35
Cream Style Sweet Corn	17 oz.	36-49
Dinty Moore Beef Stew	15 oz.	50-65
Meyenberg Evaporated Goat Milk	12 oz.	66-80

Next came the chest and shoulder exercise for strengthening the deltoid muscles (located from the top of both shoulders and extending about halfway down to the elbows). I had them sit upright on some metal folding chairs we keep in a store room for public lecture purposes. The simple instruments used for this workout were ordinary plastic milk jugs with handles. I filled each with only so much water according to the age capacity of each secretary. They grasped their jugs and slowly raised their arms forward and up until their elbows were straight. Then I had them stop momentarily when their arms were fully extended over their heads and slowly count to five before returning them down slowly to their starting positions. This maneuver was repeated a few more times with the entire procedure lasting no more than 6 minutes. Below is another table showing the measured portions of water put into each jug for the different age categories present.

CHEST AND SHOULDER EXERCISE

1-gal. jug	Capacity Filled	Age Bracket
Empty	Completely	20-35
Empty	Three-quarters	36-49
Empty	One-Half	50-65
Empty	One-Quarter	66-80

Sitting in the same chairs, they next performed an upper-arm exercise for strengthening their triceps. I had every participant hold a food can in *each* hand to correspond with their age group-ings and then raise both arms over their heads. They bent one elbow back as they lowered one hand behind their heads. Then they raised it back overhead, joining the other hand. After which they repeated the same motion with the other arms. They kept alternating between each arm for upwards of five minutes. (Consult the table under the Arm/Biceps Curl to find out the appropriate can weight for your age bracket.)

I mentioned to them that if they intended doing these proce-dures at home, they should go through each exercise about three times. For instance, they were informed not to do eight to 12 arm curls and then go on to the next activity believing they were done with arm curls for the day. I said they should do three "sets" of eight to 12 arm curls, waiting a little between each set, and then proceeding on to the next exercise. Or, they could perform one set of eight to 12 arm curls followed by one set of all the other exercises and then repeat that multi-exercise sequence two times.

Fortunately, those attempting to do isotonics will discover that it takes far less time than aerobics. If an individual is com-mitted to exercising both the upper and lower body at every ses-sion, all that person needs is two to three sessions a week. Each session should last somewhere between 20 to 30 minutes, for a total of 1 to $1^1/_2$ hours every week.

I mentioned that regardless of which exercise was done, it was important for them to perform each repetition slowly, taking as many as eight to 12 seconds. "Haste makes waste," I noted, "and you're not training your muscles as you ought to."

Breathing properly is also very important when doing these kinds of exercises. "Inhale before you lift or push, exhale as you lift," I admonished. "And inhale again as you slowly return to the starting position." What is to be avoided is swinging a can or jug fast or bounce it at the end of a repetition. And a person should not exercise the same muscle groups in more than one session per day. "Your muscles require sufficient time to recover," I observed.

Following this brief lecturing, I had them do a couple of iso-tonic maneuvers intended to strengthen the quadriceps. The only equipment we used for these were the same straight back chairs and zip-locked plastic bags filled with sand that could be strapped to their ankles with some adhesive, electrician's, or duck tape. One Glad-Lock plastic sandwich bag filled three-quarters with sand was taped around the ankle of each woman. They were instructed to extend this one leg so it was as straight out in front of them as possible. "Lower your leg back to its starting position," I continued, "but rest no more than 3 seconds before repeating." After eight to 12 repetitions (one set), I had them switch their sandbags to the other leg.

The final exercise was a hip and knee extension, especially designed for the quadriceps as well as a set of muscles called the hip extensors. For this they used the backs of their chairs for support. I led them through this last procedure myself. "Let's stand straight and point our toes outward. That's good. Now let's bend our knees slightly, directing our body weights over our toes but without doing any deep knee-bends. Be sure, ladies, to keep your heels on the floor at all times." I pointed out in passing that a pack strapped to someone's back would tend to increase the difficulty of this exercise.

When we finished and were resting, I mentioned a few safety tips to be cognizant of. "A 10-minute warm-up should be done before attempting each exercise session. The first five minutes should consist of low-intensity aerobics like walking. The next five should consist of gentle and relaxing stretching maneuvers. Sit on the floor and extend a leg straight out in front of you (with the other leg bent in toward the outstretched one). Then grab your ankle with both hands and slowly pull your body forward as far as possible, being sure to keep the leg straight all the time. Then maintain this position for about 12 seconds. Always keep your back relatively straight, since bending it could initiate an injury in those subject to a lot of back pain."

The same warm-up, incidentally, is suggested for aerobic exercise, which is why some people combine their aerobic and isotonic exercise sessions. The recommendation for this is as follows: warm-up, aerobics, isotonics, and a five-minute cooldown or five minutes of walking around to keep from shifting the body too suddenly back into low gear again.

One other thing about isotonics should be cited that you may not be aware of. The average sedentary 25-year-old woman is about 25% fat. But by the time she reaches age 65, fat accounts for some 43% of her makeup. Sedentary men go from being about 18% fat at age 25 to 38% fat by the time they start collecting Social Security. Isotonics, for the most part, can reverse that trend. It accomplishes this not so much by replacing lost muscle as in building up the muscle cells that remain. Put another way, age-related muscle loss and all the accompanying problems which go with it, don't have to be accepted passively anymore. Now, anyone whether 25, 45, 65, or even 85, whether male or female, can build up individual muscle strength. In their book, *The 10 Determinants of Aging You Can Control* (New York: Simon & Schuster), Drs. William Evans and Irwin Rosenberg mentioned putting a 101-year-old patient on isotonic exercises when he turned 97. After four consecutive years of faithful weekly sessions, the fellow ended up having the strength of a sedentary 60-year-old.

I am deeply indebted to the editors of *Tufts University Diet & Nutrition Letter* for generously letting me use some of the material contained in their July 1993 issue, which much of the foregoing was based upon. For new subscription information write to: Tufts University Diet & Nutrition Letter, P. O. Box 57857, Boulder, CO 80322-7857. (Subscriptions are $20 U.S. per year for 12 issues.) It is one of the better university-associated health newsletters around.

TRY YARD WORK FOR A HEALTHIER LIFESTYLE

Low-intensity exercises like slow-paced walking and yard work may not yield as much benefit as more intense activities like jogging, bicycling, and swimming. But they certainly have their place for certain conditions and age groups. Women who are pregnant and unable to do much heavy lifting or bending, will find raking the lawn, cutting grass with an old push handmower, or pruning back bushes to be ideal and fairly safe exercises. Studies have shown that the placenta—the filter for nutrients for the baby—is always much larger in women who have exercised *moderately.* Adaptations to exercise in the mother's body seem to nurture the fetus and produce a healthier, leaner baby.

Seniors who aren't bothered with arthritis in their hip, knee, or ankle joints will enjoy gardening, which always requires a certain amount of bending, stooping, and getting up and down different times. Other research has shown that older people who go through such gardening motions on a fairly regular basis tend to have a noticeable improvement in the ratio of "good" HDL- to "bad" LDL-cholesterol. And both yard work and gardening kept their body weights down and controlled or prevented the development of diabetes. Also, in many older folks, a reduction in hypertension was evident.

But probably the best result of all that comes from yard work and gardening is a definite feeling of exhilaration in having accomplished something purposeful and useful. Those who regularly engage in both activities claim their anxieties and depressive moods vanish after awhile, leaving them with increased feelings of well-being.

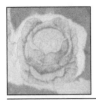

Fatigue Fixers

"WHAT HAS KEPT TALK SHOW HOST PHIL DONAHUE
GOING FOR ALL THESE YEARS?"

A TELEVISION PIONEER

Twenty-nine years ago Phil Donahue became a virtual pioneer
in the television industry. In 1967 he started the very first talk-
back show and maintained that lead until somewhere in the
mid-80s. He felt that it was important to his act to invite the
audience into it, by asking for their comments during each program. His was a mixture of earnest public-affairs chats with the
strange-but-true confessionals of ordinary women who loved
too much.

During his nearly three-decades long reign, Donahue won a fireplace mantle full of Emmys (20) plus one Peabody award. He interviewed everyone from presidents to prostitutes with equal curiosity and bluntness. At the height of his popularity he was seen in more than 211 different markets. Donahue insisted that what he did was journalism, not just entertainment. In 1981 he managed to persuade the Federal Communications Commission to declare his talk-show to be a true and "bona fide news program."

Unfortunately for him, though, his format was very easy for imitators to copy. Oprah Winfrey became his first serious threat and knocked him from his top-seated perch sometime in 1987. From then on "Donahue" was always in a gradual and steady rating slide. In 1995 he lost his valuable New York City outlet and would soon disappear from the California scene, being removed from the air in both Los Angeles and San Francisco.

BOUNDLESS ENERGY

Donahue brought a wide-eyed Midwestern charm and "apple-pie-goodness" to the talk-TV format. Trailing his microphone cord, he would bounce around the audience with seemingly endless energy and confront his guests with questions taken directly from those seated in the television studio. Many of his viewers at home probably wondered where he got all the vigor for such a hectic and demanding program.

Donahue's secret to almost "unlimited energy," has been not only in *what* he eats but in the *way* it has been consumed. Surprisingly, his secret isn't all that complex; in fact, it's quite simple when you get right down to it. The *what* part is mainly a dietary focus on salads, legumes, fresh fruits and vegetables, juices, whole grains, chicken and fish, with very *limited* red meat intake.

The *way* he consumes these items is the more interesting part, however. First of all, those items which must be cooked are usually done so by steaming, baking, broiling, or boiling them; very little of what he eats is fried or deep-fried. Also, the *number* of times he eats each day is equally important to consider here. Traditionally, most of us are used to eating three square meals a day in the forms of breakfast, lunch, and dinner. But Donahue found years ago that when he would consume 4 or 5 *smaller* meals each day, he had a lot more energy. Even his physical endurance was more intensified, enabling him to do some 6,000 shows before finally calling it quits.

At age 60, he still has that boyish look about him even if his hair has long since turned vanilla. His claim to fame will be long remembered by devoted fans for years to come.

ENERGY DRINKS

The following beverages will give an older person lots of energy. Besides this, they are healthy and good for the body. NOTE: For those with suspected or known blood sugar problems, it may not be wise to drink these very much. Instead, they might want to rely more on the carrot and tomato drinks, which won't aggravate existing diabetic or hypoglycemic conditions.

Dominican Refresco

2 cups coconut milk

2$^1/_2$ cups chopped fresh or canned pineapple

1 tbsps. pure maple syrup

$^1/_6$ tsp. almond extract

COCONUT MILK

One-half a coconut usually yields 2 cups of rich coconut milk or 4 cups of mildly flavored coconut milk. To open a coconut, place the coconut, eyes down, on a hard surface and crack with a hammer several times. Pry the meat loose from the shell with a blunt knife. Then cut the meat into small pieces and grate in a Vita-Mix Total Nutrition Center, being sure to **use the extra container with the stronger blade in it for grinding wheat into flour.** Moisten with some plain boiling water, then liquefy for 1$^1/_2$ minutes on high speed until the matter becomes extremely fine. Then pour more boiling water on this liquefied coconut and permit it to stand in a bowl for 45 minutes, before passing through a fine wire sieve to separate the milk from the solids; discard the solids.

MAKING THE DOMINICAN REFRESCO

Combine all of the items in the ingredients list in a Vita-Mix blender and puree for 1$^1/_2$ minutes. Then strain, refrigerate and chill for an hour. Tastes better when you drink it from a frosted mug or glass. Yields 4 cups.

Carrot Drink

6 *large carrots*

1 *cup mineral or tonic water*

1 *tsp. lime or lemon juice*

3 *tbsps. honey*

3 *tbsps. pure maple syrup*

2 *cups extra-rich milk*

Grate the carrots in a Vita-Mix Total Nutrition Center for about 2 minutes. Then mix with water and press through a sieve or colander. Strain and add the lime or lemon juice to the carrot and water mixture. Then add the natural sweeteners and milk. Mix well in the Vita-Mix container again, then chill before drinking. Yields about three (8 ounce) glassfuls.

Tomato Drink

3 *cups ripe tomatoes, quartered*

$1/3$ *cup carrots*

$1/4$ *cup sweet green bell pepper*

$1/3$ *cup celery with leaves*

$1/4$ *cup onion*

$1/4$ *clove garlic*

$1^1/2$ *tsp. lemon juice*

$1/2$ *tsp. honey*

$1/6$ *tsp. black pepper*

$1/6$ *tsp. salt (optional)*

Place all of the ingredients in a Vita-Mix Total Nutrition Center container. Secure the lid in place by locking under both tabs. Turn on to high speed and mix for 2 minutes. Refrigerate and chill for an hour before drinking. Yields 3 cups.

Papaw Drink

4 cups ripe papaya

4 cups water

1 (14-ounce) can sweetened condensed milk

$^1/_4$ tsp. Angostura bitters

Puree the papaya in a Vita-Mix blender for about one minute. Strain and combine with the water and milk. Mix well, add the Angostura, and serve over some ice cubes. Yields about 2$^1/_2$ quarts.

Caribbean Punch

1 cup orange juice

1 cup pineapple juice

1 cup grapefruit juice

1 tsp. pure maple syrup

1 (12-ounce) can ginger ale

Mix everything together in a pitcher except the ginger ale. Add it last of all just when you're ready to drink some of this. Pour over ice cubes, if desired. Yields 4$^1/_2$ cups.

 SUPPLEMENTS TO BOOST YOUR ENERGY

Items from the beehive have always been considered by some cultures to contain the elements necessary for promoting the production of energy within the body. Bee pollen heads this list for those who aren't allergic to flower pollen. One teaspoon of granules every morning with food usually increases energy in a rather dramatic way. Then there is royal jelly; one capsule is enough of this. Also $^1/_2$ teaspoon of honey stirred into 6 ounces of boiling water, permitted to cool a little, then restirred before drinking, can help as well, provided, of course, the person doesn't have any blood sugar problems.

Iron has always been an important mineral for giving the body the stamina it needs. Women especially seem to require more of this nutrient than men do. But continuous supplementation with iron tablets can sometimes lead to constipation. It is better to obtain the iron needed from dark leafy greens, certain organ meats like liver, and herbs such as alfalfa, burdock, parsley, and yellow dock. The leafy greens can be juiced in a Vita-Mix food blender then combined with an equal amount of tomato or carrot juice. If one doesn't prefer eating fried or baked liver, then it can be taken in the form of two desiccated liver tablets each day. One or two capsules of any of the herbs cited above is sufficient.

Finally, a high-potency B complex (200 mg. twice daily) along with a good protein supplement will put more vigor back into a tired out lifestyle.

Fighting Boredom

"VARIETY IS INDEED THE SPICE OF LIFE TO FIGHT TEDIUM"

 ### ENLARGING YOUR VOCABULARY

There is one thing I've noticed that is *totally absent* from *all* of the recent books devoted exclusively to longevity: not a single thing appears on the subject of boredom. In fact, the word itself isn't even there in them. Usually, we're accustomed to having it associated with young children or teenagers, who get restless very easily when they are *bored.*

But, from my association with hundreds of senior citizens in the last six years, it has been my own experience that they too get bored. But usually theirs is more far-reaching and deeper because it always involves life itself. Due to their advanced years and often confined because of physical or mental infirmities, their lives have ceased to hold much meaning. And they while away their time waiting for the grim reaper watching lots of television or else just sleeping. At least that's what numerous elderly folks have told me in the years that I've been associated with *Utah Prime Times* as its editor. Because the Intermountain West's largest monthly free distributed newspaper is devoted exclusively to seniors, I've had to make the rounds from Logan on the north to St. George on the south, interviewing countless older folks for this, that, or the other.

In the course of my journalistic duties, I've often switched hats different times during interviews and moved from the newspaper side of things over to the scientific side as the trained anthropologist that I am. I've routinely asked many of these older men and women what some of their major concerns are. Invariably, boredom will always surface somewhere near the top among other things like illness, loneliness, confinement, poverty, and loss of dignity and self respect. So, it's an important issue that seems to be on the minds of many seniors at one time or another, even though it isn't considered such by all those authors of anti-aging books galore.

To fully understand boredom, though, you need to know that it is equated with two other words in the dictionary that we seldom ever hear about. Boredom is defined simply as "a state of ennui or tedium" in *Webster's Seventh New Collegiate Dictionary* from a quarter-of-a-century ago. Ennui (pronounced än-wē) is "a feeling of weariness and dissatisfaction" with things or life in general. And tedium can best be described as "the quality or state of being tiresome due to *dullness.*"

How One Family Line Beat Dullness to Death

It is that last word *dullness,* associated with tedium, that I like the best of all. Because it pretty well describes many of the same old routine patterns in our own lives, not to mention those in the lives of the elderly. I asked several people from very diverse backgrounds what they have done to fight boredom in their own lives. The first was Donna McCool of Sunman, Indiana, age 54, who responded by letter; the second was my own father, Jacob Heinerman, age 82, whom I interviewed in person; and the last was Clara Rose Worden, now 100, whom I interviewed in person in 1995 when she was 99 years old. Each of them offered different insights for solving this pervasive lifelong dilemma.

Donna's letter reflects several generations of life on both sides of her family. And while there is an obvious sameness to much of what her ancestors did, it will be noticed that they did have a *variety* of activities to keep them busy all the time. As she herself put it in the letter, "we've learned how to beat dullness to death by keeping ourselves busily occupied." Most of her handwritten letter, dated March 13, 1996 is presented here in its original form without any editorial corrections or changes.

"It was my grandfather who lived 104 years. My father was still alive at 79. I am 54.

"Grandpa Edwin Richter lived on a farm and worked the land. Very hard tiring--rewarding work. He grew everything he ate. There was nothing thrown away on a hog that was butchered but the 'squeal.' They pickled the feet, used the intestines for casings for the sausage, made soup out of the stomach, ate the brains-- sweet breads and yes, even made blood sausage (by the way, I *love* blood sausage!). He always ate the fat. They always used lard to cook with. Also butchered beef and ate all of it but the hide.

"They had nothing to be bored with. There was always things to do and things to keep their minds on and hands occupied with. They always had a big garden—fruit trees, grapes, and berries. They never sprayed the crops for bugs. We just washed them good and cut the worm holes out of the fruit. All the meat was either canned or smoked to keep it. In later years they had a freezer. They used honey, molasses, sugar, and salt. They ate as many eggs as they wanted but they had their own chickens running outside eating what they chose—even let them pick corn out of the cowpies. And ate the chickens, too! Imagine that, will you! Fertilizer was manure from the hogs, cows, chickens. It made great mulch when spread on the fields.

"They rose at 4:00 A.M. and went to bed 9:00 P.M. Grandpa lost his sight at about 90 so he could not watch TV. Never took time for it anyway. His wife was Mae and lived til 81.

"My grandparents on my mother's side were Ida, 98, and Oliver Boas, 94. They were farmers also and ate maybe a bit better, because grandma baked bread and pies. The other Grandma Richter had crippling arthritis so could not knead the dough.

"They both made their own wine, and drank 1 small glass 2 times a day. Always at the same time everyday, 3:00 P.M. and at bedtime. They grew herbs and ate them—parsley, garlic, etc. When they fried meat (ham, etc.) they used water to start with. They also used the old black iron skillets and lard.

"They gathered nuts and berries and canned or dried them for the winter for pies and snacks. Most people in today's society would not consider working so hard to feed their family properly. It's easier to pop in a pizza or eat some artificial stuff from the local McDonalds than to do what my people did.

"Edwin and Mae Richter had 5 children. Oliver and Ida Boas had 11 children. Between them and their 16 children I don't believe they ever got bored. Tired at times maybe, but never bored.

"I base the long life to early to bed and early to rise, and all natural food and 'NO STRESS' as we know it. I'm sure raising that many kids wasn't easy for them. The kids of today have no manners, could care less if mom and dad had a dime as long as they can have a car and money to run on. My own boys, Thank God, are very good to us and work hard to feed their families.

"You gotta keep yourself busy. The mind always occupied and them hands doing something *productive*. Musn't let the devil in since 'idleness is his workshop' as they say. My people were never bored, didn't even know the meaning of the word I suspect. They just learned how to beat it to death by working and playing and living hard is all."

❧ MY DAD THINKS YOUTHFUL TO AVOID BOREDOM

Jacob Heinerman had the following things to say to his son on the night of Monday, March 18, 1996 between 7 and 8 P.M. Utah time, during a short interview for this particular section. At the time he was 82.

"Well, for an older person to fight boredom the mind has to revert back to young thoughts. You don't think of this that you're going to get older a year from now. But you kind of look back on what you had been doing before and try and get into the mental frame. And then also, if the physical will let you go and have or carry those mind thoughts into activity, and do that too.

"When you think of things you've done, then kind of dream about it—even though you're handicapped and maybe can't do much—but you dream about it and think about it. When you do this you're then giving your mind or you may say filling it with some good thoughts that bring you into a state of physical condition where you know that you're not getting old because your mind is *young!* When your mind is *young* then it transfers it to the body to a degree and then you're benefited all around.

"Of course, this is over a period of time. It obviously doesn't last forever. So you have to have your mind dwelling upon things that you have done before or that you had wanted to do and were dreaming about back there when you were younger. And now you're thinking about them again in old age. And this will, surprisingly enough, influence your attitude to what it was when you were much younger.

"And also get into a cheerful framework of what tomorrow will bring. And don't let it be more of what we're having now, our aches and pains and other unhappy things we tend to gripe about when the years creep over us. But you should be looking forward to a state tomorrow that will give you a youthful outlook so that you feel like what you're gaining from all this is uplifting and cheering. On a day-by-day-by-day basis you always want to have positiveness—we call it faith but the world calls it positive outlook—then whatever is done will be encouraging and hopeful and something to always look forward to. Then there will never be any room for getting bored.

"You also need to have different things to do. For example, if you have a hobby of some kind to keep you busy. Keep your mind engaged and hands active. Whether it be gardening, woodworking, or something else, it doesn't matter so long as you stay busy with something you enjoy doing. These things have a tremendous therapeutic effect on everything—mind, body, and spirit is all affected in a good way. So you're doing things of a youthful nature and never let your mind bog down in things that have to do with oldness. Instead you're always bringing new, youthful things into your life.

"And so that's how your old man here keeps himself young, even though my body keeps getting older with each passing year." I then reminded my father that he had raised my younger brother Joseph and I up to *never* refer to him as "the old man." "That's correct," he chuckled. "And you have both done well in that respect. But I guess it's my prerogative at my age to use that term if I want to on myself."

I replied, "I still see you've managed to keep your sense of humor through all of the heartache and sorrow you've been through over the many years."

"And that, too," he finished, "is also what has kept away from me the monotony of life sometimes."

A REAL PIONEER IN SPACE-AGE AMERICA

I sat in the ramshackled house of Clara Rose Worden sometime in the Spring of 1995, shortly after she turned 99 years of age on March 5th. I was then looking at an early photograph taken of her. She gave a wide, nearly toothless grin and cackled, "I was a tough old broad in my youth and, by golly, still am!" There was no denying that, for sure!

When she first moved into the little house in Touchet, Washington, she had already raised two kids and had three more still at home. She took care of the garden and fed chickens and cows while her husband, William Worden, traded horses. But that was many decades ago, in another time and era. But as of the Spring of 1996, she was still going strong, albeit with the help of a walker, in the same little house on the lane that now bears her name.

This petite woman with the great shock of thick white hair brushed back from her face, was a little smaller than in former times the day I met her, and a little unsteady sometimes on her feet. She had outlived her husband, half of her kids, and all of her friends the same age. The world had moved on without her, but there in that house, she still controlled time and her own destiny.

Her house would never make any of the slick town and country home magazines devoted exclusively to genteel living. But it was home, nevertheless, in spite of its rather homely appearance. The white exterior paint had worn down to weathered gray board, and the windows were covered with plastic. Inside, bare lights hung from the ceilings *with shoelaces* tied to the switches. The once-bright wallpaper was stained dark by time and wood smoke. In places it had even buckled and torn, revealing bare boards underneath.

But the strangest of all discoveries was what wasn't within, but located outside her premises. She had absolutely *no* indoor plumbing for a toilet. On warm days, some of her neighbors later told me, they could see Clara Rose using her walker to reach the outhouse in the front yard. But on cold days, she resorted to a hospital-style potty chair *inside*.

"Right up until I was 98 years old," she firmly stated, "I was still chopping my own wood to heat this place with." Her home had never been insulated. "My son Claude—he's 67—made me stop chopping on account I kept skinning myself so much whenever I hauled the wood in. He made me put in electric heat. That got my dander up good, but I had no say in the matter."

She scoffed at modern comforts such as the electric stove and electric fridge. "Don't have no use for any of them," she snapped with a fuss. "Ought to throw those things out with the trash where they belong." That's exactly what she did with the automatic drip coffeepot that Claude got her awhile back. (He retrieved it from her garbage can and now uses it himself.)

Another thing which "really got me fighting mad," she hissed in anger, "was when my family brought running water into my kitchen here to replace the hand pump I had been using since the time I got married. Working that thing every day like I did kept me fit. Now, I feel kind of lazy without it."

Her whole point to opposing modern conveniences was that "they tend to make you lazy and sassy, make you not want to do as much. Then what will you do with your time?" she asked, while pushing up her thick glasses that greatly magnified her still beautiful blue eyes.

"How do I keep from getting bored?" she said, repeating my question nearly word-for-word. "Well, it's like this. I've always been a very determined person all my life. William and I worked together to make a good home for our kids. But no one's ever been able to tell me how to run my life. I run it for me. When I set my heart and mind on something, I never change."

Here she temporarily paused and gave that last statement a moment's thought. "Well, *almost* never change," she corrected herself. "You fix your eye on something you want or something you believe in very hard, and never take it off that, you won't ever get bored. 'Sides, when you don't have them modern conveniences, you're always keeping yourself busy chopping wood, cooking dinner, washing dishes and clothes by hand, and traveling back and forth to the outhouse." And then with another throaty chuckle, she added, "When you're doing all of this and more, your mind don't have time to stray very far or become very useless."

Her longest period away from home was back in 1988 when she suffered a heart attack and was placed in a nursing home for several months. "I became real unhappy there," she recalled with an edge of bitterness evident in her voice. "I told Claude [her son] that if he didn't get me the hell out of that place, that I would soon be a goner. And then I'd come back haunt him till doomsday. He knew I wasn't kidding and brought me back here to the only place I've ever known as home."

Mrs. Worden didn't know why she had lived to be so old. She never drank alcohol or smoked, of course. But "I wasn't into any of that funny health food that everybody today seems to be getting so crazy over," she opinionated. "Lunch most days for us was a fried feast of bacon, breaded fish, and potato wedges. I didn't start seeing a doctor until I was 95."

And what was Clara's "secret" to keep from getting bored? "Keep your life simple, work hard for everything you get, be satisfied with what you have, remain true to your principles, and don't take sass from no one!" she finished with a jocular finality.

Forever Young

"SECRETS FOR PRESERVING YOUR HEALTH AND VITALITY"

🌾 SELF-HEALING FRACTURES

Mary A. Wolf who resides on Palmetto Street in Philadelphia, PA, wrote the following letter of interest to me on May 15, 1996. In it, she spelled out the course of food therapy she selected to promote self-healing of a serious leg injury.

Dear Dr. Heinerman:

Last December I fractured my left leg and had to spend 6 weeks non-ambulatory. Luckily enough the ad mail came despite the worst snowfalls in our Northeast region. I was fascinated with the ad literature [from Prentice Hall Direct] on your *[Heinerman's] Encyclopedia of Nuts, Berries and Seeds*. Well, I ordered the book and read it with the greatest of interest from cover to cover.

Needless to say, I greatly modified my diet at once to include all those delicious foods that have been called snack foods or fattening. The doctor that I saw at that time asked me if I took any vitamins and wanted to know which ones I took so he could recommend them to some of his other patients.

I told him about the foods you suggested in the book. I told him I regularly munched on nuts and seeds of all kinds. He was absolutely amazed by the progress of my injury. The tibia and fibula I broke are mending with bone callus, glowing white, and the diameters [thereof] have increased substantially as [the] x-rays have shown. He remarked in astonishment that he didn't know such snack foods had any healing power to them.

I am now walking well but cannot seem to give up the foods that were so good to me during my convalescence. Particularly, pistachios are my favorite with almonds second, and seeded rye the third. The list goes on and on as I am a complete convert to nuts and seeds, and also berries whenever they are in season.

Thank you for writing such an insightful book for consumers like myself. I'm sure that these kinds of foods will keep someone like myself vital and energetic for years in spite of how old we may be.

Sincerely,

/s/ Mary A. Wolf

 ## Making Your Beauty Truly Skin Deep

The skin happens to be the single largest organ of the body. It comes in many different colors and wonderful textures. Weighing in at roughly six pounds, the skin is about one-eighth of an inch thick, varying at different places on the body. Skin is continually growing from within, creating new cells that push their way outward. Yet the skin, perhaps more than any other part of the body, tells the world how you feel about yourself mentally, emotionally, and physically.

In consulting with some of my medical colleagues who are dermatologists or skin care experts, they came up with some things that they felt would help improve our body's outer covering, no matter what age a person might be. If faithfully followed, these items should guarantee radiant-looking skin for years to come.

Sun Protection. Contrary to what most doctors advise about wearing some kind of sunscreen protectant or clothing during hot weather, the skin actually benefits from *moderate* amounts of sunlight. The sun is the greatest source of the "sunshine" vitamin D. The sun's ultraviolet rays convert a form of cholesterol present in the skin to vitamin D. Most of the body's need for vitamin D can be easily met by *some* exposure to *modest* amounts of sunlight. The best times for this are usually in the morning or on a cloudy, overcast day, when the heat of the sun isn't so intense, and the risk of getting a sunburn much lower. Also the consumption of vitamin D-rich foods, like sunflower and sesame seeds, sprouted alfalfa seeds, and salmon, tuna, and mackerel helps create beautiful skin. The sun benefits us in others ways too: it clears up acne, relaxes aching muscles, and eliminates depression.

The secret here is *moderate* amounts of sun at the times suggested. Too much sun can break down collagen and elastin components of the skin, causing loss of moisture, flexibility, and tautness. Sunscreens are good to use when you're out during the hottest part of the day for any length of time. They also help to prevent melanoma, a form of skin cancer, due to overexposure to sunlight.

Oil-Rich Foods. Don't confuse this with greasy foods that are fried or deep-fried. I'm speaking here of those things found in nature which have *naturally-occurring* oils and fats in them. Heading the list is avocado: societies in tropical settings where it grows and that make abundant use of the same, always seem to have smoother-looking skin than those cultures which don't take advantage of Nature's own "natural butter." Then there are those nuts and seeds, which a fan, Mary A. Wolf, wrote to me about and mentioned in the very beginning of this section. One portion of her letter, which I edited out because it didn't fit with fractures, is presented herewith:

> An unexpected and beneficial side-effect happened during those several months that I was munching down my pistachios, almonds, and sunflower seeds. I noticed that the surface of my skin was actually beginning to look *younger* than it used to. Maybe I'm losing it, Dr. Heinerman, but I could actually swear that my complexion was improved. Am I crazy or is there really something to this?

I wrote back reassuring her that her sanity was intact and that she was not suffering from an overactive imagination. I explained how the fats and oils in such nuts and seeds were replenishing the very nutrients her skin was lacking in. In her case, as with anyone else, the skin beauty was within and coming out, instead of being the other way around.

There are also a number of other foods with natural fats and oils. Whole raw cow's milk or goat's milk are options to consider. Also the vast array of seafoods readily available. Fresh-water fish are especially rich in natural oil content; also sardines, salmon, tuna, trout, mackerel, and haddock to name just a few. When preparing them for eating, try steaming or baking instead of frying or broiling. That way, more of their oil contents will be preserved intact.

Moisturizing Foods. The skin is in constant need of moisture due to different factors that tend to dry it out all the time. These can range from too much sunlight and exposure to the wind to excessive consumption of alcohol, coffee, colas, and soft drinks to use of lotions, perfumes, and scented soaps. The best foods to consume for vibrant looking skin are things with high-water content: any melons or berries or cucumbers when in season are great for this.

But the *very best* moisturizing agent of all is just plain *water.* Be sure to drink plenty of purified water—a minimum of seven cups per day in between meals is advised. Water moisturizes your skin from the inside out and helps to eliminate poisons from within that make your skin look old.

Moderate Exercise. I've already discussed exercise a lot in other parts of this book. Its importance to human health cannot be underestimated. Old people who look quite young for their ages, *always* are engaged in some form of physical activity.

The best kind of skin exercises are those that involve a lot of stretching. That's probably why yoga enthusiasts always feel and *look* so much younger. All of that stretching, combined with mental exercises to calm the agitated spirit within, not only furnish an outer glow of health but also radiate a serenity that actually *enhances* the beauty of their skin in a subtle way.

Don't forget, though, the obvious benefits to be derived from aerobic and endurance activities. These actions promote faster heart beat and improved circulation. Which means that the body perspires more often, thereby eliminating accumulations of poison from within that tend to make the skin appear much older than it really is.

Soft-Heat Sauna. Native American tribes throughout the Western Hemisphere have understood for many centuries the therapeutic benefits that come from frequent use of sweat lodges. In different tongues and dialects the adage was pretty much all the same: "There's nothing like a good sweat to make you feel fit for the day." Lodge sweating stimulates and speeds up the metabolic processes and inhibits the growth of pathogenic bacteria and viruses. Many toxins that have built up in the system over a period of time are shed through perspiration. There are some excellent books on the subject of lodge sweating. One can usually find a Native American shaman somewhere who is skilled in such a thing and can instruct you on how to do it.

For those unable to make such connections due to age, economic or geographical limitations, there is available something else that is a good substitute. A soft-heat sauna (also known as a radiant or infrared sauna) is wonderful for the system. Unlike the older, outdated technology sauna of the past, which raised air to high temperatures, a soft-heat sauna warms the muscles and skin directly. It accomplishes this by warming air to only comfortable level, permitting for fresh air ventilation so that a person never feels suffocated. Because an individual can use this type of sauna over an extended period without complications, he or she can reap greater health benefits than through a high-temperature sauna.

Dry-Skin Brushing. During the writing of this book in the first half of 1996, I consulted often with my father Jacob Heinerman for some of his advice that is scattered throughout the text (besides the lovely foreword he wrote especially for this book). Then he was 82 years of age. I had never paid much attention to the many compliments he's received since he turned 70 about how youthful he looks for his years. But now, with the writing of this book, I began to focus more sharply on that and recalled some of the comments made by others who see him often.

Not meaning to brag, but my dad *really does* look about 15 to 20 years younger than his actual age. And what has been his own "beauty secret" (if I dare call it that) for looking so youthful? Why nothing more than dry-brushing his body with a natural bristle brush morning and night. This daily going over that his skin gets helps to slough off dead cells on its surface and gives him a healthy glow.

Now, dad prefers to brush in circular motions, always moving towards his heart. He uses common sense, of course, and avoids brushing patches of eczema, skin eruptions or any other infected area that may show up from time to time on skin. This is so as not to irritate such problem areas until they've fully healed or cleared up. His brushing strokes are very gentle and never aggressive or hurried. And, he *never* brushes his face. My younger (by one year) brother Joseph always wipes the top of our father's bald head with a slightly wet towel to remove dead skin cells from there and to stimulate circulation to the scalp.

Omega Fatty Acids. Dry skin is usually a sign of a deficiency in omega-3 fatty acids. Essential fatty acids (EFAs) are nutrients the body is unable to synthesize; these must be supplied by the diet and are the basic building blocks of every cell in the body. The two EFAs are omega 3 (alpha-linolenic acid) and omega 6 (linoleic acid). Four of the very best sources for such omega-3 fatty acids are: cod liver oil (1 tbsp. daily), flaxseed oil (2 teaspoons daily), olive oil (1 tbsp. daily), and evening primrose oil (4 capsules daily).

These are best taken with 1 or 2 capsules of the Complex C-3 turmeric product manufactured exclusively by the Sabinsa Corp. of Piscataway, NJ. Sabinsa's remarkable antioxidant product works wonderfully well with any of these omega-3-rich oils to create beautiful and luxuriant skin tone.

NUTRITIONAL BRAIN BOOSTERS

Some two decades ago, few if any of us had ever heard of Alzheimer's disease. Most seniors back then just suffered from the inevitable Oldtimer's disease but nothing else that disturbed brain function. Today, it's one of the diseases feared most by older folks. In fact, in some areas of the country, it even outranks heart, cancer, and AIDS in terms of the fear it engenders in the middle-aged and elderly. Currently, about 4.2 million Americans suffer from varying degrees of Alzheimer's. And if no cure is found for it soon, the Chicago-based Alzheimer's Association predicts this number could escalate to 14 million by 2050.

I asked Miklos Boczko, M.D., by phone what he attributed this sudden increase to. He is a neurologist working out of White Plains, NY. "You can't pin it down to just one or two things," he stated. "Alzheimer's results from the confluence of many factors. Dementia has a definite familial aggregation. If someone in your family has the disease, your risk is obviously going to be much higher. Therefore, you should be tuned into its likely causes and treatments."

I then asked the good doctor a very direct question. "I have a dear friend about my age, who recently buried his mother, who had acquired Alzheimer's. Should he be worried about being at a greater risk for this disease than say I might be, since neither of my folks or their grandparents ever had it?" His response was, "Yes, he is definitely at higher risk than you would be. And your friend should become better acquainted with the problem long before he might become subject to it."

Boczko thought that the cumulative stress of an inadequate diet, a poor intake of particular nutrients vital to brain function, and long-term exposure to toxic chemicals, combine together to cause Alzheimer's. Two of his suspected causes set me to thinking about my own research, not so much into Alzheimer's as into other topics like longevity and folk remedies. In the many years that I've interviewed thousands of people, I've discovered one very interesting thing: those who are agrarian-based and rural-dwelling have far *less* incidence of Alzheimer's than do those who work and reside in large metropolitan areas.

Although it's only a hypothesis for now, I'm inclined to think that big city *smog* is one of the real culprits for turning so many otherwise normal older people into mindless vegetables in the course of time. This doesn't mean that a few years of city dwelling will do this. But it does *infer* that long-term residence could, in fact, put enough lead, nickel, and other heavy metals into the brain to make it inoperable after awhile.

There now arises an even more intriguing matter relative to all of this. How about those older folks who've moved between rural and urban neighborhoods in the course of their lives? My own father Jacob Heinerman is one that I know of who fits into this category. He was born and raised in a large city (Salt Lake, of course). But when he married, he relocated to the country and raised my brother and me on a farm with an orchard on it. Then after some years of this, he sold the farm and moved back to the big city to work in an antiquarian bookstore and in retail selling. He eventually got out of those occupations and went into painting houses, which required a lot of outdoor labor with a fair number of his customers being located in rural areas. Our family later moved to a small farm in south-central Utah, where we resided for a decade or so before returning again to Salt Lake City, where we were as of 1996. Our intents and desires are to make one final move to a large family ranch located in the desert wilderness of southern Utah, where the air is pure and clean and entirely devoid of heavy metal pollutants. We anticipate this should be accomplished sometime in the 1997 or 1998 period.

The point I'm trying to make here with this short rehearsal of facts is that my dad, who was 82 when this book was written, has *never* showed any signs of dementia. Oh yes, it is true that he becomes occasionally absentminded in some things, but then, so do both of his sons, who are decades younger than he is. In my father's case, his back-and-forth moving between city and rural life, has apparently helped him to avoid large amounts of poisonous metal toxins accumulating in his brain tissue.

Also, there is the matter of stress. Rural-induced stress is quite a bit different than urban-caused stress. Country living with its own set of problems doesn't promote anywhere near the frenetic pace of things that city dwelling does. The latter, in fact, is at such an accelerated pace that the body is forever pumping out inordinate amounts of adrenaline and other hormonal substances which can build up to toxic levels in a matter of years. Also, rushing through life can cause the blood vessels to experience a *gradual shrinkage*, thereby limiting circulation to the brain. And don't forget that the sights, sounds, lights, colors, and actions of a big city definitely assault the human senses with greater *negative* impact than country things do. I mean, wouldn't you trade gray smog any day for a whiff or two of cow or pig manure? Granted that the latter may not be the most pleasant aromas around, but they certainly are a lot healthier for your brain than are the vehicle exhaust and factory smokestack emissions being breathed in everyday by tens of millions of people nationwide.

While the majority of the population could never relocate to the country, there are still some nutritional things which can be done to boost your own brain's mental capabilities and, more importantly, to help *prevent* the possible onset of Alzheimer's disease in later years. There is a class of so-called "smart nutrients" that have been a boon to younger people for memory enhancement and thinking. It is believed that they might also have considerable merit with older folks as well. These nutrients include choline, which is related to the B-complex family, vitamin B-12, carnitine and antioxidants like the Complex C-3 from turmeric put out by the Sabinsa Corp.

But choline, B-12, and carnitine work in concert with each other as opposed to being taken alone at different times. Choline is the principal precursor in the formation of lecithin. Choline-rich foods include certain animal organs (brain, liver, and kidney), eggs, brewer's yeast, wheat germ, milk, cheese, fish, and soybeans. But studies have often shown mixed results from choline supplements alone, whether used for memory enhancement or for treating Alzheimer's. Sometimes they help, and sometimes they don't. One reason could be that the conversion of choline to acetylcholine is dependent on vitamin B-12 and carnitine. Most older people are usually deficient in both of these nutrients.

Gregory E. Gray, M.D., Ph.D. of the University of Southern California School of Medicine, told me in a phone conversation sometime ago that he discovered low B-12 levels in a third of senile patients he tested. But when he gave Vitamin B-12 to 13 such individuals, eight promptly recovered and three experienced partial recoveries. He directed my attention to the *Journal of the American Dietetic Association* (89:1795-1802) for December 1989 for his full report on the matter. Foods with respectable amounts of B-12 in them include beef, eggs, fish, milk products, organ meats, pork, and cottage cheese. *But beware that alcohol, coffee, and tobacco can rob the body of this important nutrient in a hurry!*

Carnitine is the other ingredient in this nutritional trio to boost brain activity. The highest carnitive-containing foods are beef steak, ground beef, and bacon. Medium levels of this nonessential amino acid occur in fish, chicken, whole milk, and American cheese. The poorest foods for it were cereal grains, vegetables, and fruit.

Carnitine can be purchased in health food stores as L-carnitine and can be taken in doses up to 2–3 grams per day without causing any side effects, except maybe for slight and temporary diarrhea.

Quite recently, Jay W. Pettegrew, M.D., of the University of Pittsburgh School of Medicine, wonderfully demonstrated the amazing action of this amazing nutrient on Alzheimer's patients, Writing in the January-February 1995 issue of *Neurobiology of Aging* (16:1–4), he mentioned giving 3 grams of acetyl-L-carnitine daily to seven probable Alzheimer's patients for one year. Five other probable Alzheimer's cases received a placebo, and 21 healthy patients were used as a control group. Tests to assess cognitive function were given to all the patients at six and 12 months, and a number of neurochemicals were also measured.

Although the acetyl-L-carnitine and placebo groups had virtually identical cognitive scores at the beginning of the study, the acetyl-L-carnitine group ended the study with "significantly higher" scores. That was because they had maintained their cognitive function, whereas the disease got worse in the placebo group. He also noticed that deleterious chemical changes in the brain occurred at a much slower rate among patients taking acetyl-L-carnitine. These findings are particularly noteworthy because the patients treated with acetyl-L-carnitine were older, and presumably more resistant to treatment, than the placebo group.

The advantage of combining a curcuminoid complex with choline, B-12, and carnitine, is to prevent free radical destruction of existing brain tissue. The Sabinsa Corporation of Piscataway, New Jersey has developed the *only* working curcuminoid complex from turmeric root capable of preventing this from happening. Generally 2–3 capsules daily of Complex C-3 in conjunction with the other nutrients is good enough for this. (See Product Appendix for more information on Sabinsa's fine products.)

🎇 Multivitamins for Your Personality

One of the more obvious signs with the attainment of old age is that the disposition gets crankier and the personality becomes more ornery. To help alleviate this from ever happening, take a high-potency multi-vitamin of some kind. The best kind I recommend happens to come from the Great Salt Lake and is a unique blend of both vitamins and minerals alike. It is Pure Inland Sea Water marketed by Trace Minerals Research of Ogden, UT (see Product Appendix).

A recent study proves that you may not have to make major lifestyle changes after all in your diet or behavior to improve your mind or mood. A team of British scientists gave college-age men and women a high-potency multivitamin supplement, containing 10 times the Recommended Dietary Allowance (RDA) for vitamins B-1, B-2, B-3, B-6, B-12, C, E, and biotin, and RDA levels of vitamin A.

David Benton, M.D., of the department of psychology at the University College of Swansea in Wales, asked 129 healthy volunteers, ages 17 to 27, to take either the vitamin or placebo each day for an entire year. People taking the vitamin had better moods, improved thinking, and faster reaction times, according to two articles by him published in *Biological Psychology/ Pharmacopsychology* (32:98–105, 1995) and *Psychopharmacology* (117:298–305, August 1995). Both men and women improved, but the women seemed to have the greatest benefits. It took a year of supplementation before the improvements became statistically significant.

Benton contended that psychological symptoms are usually the first sign of a vitamin deficiency of some kind. The reason, he explained, is that many of the B vitamins and vitamin C are involved in the production of neurotransmitters.

🎇 Having the Energy of a Kid Again

Wednesday, May 29, 1996 was a busy day for me. The phone began ringing at 7 A.M. Mountain Standard Time. My first call came from Mark Douglas of WJON-AM in Saint Cloud, MN, who taped a 20-minute interview with me. In it I recommended what I term "The Three D's for Getting Well"—DESIRE, DISCIPLINE, and DO IT! Then came a call from Scott Sands of WNSL-FM radio serving the Hattiesburg-Laurel area of Mississippi. He and his co-host Allyson Scott enjoyed me so much that they asked me to stay into the next hour; I was on their rock music program from 7:30-8:10 A.M.

I had just barely hung up after that when Donna Mason called from station WDNC-AM in Durham, NC. "Sounds like a disease, doesn't it?" she joked about her station's call letters. We went live for one solid hour, taking a number of phone calls along the way. I wrapped up her show at 9:15 A.M. But before doing so, she asked me in closing (and partly out of curiosity): "Say, Dr. Heinerman, how is it that you have so much energy and zip to you this morning, considering that you've done three fast-paced radio shows back-to-back within a two-hour time period? Other guests usually need a break in between, but you seem to keep going without a let up in your stamina."

I explained to her that I took Mighty Greens every morning. "This is a product from Pines International of Lawrence, KS (see Product Appendix). It includes over two dozen vegetables and herbs in a concentrated powdered drink mix. I take $1^1/_2$ tablespoons and stir it into a glass of tomato juice to make it more palatable. This gives me sustained, time-released energy for up to six hours at a time. It *is* the most *potent* green vegetable drink mix on the market today." She responded with a laugh: "Well folks, you heard it from the good doctor himself—*Mighty Greens* is what it takes to feel good again!"

I met retired advertising executive Jack Shapiro, age 71, of Salt Lake City at a dinner engagement recently. He recalled my name during my 5-year editorship of *Utah Prime Times* (a monthly seniors newspaper). His agency occasionally bought ad space from us for various political candidates they were representing.

Jack and I got involved in a serious discussion about health. He told me that when he was a young man he once worked at a job cleaning floors that required use of toxic chemical solvents.

The ventilation was poor and he apparently ended up poisoning himself by breathing in some of their toxic fumes. But the effects upon his system were very subtle and it wasn't until some years afterwards that he finally realized the full extent of the damage that had been done to his respiratory system. "I always felt kind of tired in the afternoons without ever knowing the real reason to it," he recalled. "My doctor told me that I had contracted chemical bronchitis, which brought this other condition on."

So, he started taking Ginkgo Biloba Plus from Wakunaga of America. (This is a unique blend of ginkgo biloba leaf extract, aged garlic extract, and ginseng extract.) He averaged the equivalent of 4 capsules daily and took it with either juice or water. He declared at the dinner table in the home of our hosts, Max and Bernice Eisen: "This stuff has helped give me more energy than I ever had before, and has helped me to think a lot more clearly, too." Jack belongs to the E1 Kalah Shrine Temple and is a member of a special club within that group called The Jesters, who are made up of prominent civic officials and professional people (both active and retired). He arranged for me to speak to this group of about 40 at the prestigious Alta Club in downtown Salt Lake City on Monday, June 10, 1996 on the topic of "Ancient Nutritional Healing Secrets for Modern Man."

Older people may not immediately recognize the name of Jean-Claude Van Damme, but those of a much younger generation certainly will. This 33-year-old ex-middleweight champion of the European Professional Karate Association has appeared in a number of action-adventure movies such as "Lion Heart" in the last decade. The 5-foot-10-inch, 185-pound actor still exhibits the charisma and well-poised kicks and punches that have earned him status as one of the kings of such films.

But how has he managed to keep his body and mind in such youthful shape for such demanding movie roles? Believe it or not, it isn't some kind of special diet or secret Oriental herbs which he credits his teenage agility to. It's in *stretching* and *imagination*. Van Damme was once a skillful ballet dancer before he hit it big-time in his fast-paced action thrillers. Of course, no one in his right mind is going to ever question the manliness of this guy, unless he intends spending his vacation in the intensive-care unit of a local hospital somewhere!

But Van Damme asserted in an interview that the daily sessions of required stretching exercises helped to keep his body more limber and spine flexible. In fact, medical researchers now know that *the spine is one of the fastest aging parts of the human body.* Van Damme doesn't intend letting his ever get old by any means. Stretching also helps to keep his back and leg muscles elongated (they tend to shrink with age). Afterwards, he spars to keep his legs flexible and does karate movements to keep in cardiovascular shape. "I train my heart, muscles and flexibility, so my workout is an overall one," he reminded his interviewer.

But "the 'theater of the mind' also needs to see positive daily workouts to keep everything in shape," he continued. "I prefer imagination to anything else for keeping my brain reflexes alert. Whenever I work out my body in a gym, I'm also running my mind through some pleasant routines as well. I think of things that are agreeable and pleasant to me; nothing negative that is going to weigh me down while I'm exercising my body."

"Imagination for here," he said, pointing a forefinger to his temple, "and stretching or karate for this," while directing the interviewer's attention to a bulging arm bicep. "If you do *both*—the body and mind *together*—then you'll always feel youthful, even if you get older. Oh, and one more thing—remember to always drink *a lot* of water *before* and *after* each physical workout. This gives the body a better chance to recoup."

🌱 Forever Young

The things which have been presented in this section will definitely assist you in preserving your own mental and physical vitality. Some of the things mentioned herein, are elaborated on in other parts of the book; still others are unique only to this section. But their combined efforts certainly do more good than if they were done individually at different times.

Also, a significant piece of philosophy in passing: Pride and arrogance tend to make you older, while being meek and humble as a little child can preserve your youthfulness for many, many years. *That is a fact of truth revealed from Heaven above;* the wise will heed it, but fools will not!

Fountain of Youth Revisited

"UNIQUE TIPS FOR NEARLY AGELESS BEAUTY"

 PONCE DE LEÓN AND THE FOUNTAIN OF YOUTH

Following the discovery of the Americas by Cristobal Colón (anglicized to Christopher Columbus) in 1492, there was a mad rush to the Western Hemisphere from the Old World by numerous conquistadors and explorers. Many of them, like Hernando Cortez and Francisco Pizarro and his brothers, were after gold and left their bloody marks in the annals of history by conquering great Indian empires such as the Aztecs and the Incas.

Not all of these explorers were after material wealth, however. Some of them were chasing dreams of a different sort. Among the more noble was one Juan Ponce de León. He started out as a page in the royal court of Aragon, then later began his career of exploration in 1493 as part of Columbus' second expedition to the New World. It was on this expedition that he first heard rumors from the natives of a mythical pool of water that could keep a person forever young if such an individual drank from and bathed in it. Nine years later he traveled to the West Indies under Nicolás de Ovando, who served as governor of Hispaniola. As Ovando's deputy, in 1508–09 Ponce de León explored and settled Puerto Rico, founding the colony's oldest settlement, Caparra, near what is now San Juan.

Here the legend became more frequent and expanded. From the lips of different island natives, he heard rumors about a "Fountain of Youth" to the east somewhere, that turned old, crippled people into young and healthy individuals again, once they had partaken of its holy waters and dipped themselves in it accordingly. Royal orders were soon forthcoming for him to search it out. It was while on this earnest sojourn that he accidentally discovered Florida in the spring of 1513, though at the time he didn't realize he was on the mainland of North America.

The region was so named because it was discovered at Easter time (the Spanish, Pascua Florida).

After landing near the site of modern St. Augustine, he coasted southward, sailing through the Florida Keys. Along the way he encountered some Seminole Indians who told him through an interpreter that his desired Fountain of Youth was not too far away. He ended his search near Charlotte Harbor on the west coast and sampled a lot of water taken from many local streams, ponds, and lakes. But none of them made the wrinkles go away, the gray hair disappear, or the step become more lively and energetic. In the end, he gave up chasing his phantom miracle water and turned his attention to other pursuits.

While Ponce de León's Fountain of Youth was obviously a mythical one from all appearances, it is quite possible to realize *some* of the benefits it was purported to have contained. These can be achieved, not by dipping yourself in some magic water or even drinking it, but simply by following a few wise suggestions that will definitely roll back the years for you to some extent.

VEGETARIAN-FITNESS CONNECTION

A consistent, diverse exercise program done properly can help defy the consequences of aging. Scattered throughout this book are a number of different exercises designed to help you achieve that very thing. But combating the degenerative cycle requires a healthy diet, too.

Practicing vegetarian eating habits can make a real difference in how you feel following moderate to rigorous exercises. Since the mind, body, and spirit can't be disconnected, neither can our body be separated and unaffected by what we eat. Inactivity is a major health risk, as is a high-fat, low-fiber, high-cholesterol diet, which most vegetarians and especially vegans, obviously try hard to avoid.

Doctors who've treated vegetarian patients have discovered that their rates of recovery from illness or surgery are usually quite a bit faster than their non-vegetarian clients. Those assigned to work in intensive or critical care units or emergency rooms of different hospitals have reported that vegetarians *always* recover much more quickly from serious injuries. As one critical care specialist observed: "Their [meaning vegetarian patients] outward healthy appearances reflect what is going on inwardly."

Meat consumption (fish excluded) has always been a drag on the human system and greatly contributes to the aging process in general. But a vegetarian diet (devoid of animal flesh except for fish) combined with appropriate and sensible exercise can make you look and feel good, and reverse many of the symptoms of aging.

SOUPER SALAD TO MAKE YOU LOOK AND FEEL YOUNGER

Obviously no single recipe is going to make you feel younger overnight. But multiple recipes that are meatless and contain healthy ingredients will, over the course of time, make you look entirely different than you now are. By consuming mostly vegetarian dishes, you will become the envy of relatives, friends, and neighbors around you, who will curiously inquire, "What's happened to you lately . . . you look *so* young?"

The following pair of recipes are only meant to serve as a guide in this direction. There are plenty of books on the market devoted exclusively to vegetarian cooking. You are encouraged to buy some of them and try the many wonderful recipes they contain. One thing you'll discover upon rotating between the following soup and salad, is how much better your digestive tract will feel after eating one of these at different periods of the day. You'll not only experience a lighter sensation within your body, and more of a clearer thinking ability, but also will be pleasantly surprised to see just how much more energy you can get from relatively simple meals.

Lentil Soup Age Saver

2 large onions, chopped

2 tablespoons, olive oil

3 cloves garlic, minced

$1/_2$ teaspoon each, turmeric and coriander

4 cups chopped fresh tomatoes or 2 16-ounce cans

1 pound (2 cups) red lentils, rinsed

8 cups vegetable stock

$1/_2$ pound green beans, ends trimmed, cut into 1-inch pieces

2 tablespoons chopped fresh oregano or 2 teaspoons dried granulated kelp to taste (a seaweed available in health food stores)

In a stainless steel pot (never use aluminum for cooking anything), sauté the onions in oil over a medium heat until they become somewhat clear (appx. 5 minutes). Then stir in the garlic, turmeric, and coriander, and cook for 45 seconds. Next, add the tomatoes, lentils, and stock and bring to a boil. Then reduce the heat and simmer, partially covered, until the lentils are tender, for about three-quarters of an hour. Add the green beans and oregano after this, and continue cooking some more until the beans are tender (about 12 minutes). Finally, season with some granulated kelp to taste. Serves 8.

 ## "SHE BECAME A TOTALLY NEW WOMAN"

The following is true and correct information, just as I try to put in each one of my many health books. It came to me courtesy of Nancy Ross, age 45, who resides in Brooklyn Heights, New York. She is in marketing and public relations and is an adjunct professor at the Fashion Institute of Technology in the borough of Manhattan.

Simple Salad Youth Restorer

1 medium red cabbage, cut into chunks

2 cucumbers, peeled and sliced

4 ripe, firm tomatoes, cut into wedges

6 tangerines or oranges, peeled and segmented

1 red onion, thinly sliced

1 green pepper, seeded and thinly sliced

2 tablespoons each, apple cider vinegar and lemon juice

3 tablespoons olive oil

2 teaspoons oregano

granulated kelp to taste

In a large bowl, toss together the cabbage, cucumbers, tomatoes, tangerines, onion, and green pepper. In a small bowl, whisk together the vinegar, lemon juice, oil, oregano, and kelp. Drizzle dressing over the salad and gently toss. Makes a dozen servings. NOTE: This salad contains a number of antioxidant ingredients, which help to control free radical activity that is known to be responsible for accelerated aging.

She was part of an audience of almost 100 people who gathered in the basement of the big Barnes & Noble bookstore at Rockefeller Center (600 Fifth Avenue) on Thursday, April 11, 1996 to hear me speak on anti-aging issues for about 45 minutes. Afterwards, I signed a lot of books and answered a number of questions from those who stood in line to meet me.

When Ms. Ross' turn came, she shared the following information with me and gave her kind permission to use it as I saw fit. Nothing has been altered or changed from the way she presented it then.

"My grandmother, Kate Wolpin, lived to the age of 105. Her mother lived to be in her nineties. My own mother is still 'a kid' in her seventies. I hope to follow in their steps eventually.

"But mom's health wasn't always so vibrant. When she turned 69, she was struggling with a virulent strain of hepatitis. Doctors gave her a very poor prognosis and said she wouldn't live past six months the way she was going. This was quite discouraging to hear.

"At the time I happened to be training with a fellow in a local gym, whom I mentioned mom's condition to. He expressed himself to the effect that he thought he could help her. I introduced them to each other soon thereafter and he went to work.

"He put her on a program that included *a lot* of beet juice mixed with different kinds of greens. I don't know the exact ratio, but know that there were more greens than beets to the juice mixture. This combination was made fresh every day. I think that for every two small beets, he used double or even triple the amount of greens: parsley, celery, Romaine lettuce, spinach, watercress, and so forth.

"The beet-mixed greens juice was the heart of his program. But he also had her take capsules of milk thistle and dandelion every day." (Ms. Ross didn't know the exact quantity of each, but I will suggest two capsules of each herb daily with water or juice.) "She ate steel-cut oats soaked overnight and lightly cooked, every morning for breakfast. Very little milk was used on it. There were some other things that I can't recall right now, but these are the essential things I've given you.

"In just a few months, she had gained back 20 pounds. Her natural color returned and she became vigorous once again. And she did it all naturally without any drugs or chemical additives. She now plays tennis, swims, jogs, and has a full life once more. *She became a totally new woman* [from this regimen]!"

❧ "EVEN WEAR" FOR LONG LIFE

Some years ago I had the good fortune of meeting and visiting with the late Canadian epidemiologist Hans Selye in his research center at McGill University in Montreal, Quebec, Canada. He had devoted many years of his life to studying the effects of stress on the human body. I asked him how he would capsulize all of his findings.

Dr. Selye informed me that old age is nothing more than what he called "uneven wear" on some body parts. The ideal, he noted, would be to have "everything wear more evenly." Then "people could expect to live a lot longer" than they presently do.

He used as an analogy the four tires on an average car or truck. If they are properly mounted *and balanced*, then "they will wear evenly for a long time," he noted. But "if one of them should not be in perfect balance, then it will show wear a lot sooner than the others will."

"Our lives are the same way," he continued. "Everything should be in harmony and balance between the mental, emotional, physical, and spiritual. Then all of our internal organs will pretty much wear out the same." Otherwise, as we now have it, the heart may go first, or the kidneys, or the eyes. When this happens, then additional strain is placed upon the other organs and death ensues more quickly.

He stated unequivocally that "our lives need *balance* to them. Doing things in *moderation* and especially having *variety*, along with a sense of the sublime and contemplative, should give our lives all the balance they'll ever need!"

Love Makes You Live Younger

The greatest attribute we can possess within ourselves is *love*. As defined by the folks who give us dictionaries (called lexicographers), it is "a fatherly, motherly, brotherly, or sisterly attachment to others besides ourselves, with a genuine concern for their welfare and good at all times." Put another way, it is "an unselfish affection to promote good in the behalf of others." It is the ultimate personification of what constitutes the Great God of Heaven and Earth Himself and certainly transcends our own lowly and base sexual embraces by a wide margin.

I have had many opportunities the world over to see this principle in action time and again, irrespective of the belief systems of the individuals thus motivated and being studied by myself at the time. I shall cite just a few that are near and close to me, which can serve as effective role models for the rest of us.

The first of these is my own esteemed father Jacob Heinerman, who as of this writing in mid-1996 was himself 82$^{1}/_{2}$ years of age. His childhood and upbringing was in a Mormon home with European standards of parenting. The love demonstrated to him was a wonderful admixture of fatherly austerity comingled with motherly benevolence. Those years were wonderful—the best of times—and left him very normal.

However, his married life was sheer hell, to put it mildly. His mate, Jennie Faith Davidson came from an extremely unfortunate background filled with prejudice, cruelty, abandonment, violence, and hatred. Her warped values nearly ruined the lives of her two surviving sons (my brother and I, three other children having died in their infancy), before her own life ended quite tragically at the point of a gun. But through it all, my father remained true to her and attempted to help her become a better person. His efforts, though, never met with much success. However, his own love became considerably enlarged with the huge amount of patience and long-suffering that was acquired throughout this entire ordeal.

That, coupled with considerable meekness and humility, shaped his own compassion into something almost approaching the godly, I would have to say. Today this octogenarian is revered and adored by his two sons for the special love he has shown them through the years. But, more importantly, *this love has allowed him to live longer than expected.* My father has had a number of major health problems in his lifetime ,which he has attempted to treat naturally. These include: asthma, diabetes, heart murmur, hernias (3 of them), hypertension, hypoglycemia, insomnia, nervousness, and rheumatism.

But above and beyond the herbal and vitamin/mineral supplements that he routinely takes for all of these things, has been his steadfast *love for others* that has carried him through the worst and most difficult moments of each of these problems. Love has been the "magic potion" that has brought a renewal of sorts to his time-worn frame, giving him an unbelievable youthful vigor that amazes those around him who know how hard and difficult his lot in life has been.

The second person who comes to mind is my dear friend, Linda Steele. She is in her mid-thirties and works in the Human Genetics/Epidemiology Dept. of the University of Utah Medical Center as a medical researcher. In order to protect her privacy, I'm not going to delineate for the reader the many traumas and abuses this good woman has received in her life. Suffice it to say, hers has been an emotionally battered existence that came close a couple of times to being terminated by her own hand.

But Divine Providence overruled each time in her behalf and she somehow managed to surmount the herculean obstacles thrown in her path quite often. The secret to her survival success has always been *to forget herself in the service of others*. I have watched this woman in the action of rendering untiring kindness and have marveled every time at just how well she has held herself together. She maintains that "when you sacrifice your own time, energy, and efforts in behalf of the truly needy, then your own burdens seem to become much lighter to bear."

When she used to fret and worry all day long about her own dilemmas, she felt physically uncomfortable. In many ways her own self-pity was taking its toll on how she looked, felt, thought, and behaved. "It's as if I was aging by the hours instead of by the years," she recalled one time for me in a telephone conversation we had together. But when she reached that point in her life that self-love became translated into *love for others*, then a most wondrous transformation gradually began to unfold within her. "I felt younger in heart and spirit than I had in years," she said. "It's as if I was suddenly freed from a prison of self-containment. *Selfishness aged me, but compassionate service to others has revitalized my being for the better*," she insisted.

My third and final example is a family consisting of nine people. I've known Merrill and Shauna Gee and their kids for awhile now. They belong to the Haven Ward of the South Salt Lake Stake of The Church of Jesus Christ of Latter-Day Saints, to which I also belong. They live in a very modest home in an ordinary neighborhood and like so many others, struggle each month to get by on what he brings home as a low-paid engineer.

They have seven children, ranging in age from 17 all the way down to age four: Gardner, Gavin, Nathaniel, Austin, Natasha,

Andrew, and Rebecca. These are bright and beautiful children, secure and happy in a knowledge that *their parents love each other dearly*. And yet the love I've seen exhibited between Merrill and Shauna on many an occasion isn't so much a "clinging," "hand-holding," or "smooching" kind of sensual attraction, as it is a practical and working affection.

They make a fine team and together evenly split the duties of parenthood. Each one works without complaint in his or her respective domains of authority—he at his computer work and she within the home. This arrangement, of course, goes against the present trend of both parents working outside the home to make ends meet. But their attitude and outlook on parenting is quite unique: They see their seven children as their primary investments, and as such are willing to pour their whole hearts and souls into that endeavor by giving up the opportunity for an extra income and farming out some responsibilities to baby-sitters along the way.

In early childhood, everyone of their kids has received his or her fair share of hugging and sitting on mommy's or daddy's laps to hear a bedtime story of some kind. There is a definite contentment in the home, which all partake of equally. No violent TV shows or movie videos are ever allowed to pass their eyes. They are kept busy with room cleaning, dish washing, yard raking, lawn cutting, newspaper delivery, swimming and acting classes, ballroom dancing, and numerous church activities.

As the parents have shared their own lives and responsibilities, so too have the children, one by one, picked up on this as well. The oldest of the old has been known to tuck the youngest of the young in bed at night, when the covers were absent-mindedly kicked off during a cold, winter night. And the middle ones care for their younger siblings by holding their hands when crossing busy intersections or seeing that they got fed at suppertime.

I have been in the Gee home on numerous occasions and under many different conditions. And I have yet to see the type of sibling rivalry that is almost universally known elsewhere. There is no real fighting, quarreling, bickering, or teasing among the lot of them. This isn't to say that they are perfect kids, for they do have their occasional moments of laziness, stubbornness, or indifference that are common to human nature. But the sassiness and arguing you automatically expect from today's youth is virtually absent here.

It all gets back to one very simple philosophy: both parents love and respect each other a lot. It has been said that if a man loves the mother of his children, that the children, upon seeing that demonstration of love, will naturally emulate it themselves as they grow up. That is what has been at work here and left its indelible imprint of harmony everywhere I look. To visit them day or night, rain or shine, organized or in "wonderful confusion," is to come away with a *genuine* peace that leaves you feeling younger and like a kid all over again.

Free Radical Cell Aging Reversed

"CONTROLLING SCAVENGER MOLECULES THE QUICK AND EASY WAY"

WHAT'S NEW WITH GETTING OLD?

Mounting research in the last few years points to aging as being caused by the body's cells being repeatedly assaulted by free radicals. In an article entitled "Oxidative Stress and Human Aging," which appeared in a supplemental issue of *Biochemical Society Transactions* (23:375S, 1995), the authors reported free radicals deplete cells of the energy they need and, as a result, *less* new cells are produced. When cell multiplication slows down, old cell death *increases;* this could literally be termed "old age" but by broad definition.

Think of free radicals as similar to youth gangs roaming at large in big city metropolises like Los Angeles. They wreak havoc and destruction wherever they go. Nothing that was normal *before* their visit remains so afterwards. These free radicals are errant molecules lacking electrons and busily going about in search of them. Anyone who has ever played the video game of Pac Man knows that the object of the game is to see how many items the circular head can gobble up in the shortest length of time. With free radicals it's pretty much how many healthy cells they can injure while on their rampages.

Certain methods of preparing food can *dramatically increase* the amount of free radicals. Grinding up beef, forming it into hamburger patties, and then frying them probably adds *more* free radicals than many other foods I know of. Also, meat which is fried, broiled, or charbroiled tends to have a greater increase of these nasty molecules in them than foods which are baked, boiled, or steamed.

Throughout much of our lives, our body cells are being constantly bombarded by free radicals. There is sufficient scientific evidence now to suggest that most of the degenerative diseases associated with aging have their origin in damage from free radicals. These diseases include cancer, inflammatory joint disease, asthma, heart disease, senile dementia and Alzheimer's disease, Parkinson's disease, and degenerative eye disease.

 ## HEALTHFUL AGING

Fortunately for us, these molecular sharks zipping around in our cellular seas can be effectively neutralized with a class of compounds collectively known as antioxidants. They are produced in the body and found in many of the things we eat. But as we get older, our systems make fewer antioxidants and we absorb them less efficiently from what is consumed. So, it just makes perfect sense to frequently eat those foods that are naturally rich in antioxidants—especially those high in vitamins A, C, and E.

Fish and fish oil, green and yellow fruits and vegetables, goat milk and cheese, carrots, spinach, and beef liver are just some of the foods containing generous amounts of vitamin A and beta carotene. Many fresh fruits and vegetables are high in vitamin C. They range from berries and citrus items to bell peppers and mustard greens. Members of the cabbage family tend to have some vitamin C in them as well: cabbage, kale, kohlrabi, Brussels sprouts, and cauliflower. Potato, sweet potato, tomato, turnip greens, and melons also contain some vitamin C. Vitamin E is represented by a class of tocopherols, the most important of which is alpha-tocopherol. It occurs principally in products derived from plants, particularly cold-pressed vegetable oils (such as wheat germ oil), leafy green vegetables, and whole-grain cereals. And even though animal products contain very little vitamin E per se, still the best sources for what is available are liver, heart, kidney, and eggs. (Elsewhere in the text I've mentioned the health benefits to be derived from taking Rex's Wheat Germ Oil. This product is primarily intended for animal use only, but won't hurt humans. It is somewhat difficult to obtain unless you're in veterinary medicine. An amount of one tablespoon per day *with* a little food is suggested. It is best taken at night. To obtain a quart can of this for your own needs, send $65 to: Anthropological Research Center, P. O. Box 11471, Salt Lake City, UT 84147.)

🐉 Lengthening Your Lifespan with Nutrients

There are some other important nutrients worth examining that have impressive antioxidant powers to them. They include melatonin, curcumin, glutathione, and a trio of B vitamins (pyridoxine, folic acid, and choline). Each of these in their own unique way play an important role in *slowing* down free radical cell aging.

Melatonin is a life-giving hormone produced by one of the body's "master glands" (the pineal). As we get older this gland shrinks from the size of a single corn kernel to something even smaller. As a result, our melatonin productions drop accordingly.

An entire book on the subject has been written by one of the world's leading melatonin researchers, Dr. Russel J. Reiter. Entitled *Melatonin: Your Body's Natural Wonder Drug* (New York: Bantam Books, 1995), it praises the many virtues of this multi-purpose hormone. A quick check of the table of contents revealed to this author that melatonin may be good for the following things:

- Boosting the body's own immune defenses (Chapter 4).

- Helping combat HIV infection in AIDS patients (Chapter 5).

- Affording possible protection against cancer (Chapter 6).

- Assisting in the reduction of cholesterol and blood pressure (Chapter 7).

- Enabling hopeless insomniacs to get a good night's sleep (Chapter 8).

- Getting your body's time clock resynchronized (Chapter 9).

- Extending personal sexuality in the later years (Chapter 10).

- Improving mind, memory, and mood as you grow older (Chapter 11).

Melatonin is the latest health food fad and the rage of all those seeking to keep themselves young for as long as possible. You may not know it, but bad lighting and electromagnetic fields generated by power lines and numerous electronic devices can severely deplete melatonin reserves in your body *in a hurry.* So some supplementation seems to be in order here, but I'm opposed to long-term use since we don't know what the effects will be. I recommend 3–6 mg. of melatonin every *other* day or 3 times weekly at the most. Just because it may be the "miracle substance of the mid-90s" right now, doesn't mean you have to go hog wild on it. There should be moderation in all things, *especially* when it comes to nutritional supplementation!

Curcumin, a derivative from turmeric root, stands tall in my book of useful things to take. Not just because it is a great antioxidant or a wonderful liver protectant against diseases of that organ, but because I've seen it *delay* the onset of aging in some Third World nations I've visited where turmeric is extensively used in the food supply. From India to Indonesia and points in between, curry powder is used by several *billion* people in many different kinds of foods. Turmeric is one of a dozen key ingredients that go to make up this stuff; its principal function is to give curries their lovely golden colors.

And I discovered a strange thing as I traveled over the earth to those places where curries ranked supreme in meal preparations: many of the people who consume them on a regular basis take *longer* to get old than we do! *That's a fact* that you can take to the bank and deposit or put in your pipe and smoke. (Consult the entry under WRINKLES for more about this startling but wonderful phenomenon.)

The very best standardized turmeric extract on the market at present is Curcumin C-3 Complex from the Sabinsa Corp. It goes one step beyond vital cell protection by *preventing* the formation of free radicals as well as knocking out those that already exist. (Call 1-800-248-7464 or 908-777-1111 for more information.)

Glutathione is another potent cellular antioxidant. It fights free radicals that are generated both biochemically and environmentally by pollutants. However, it is not present in the body in unlimited supply and needs to be replenished every so often. Foods that contain glutathione include asparagus, winter squash, tomatoes, potatoes, avocado, peaches, and watermelon. Herbs that have this tripeptide include marshmallow root, fenugreek seed, comfrey root, and slippery elm bark.

Glutathione is a component of glutathione peroxidase. Scientists have noticed that seniors past 60 with high levels of glutathione in their circulating plasmas, have fewer health problems and more normal weight patterns than do those with lower levels. Those already in their 70s with low levels of glutathione are at greater risk of incurring arthritis, coronary artery disease, and diabetes.

A trio of B vitamins—B-6, folic acid, and choline—rounds out our short list of nutrients that will pump "new life" into your tired body's many worn-out cells. Pyridoxine helps to prevent atherosclerosis by lowering "bad" cholesterol and improves fading memory by bringing more blood sugar to an energy-starved brain. Folic acid plays a critical role in combating cloudy thinking and numbness of the extremities—both associated with old age—by enlarging the blood vessels for improved circulation. And choline—a necessary precursor for lecithin formation—helps improve nerve transmission by repairing damaged myelin sheathing (the fatty protein substance in which the nerves themselves are encased).

Food sources for all three B vitamins are plentiful. Vitamin B-6 may be found in large quantities in muscle meats, liver, vegetables, whole-grain cereals, and some seeds and nuts. Folacin (folic acid) is widely distributed in plants, especially in their green parts—hence the name folacin. Rich food sources include liver and leaf lettuce, other leafy green vegetables and legumes. Choline is present in abundance in brains, liver, kidney, eggs, yeast, and wheat germ, occurring in lesser amounts in milk, cheese, beef, and vegetables. (Rex's Wheat Germ Oil, mentioned elsewhere in this section, is a rich source of choline.)

These are some of the things which can be taken on a fairly regular basis to help you age more gracefully. Think of them as the nutritional silver lining in your gray clouds of advancing years.

Frailness Prevention

"WHAT THE NEANDERTHALS DID TO GET MASSIVE BONE STRENGTH"

🌿 OLD-AGE FRAILTY

One of the most common signs of aging is the bone fragility so evident in older people. The chief cause of this is usually attributed to osteoporosis. This is a condition in which there is varying losses of bone mass due to depletion of minerals essential to bone formation (phosphorus and particularly calcium). The affected bones tend to become porous and brittle and susceptible to fractures.

The wrists, hips, and vertebrae in the spine are the most common sites of fractures due to this problem. The disorder is very common among people over the age of 70 and affects women four times more often than men, owing to hormonal changes that occur with menopause.

But bone fragility in the later years of life can be easily circumvented by adopting a diet common to Stone Age times. Certain foods eaten then contributed to bone size and strength far in excess of those standards typical for modern man. The best model by far to use for studying this are the Neanderthals.

✤ ORIGIN OF THE NEANDERTHALS

The January 1996 issue of the *National Geographic* carried an excellent article on the Neanderthal race for anyone wanting to read up on the subject more. Some of the following information has been gleaned from that reference source.

They were first brought to the attention of an anxious and curious world with the discovery of one of their skeletal remains in the Neander Valley of Germany in 1856. Men working with picks in a limestone quarry near Düsseldorf dislodged the first Neanderthal fossil, which was quickly proclaimed as being the "missing link" between apes and humans by some scientists.

Eventually more bones with the same strange features were unearthed in Belgium, France, and other places throughout Europe. Then around 1900 bones belonging to as many as 80 Neanderthals were found in a cave close by the village of Krapina in what is now the Republic of Croatia. They appeared on the scene, scientists believe, around 260,000 years ago, but became extinct as a race about 30,000 years ago with the arrival of anatomically modern humans. The Neanderthals were migratory folks and roamed as far north as Great Britain and as far south as Spain. From central Europe they went eastward into parts of central Asia and migrated into the Middle East, too. Their total population is thought to have been in the tens rather than hundreds of thousands.

✤ MAKE SCHWARZENEGGER LOOK WIMPISH

Movie fans instantly identify film star Arnold Schwarzenegger. He is the former Austrian body-builder and several time winner of the "Mr. Universe" title, who turned to acting as a second and very lucrative career. His most popular movies have always featured him in action flicks as the big, muscle-bound hunk, who managed to do the bad guys in and emerge as the strong-man hero at the end.

His well-built frame, big muscles and athletic strength have made him the stereotypical "macho man" type generally emulated by other men and adored by countless women everywhere. But, according to anthropologist Erik Trinkaus of the University of New Mexico in Albuquerque, were Neanderthal men alive today, they "would have made Schwarzenegger look like a wimp" by comparison. He handed over to Rick Gore, a senior assistant editor of the *National Geographic,* a thick, heavy rib belonging to an ancient Neanderthal man. The other hefted it in his hand and knew almost "immediately that its owner was no 98-pound weakling."

"Imagine the muscles that [were] attached to that," Trinkaus declared to his visiting guest. "[Why] if I had muscles like that, all I'd have to do is flex my pecs and I'd break my ribs. Their bones tell us they had a lot of strength and endurance."

THE ULTIMATE SUPERMEN

The fictional comic strip/TV/movie hero known as Superman has been depicted as a man capable of flying through the air in a horizontal position anywhere he wants to, leaping the tallest buildings in a single bound, crushing to dust baseball-size granite rocks with his bare hands, and having bullets bounce off his chest from a fired gun. But such a character remains only in the realm of fiction and make-believe.

However, in the real world of anthropology, Neanderthals come about as close to this mythical representation as anyone. They were and still remain to this day, the world's greatest species of super-humans.

A brief physical description of them was published in the *Smithsonian* magazine (December 1991, p. 114) sometime ago. "What makes a Neanderthal a Neanderthal is a suite of exquisitely distinct physical traits, including massive limb bones; a barrel chest; thick brow ridges; a huge, protruding face and nose; a receding forehead, the absence of a well-defined chin; and a bunlike bulge on the back of the skull." And, on average, Neanderthal brains were "slightly larger" than modern human types. "Neanderthals appeared to be supremely well adapted" to the Ice Age environs they inhabited. Their closest modern *physical* equivalents might be the Alaskan Eskimos and Inuits, but lacking the superhuman strength of the former.

Because so many Neanderthal skeletons have been found in relatively good condition over the years, scientists around the world have been able to thoroughly examine these people in great detail. So strong were the men that they could *outrun* and bring down *by hand* wild game such as stag, elk, deer, bison, and the like. They could have lifted up the front end of *any* modern car or pickup truck without the aid of a hydraulic jack. And if one of their number had been in the professional boxing ring with the world's strongest fighter, Mike Tyson, he would have literally crushed the other one's skull to pieces with one well-aimed jab or, more likely, even decapitated him.

Neanderthal women were built like Amazons (a tribe of warlike women in Greek mythology possessed of superhuman skills). According to *Current Anthropology* (Vol. 29, No. 4, August–October 1988), they had bigger hips, wider pelvic areas, and larger birth canals, enabling them to give birth to much heftier babies after a typical ten-month gestation period. Their jaws were twice as powerful as those of modern women and capable of cracking open hard nut shells without the aid of a metal nutcracker. If they had been working out in a gym they could have easily bench-pressed 400 pounds without ever breaking a sweat!

🦑 BONE STRENGTH LIKE THE NEANDERTHALS

It is not possible, of course, for any of us living today to ever get the kind of incredible strength that these prehistoric people had. But it is possible through the right type of diet to at least duplicate some of their bone mass density and thereby prevent skeletal fragility as we grow older.

Neanderthals were foragers and not farmers. They ate a variety of wild animals, fish and shellfish, edible roots, leafy vegetables, some large fruits, berries, nuts, and seeds. As a result they suffered virtually no loss of bone mass. But, as later evidence was to show, their anatomically modern replacements, who subsisted more on domesticated crops and farm animals, became prone to osteoporosis. According to the *Journal of Human Evolution* (Vol. 14, No. 5, July 1985), agricultural populations are subject to more bone loss than are hunting-gathering societies like the Neanderthals.

In an extensive article on bone chemistry in the same reference journal, the role of strontium was explored at length. It is perhaps the least known of all the macrominerals that go to make up structural tissues and body fluid—sodium, magnesium, phosphorus, chlorine, potassium, and calcium. Yet, interestingly enough, this hidden nutrient is perhaps one of the most critical for keeping bone mass intact. According to the same publication, "More than 99% of the strontium in vertebrate tissue is found in the mineral component of the bone." This strongly hints at a greater importance for it than had heretofore been recognized.

Anthropologists always report strontium concentrations in parts per *million* (ppm) per sample. But for comparative purposes, they often use a ratio of strontium ppm to 1,000 ppm of calcium in order to demonstrate the minuscule amount of the former with the greater quantity of the latter. Continual research has shown that both minerals are invariably linked together in spite of their extreme contents range.

Scientists as yet do not completely understand the mechanism by which strontium works in conjunction with calcium to keep bones strong. It is believed that strontium may act as a kind of mineral "glue" to hold calcium intact for a long time. It is thought that strontium also acts as a binding agent for magnesium and calcium, keeping them together in the skeletal frame in the right proportions.

As of mid-1996, I had never been able to find in any of the consumer health magazines or books on nutrition, any articles or information devoted exclusively to strontium. Come to think of it, there wasn't even a mention of this vital nutrient. This startling lack of data can probably be attributed to a general public ignorance of it. Only in the anthropological and archaeological literature will one ever find information concerning strontium.

In order to increase the density of your own bones to prevent future fragility, it is highly recommended that you often consume those items which Neanderthal people regularly subsisted on. Food sources most rich in strontium—measured in parts per million, mind you—are as follows:

- Berries with tiny seeds in them: blackberry, blueberry, currant, hackberry, raspberry, and strawberry.

- Nuts, especially almonds, Brazils, cashews, filberts, macadamias, pine nuts, pistachios, and walnuts.

- Seeds, particularly chia, dill, fennel, flaxseed, poppy. pumpkin, sesame, and sunflower. Also the seeds in dark red and purple grapes, but not the outer flesh.

- Tuber vegetables like carrots, cassava, parsnips, potatoes, and turnips.

- All types of squash and cucumbers.

- Both fresh- and salt-water fish and shellfish.

- Most wild game but not domesticated animals.

Include more of these things in your daily diet and you can enter the golden years of life without fear of bone frailty.

Supplemental Sources

Bone-strengthening strontium may also be obtained from several fine nutritional products. One of these is ConcenTrace Trace Mineral Drops (5 drops per 6 oz. glass of water) from Trace Mineral Research of Ogden, Utah. Two others from one company (Pines International) are plant chlorophyll drink mixtures called Green Energy and Mighty Greens (one tablespoon of either in 8 ounces of water or juice). Another nice product is a Russian herbal formula from a family of physicians who once treated the Czars; it is called Badmaev 28 and is manufactured exclusively by America's Finest Inc. of Piscataway, New Jersey (1 tablet per meal 3 times daily).

Finally, there are a pair of products manufactured by Wakunaga of America: Kyo-Chrome and Kyo-Ginseng. One capsule of each twice daily with meals is recommended. (For further information on where to obtain these fine supplements consult the Product Appendix in the back of this book.)

(See also HEALTHY BONES and OPTIMISM FOR OSTEO-POROSIS.)

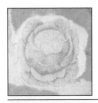

G

Gout Begone

"SOLICITATION FOR FUNDS ALSO BRINGS HELPFUL
REMEDY"

Several months ago I did some fund raising for the Lion's Club
Help the Blind Fund. I spent several hours in downtown Salt
Lake City asking for donations. After awhile I noticed sitting
close by on the edge of a cement planter box, a uniformed bus
driver with the Utah Transit Authority. He was casually smoking
a cigarette and waiting, I supposed, for his next bus route
change. At different intervals when the crowds crossing the
intersection somewhat died down, I would meander over to this
fellow and commence chatting with him.

In our sporadic dialogue, he discovered that I wrote books on
alternative health. He then volunteered some information for me,
which I found most interesting. He claimed to have been both-

ered with a bad case of gout for several years and found no permanent relief to his solution. Not until, that is, he turned to herbs.

He said he made a tea consisting of four different herbs which he purchased from local health food stores. He used equal parts (one tablespoon each) of speedwell, stinging nettle, watercress, and wood betony in one quart of boiling water. He covered the pan with a lid and simmered the ingredients for a few minutes, before setting aside to let steep awhile. He strained the contents into another container and poured himself a small glass which he drank morning, noon, and night without fail.

He stated that within a matter of weeks all of his gout had disappeared and he has never been troubled with it since then. He still drinks the tea occasionally, but not as often as he used to. He figured he must be drinking it about twice a week now as a safety precaution. He was kind enough to scribble down the herbs on a scrap of paper, since I was busy with my funds soliciting and unable to write this information myself.

I never learned the man's name, but didn't have to wait long to prove the efficacy of his own formula. An older friend of mine, who was bothered with gout himself, was given the formula a day later. He immediately started on it and within days noticed a big difference in how he felt. He said that the gouty pains in his big toes disappeared almost at once, and that the swelling in both ankles was starting to subside. He was happy to see results so quickly from a formula provided by a kind stranger.

Gray Hair Goners

"PROVEN WAYS COURTESY OF A LIMERICK WRITER, A TRUE BELIEVER, AND A SHEEPMAN"

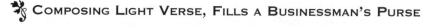 COMPOSING LIGHT VERSE, FILLS A BUSINESSMAN'S PURSE

I first read about Al Kracht's unusual talent in Section B of *The Wall Street Journal* for Thursday, March 21, 1996. At age 68, this retired advertising executive enjoys a nice, undisturbed career as a limerick ghostwriter that earns him something between $30,000 to $40,000 a year. "You aren't from the IRS are you?" he asked half-seriously when I put the question to him on annual earnings for this occupation. "The lady from *The [Wall Street] Journal* asked the same thing and I told her it was nobody's business how much I make." But when he was reassured that I wasn't from the federal government, he opened up a little more and gave me the income range previously cited.

"People don't understand that a limerick generally focuses on a fixed or given situation. Ordinarily it never encompasses a set of multiple events as say a poem or piece of prose might do. I keep having to explain this to those who want me to write something witty and clever for them or their friends or relatives."

Al figured that since 1990 he has written, on the average, about 200 limericks for people all over the world for many different circumstances. "There was this guy who called me from Uppsala, Sweden—wherever in the hell that is—who wanted me to do a limerick for his dad on the guy's 79th birthday; his father had been a sugar mapler and beekeeper for many years. I devised funny limericks to reflect both of those professions."

No Gray Hairs on His Head

Al mentioned that the funniest limericks are always the bawdy ones. He then recited a piece which we both found quite humorous, but which, he said, might offend some devout Catholics. After running it by my manuscript editor Douglas Corcoran at Prentice Hall, who himself is Catholic, I wisely decided to omit it from these pages because of its perverted subtleties.

However, one that easily passed the editorial muster was this little ditty Al shared with me:

Said the Bishop of Whittington Muse,
"I don't mind if parishioners snooze,
But it's awfully unfair
When I lead them in prayer,
To be snoring so loudly in their pews."

But what really got my attention was the announcement by Mr. Kracht that he had virtually *no* gray hairs in his head to speak of. When I inquired for his "secret" to this success, I was amazed to learn that it was *cranberries* of all things! "Ever since I was 9 years old, I've been eating cranberry sauce or drinking cranberry juice every day," he continued. "It started with the big dinners my grandmother used to fix us practically every Sunday. She was German and most of the things she cooked were quite dry and covered with a lot of gravy. In order to add some moisture to what I ate, I started eating cranberry sauce with them and got hooked on it. Now, some 60 years later, I'm still addicted to the stuff. My body just can't seem to get enough of it.

"And *that's* why my hair has remained its naturally dark-brown color all this time. When I tell this to others, they're always a little skeptical at first. So I ask them, 'Didn't the American Indians in New England eat cranberries all the time?' They'll nod and then I say, 'Did you ever see any pictures of them with gray hair?' By then I've made my point."

🌺 JESUS TOLD HER WHAT TO DO

Sometime back in 1988, a fan who avidly collects most of the health books I've written, sent me several clippings from a couple of newspapers published in Snohomish County, Washington. He knew of my lengthy and ongoing studies in longevity and felt that the subject of the articles would be worth my while interviewing.

At that time Bessie Hubbard was 102 years of age. The local community paper, *The Stanwood Camano News* had described her as being "one feisty old lady." The larger metropolitan *Everett*

Herald (published in the city of Everett) termed her "a human meteor, a real ball of fire." Not bad for someone described by a close friend as being "jest too damned ornery to die." My curiosity was piqued enough by what I read to book a flight to the Northwest and see for myself what made this "live wire" senior such a bundle of energy and nerves.

When I entered her small apartment in Stanwood, I noticed religious paraphernalia all around. Her residence surely wasn't lacking for crucifixes, Bibles, or pictures of Jesus. They were *everywhere!* Noticing my astonishment, she snapped, "Keeps the demons out!"

As she bade me to make myself comfortable, this woman of high-powered spiritual zeal suspiciously eyed me for a moment before gruffly asking, "Been saved yet?"

I looked at her and asked, "Beg your pardon?"

She retorted, "Are you deaf or something? I asked if you've been saved or not?"

Thinking I might get no where without a suitable answer, I quickly discerned that my options were limited to only three: a negative (which might have quickly concluded the visit), an affirmative (which would have been a lie), or something in between. I chose the latter and told her that I was "working towards that goal with the help of Jesus Christ."

Just the mere mention of Jesus' name quickly satisfied her that I was "a good guy" and we settled down to the purpose of my visit.

I came to find that she had subscribed to *Prevention* health magazine way back in the early 60s when it was still quite alternative-minded in its contents. This had caused her to make radical changes in her diet, excluding shrimp, lobster, crab, oysters, dairy products, and foods high in salt, sugar, or fat. Instead she opted for salt-water fish, beef or chicken, and root or leafy vegetables.

But the thing that caught my attention the most was her nearly perfect *dark* hair. I kept looking for a gray strand but couldn't find any. Noticing my gaze affixed more to her scalp than her face, she consciously raised a hand and patted the top of her head. I then asked her what she had done to keep her hair from turning gray.

Her answer came dressed in typical evangelical language. "Jesus is all I care about. Living with Jesus in my life has never made me lonely. His advice is the only worthwhile advice listening to." She then proceeded to tell me that many years ago in middle-age, while anxiously engaged in one of her fervid prayers on other matters, "I asked Jesus, for no particular reason, what I could do about my gray hair. He spoke to me through the Holy Spirit and told me what to do."

Here is the hair-darkening formula she gave me, devoid of its more exotic religious trappings. From a practical point of view it works just as well as it did from Bessie's spiritual perspective.

The necessary ingredients are as follows: $1/4$ cup sage, $1/2$ cup black walnut hulls, 3 black or green teabags, $1/4$ cup rosemary, $1/4$ cup stinging nettle, $2^1/4$ teaspoons olive oil, 8 cups Mount Olympus (the brand she used) or equivalent spring water, and a pair of rubber gloves.

Bessie boiled the spring water first and set it aside. She then added all of the aforementioned herbs, covered the pot with a lid, and let them steep for 5 hours. Then she strained everything through a fine-mesh wire strainer, added the olive oil, put the liquid into a fruit jar sealed with a Mason screw-on lid, and stored it in her refrigerator for 21 days.

Every morning when she would take her usual bath, she would shampoo and rinse her hair as usual. Then she would slip on the rubber gloves, give the fruit jar several good shakes to mix the contents up, and then pour out $2/3$ cup of this liquid. She slowly poured little amounts of it on to her scalp and began gently massaging it into her hair for about 2 minutes. She squeezed out the excess liquid and dried her hair with an *old* towel (on account of this rinse badly staining whatever it came into contact with).

She would sit on a stool and do this over her wash basin instead of in the tub, where it would be likely to stain her skin. She followed this rinse procedure with a good conditioner of some kind. Her formula, she said, gave her about 12 to 14 treatments.

"I've been doing this ever since," she loudly exclaimed with both arms raised and outstretched and her gaze heavenward. "And just look at how beautiful the color's remained. *Nothing* in my life is gray anymore since I found the Lord Jesus; no, not *even* my hair!"

🌿 Additional Remedies

An old Utah sheepman I know, whose jokes are pretty b-a-a-d, told me years ago that he could produce wool in his flock which was alternately black, then white, then black again, simply by varying the amounts of copper in their diets. I told him he was "pulling my leg" (not the "wool over my eyes").

But he absolutely insisted that this could be done. He explained that in sheep whose black wool is an inherited characteristic, the elimination of copper from their diets turned their hair white long before any evidence of anemia set in. I felt a little bit sheepish for ever doubting his word.

So I began pursuing the matter further based on the information he had given me. The Anthropological Research Center in Salt Lake City, which I've been the Director of now for over almost two decades, solicited middle-aged volunteers of both sexes who had gray hair or still managed to retain their own natural dark colors. Samples were snipped and sent off to a laboratory for analysis. It was revealed in our study that those with darker hair had significantly higher levels of zinc; also their zinc-to-copper ratios were about 2 to 1.

One lady, who had just turned 59, had considerable gray hair with a zinc-to-copper ratio of 7:5. But a 56-year-old insurance executive with black hair showed a ratio of 15:8.

Based on our own research, I have been recommending anywhere from 30–60 mg. zinc and no more than 5 mg. copper every *other* day for getting rid of the gray. **Caution:** Both trace elements are cumulative within the body, and should *not* be used all the time, but intermittently (3 weeks on and 2 weeks off).

🌿 A Confession: It's Genetic, Folks

I feel an obligation to my readers, however, to point out something else regarding gray hair. This author has had quite a bit of it for years, and all of the zinc and copper in his diet hasn't really made a noticeable difference. So what gives in a situation like this? It's not that the earlier research was flawed by any means, but simply that gray hair (like baldness) is *hereditary* in some instances. And no matter how good your diet or supplementation program may be, or how stress-free your lifestyle is, you're still going to get gray hair or go bald!

In other words, it's a *genetic* thing. But for many other older men and women who've followed my nutritional counsel and taken adequate amounts of zinc and copper into their diets, they have naturally pigmented hair without the gray! Foods rich in copper are brewer's yeast, wheat germ oil, sesame and sunflower seeds, nuts, cheese, oysters and other shellfish, fresh- and saltwater fish, eggs, poultry, and meat. As for zinc, milk, eggs, wheat germ and wheat bran, salad-type (leafy) vegetables, meat, fish, wholegrain cereals and breads, nut, seeds, and legumes. The best choice is a combination of foods and *occasional* supplementation to get enough of the zinc and copper your body needs to retain the natural color of your hair and completely do away with the gray!

Growing Old Gracefully

"HOW TO WORK IN HARMONY WITH THE AGING PROCESSES"

Society's Big Challenge: The Aging Baby Boomers

The generation born between 1946 and 1964 have been collectively referred to by the liberal news media as Baby Boomers. They married later, divorced more often, and had fewer kids—or else none at all. It appears that old age may look far different as the first of this generation start to retire in 15 or 20 years from now. Then an unprecedented "gerontological explosion" will begin to rock the nation from one end to the other.

By 2020 when *that* Grandparent Boom is in full swing, an estimated 2 in every six Americans will be 65 or older, compared with just one in eight today. That's an increase of over 20 million seniors, according to a study released on May 20, 1996 by the U.S. Census Bureau. The report was one of the most comprehensive ever done on aging in America. It provided a detailed portrait of the elderly while issuing a clarion call for government and society at large.

The report clearly expects the Baby Boomers to eventually remake the final stage of life and force new answers to questions routinely asked about quality of life and medical needs. Previously, this generation, with the sheer magnitude of its numbers, had redefined childhood and then adolescence.

Increasing longevity means fewer women widowed by their 70s, but many others living alone because they never married or long ago divorced. These new seniors will begin retirement with more college degrees and generally better health than their parents before them had. But their increased longevity ultimately could mean more chronic disability in the long run.

That spike of seniors will certainly be placing a tremendous strain on the myriad specialized services and programs now required of an elderly population. "A window of opportunity," as the report noted, currently exists for these Baby Boomers to start planning for the inevitable. This entry section has been especially designed to help them better prepare for maturity, so they can "grow old gracefully."

GRACEFUL AGING—TIP #1: DON'T FEEL SORRY FOR YOURSELF

In order to age like good wine, there can't be any sour moods to your mental and emotional states. Granted that there may be loneliness or sorrow due to the passing of a loved one. But those feelings are quite different from self-pity, which is a beggarly way of behaving. Feeling sorry for yourself all the time is the emotional equivalent of holding out a hat or tin cup on the street corner and asking passers-by to donate their pocket change to you. Such *expected* handouts of sympathy are more demeaning than beneficial, for they rob the individual of self dignity.

A great inspiration for Baby Boomers to look to in this regard is none other than screen legend Jimmy Stewart. In 1994, Gloria, his beloved wife of 45 years, died. Since then "he has never gotten over her death," a close family friend confided to reporter Jim Nelson. Even though she's been dead for that long, "he still keeps some of her clothes hanging in one side of the closet so he'll feel closer to her. And he's insisted on leaving the bedroom just the way it was when she was living."

It is true that her loss has weighed down heavily upon this man. Formerly a very active and outward-going personality, Mr. Stewart has since become a hermit within his Colonial-style estate located in swanky Beverly Hills, California. It is not uncommon for him to sit for many hours a day in the bedrooom he shared with her, with the lights off and the drapes drawn. Every once in awhile the frail actor "has his housekeeper pop one of his old movies into the VCR and he watches it." According to Nelson's anonymous source, "that makes [Jimmy] happy and he gets a dreamy faraway look in his eyes."

But in spite of the lengthy and obvious bereavement this great film legend has been going through, *he never once has shown any self-pity!* Nelson's mysterious informant declared to the *National Enquirer* reporter that "the spirited Midwesterner showed he still has the 'true grit' that would have made his buddy John Wayne" mighty proud of him.

"Don't ever cry for me," he told his close friend. "I've had a most wonderful life. I've met fantastic people and acted in terrific films. God has been good to me in many different ways." He confessed that his present depression was only due to the absence of his dear wife—"I miss her very much and look forward to being with her again very soon. I've already overstayed my welcome in this world. But now it's time for me to be on my way. I don't want anyone to feel sorry for me. *I don't feel sorry for myself,* so why should you?" he asked his friend. "I'm not a bit afraid of death. In fact, I kind of welcome it, because I know that that will enable Gloria and I to be reunited in a much better world."

This was the philosophy of one of the world's greatest cinematic heroes when he turned 88 on May 20, 1996. Except for his wife's sudden and unexpected demise which left him shaken to the core, Jimmy Stewart has lived a full and good life. And, in the process, he has shown the rest of us how to age with grace. In a period of despair, he still retained enough of that original pluck which made him so great in the first place, and *refused* to feel sorry for himself, even while his heart was heavy with sorrow and his spirit understandably depressed.

GRACEFUL AGING—TIP #2: KEEP YOUR TIME BUSILY OCCUPIED

On Thursday evening, May 23, 1996 I was officially inducted as the new president of the downtown Salt Lake City Lions Club in a formal ceremony attended by many fellow Lions and their wives, and selected friends. The inaugural dinner event was held in Brigham Young's Lion House, immediately adjacent to the LDS Church Administration Building.

The following morning I was busy performing a civic duty for the sight-impaired: I transported seven elderly people from their various homes or apartments within the city to the First Congregational Church located on 2150 Foothill Blvd. in the Holladay area. There they received a nice lunch and spent a couple of hours listening to poetry being read aloud to them by volunteers. At the appointed hour of 2:30, I was there again to pick up and deliver them safely back to their individual residences again.

In the process of doing so, I had a chance to become acquainted with each and every one of them. I put to the seven of them the question, "What single thing do you believe has helped you to age gracefully?" The answers they provided make up the rest of this section. I marveled at the uniqueness and originality of some of them, but gave verbal acknowledgment of my gratitude for everything that was volunteered with their identified permission to use here.

John Mativietch, age 81, went through some of the fiercest combat of World War II, but managed to escape without a single scratch. Then he came back home to Utah and started working in a mine. Not too long after that, he met with an unfortunate explosion that left him blind in both eyes and minus his left arm below the elbow.

But in spite of these terrible setbacks which fate had dealt him, he has managed to grow old with charm and style. He has a keen wit and charming manners that brought forth ready compliments from his other six sight-impaired friends. I could detect *no* anger, bitterness, or depression in his life despite what he has suffered. So, I asked him as we drove to the church, "John, what makes you so happy and humorous, considering your physical limitations?"

He came back with this rejoiner. "Well, sonny boy, it's like this. When I laid in that hospital bed for several months, knowing I had lost the use of my eyes and one arm, I started to thinking. I sez to myself, 'Now, John, you could go through life feeling sorry for yourself. You could even get mad at God and the world'for what has happened to you, and hate them forever. You could even end your life tomorrow and be finished with the suffering.'

"But, after running all of these things through my mind, and looking at the matter from every negative angle possible, I decided it was better to explore other options. I figured I come here to learn, to live life to its fullest. And so what, if I didn't have everything functional as it should be. Hell, at least I was still alive. So, *I seized the moment* and determined then and there *to keep myself busily occupied* with whatever I could.

"I asked friends and relatives to come by and read to me every day out of the paper. Or just to sit and talk with me about whatever was happening. I started listening to the radio a lot. I became well-informed on all matters. I took up listening to all kinds of music and began teaching myself to sing some of the lyrics I heard. I soon became rather proficient in singing a number of tunes from memory to the delight of others.

"I started using my imagination more and coming up with a number of different short stories, which I dictated to friends and had them write down for me. I ain't never had any of them published yet, nor do I expect to. But, at the very least, they have provided hours of entertainment and enjoyment for all those I know and care about.

"At one time, when I was a little younger—in my sixties, I think—I served as a volunteer for counseling troubled teens, who had been contemplating suicide themselves. I gave them some good pep talks and told them just how much life had to offer them. I told them that life was too damned exciting at this point to quit now—especially while they were ahead of things by staying alive! I've often used my own experiences to help turn them around. I guess when they saw and heard an old blind and crippled man like me, laughing and chatty in a friendly way with them, it made them realize just how much *more* they had to live for than what I had.

"By keeping myself busy all the time *in the service of others*, I have been able to grow old *with style!*" Then turning to the rest of his fellow passengers in our vehicle, he asked, "Don't you just hate old people who gripe and bitch and whine all the time? Gad! I feel like a kid when I'm busy." Everyone else nodded and gave their whole-hearted verbal agreements to the things he had said.

🌱 Graceful Aging—Tip #3: "Don't Sweat the Small Stuff"

Fredda Cohen from the Avenues section of Salt Lake City may be sight-impaired, but is pretty darned smart for a 69-year old. She was one of those I transported back and forth to the first Congregational Church on May 24, 1996. Her philosophy on life in general may help to improve the outlook of others much younger than herself who have a lot less problems to contend with.

"I never sweat the small stuff," she spat out with obvious intensity. "To me, the small stuff is anything that isn't big enough to worry about. Now, earthquakes, floods, tornadoes, lightning storms, and bubonic plagues—them's B-I-G things to do some mighty serious worrying about. But the rest is just small potatoes!"

And, what in her estimation, were "the small potatoes"? "Well, just look at me dearie," she chirped from the back seat.

"I'm blind because of muscular degeneration. Got arthritis so bad in my hips it pains me to move. And I'm barely getting by on Social Security. But, that's nothing compared to how bad things *could* really be. I could be in a nursing home strapped to a danged wheelchair, drooling all over myself and not even knowing my name. I could be in a hospital Intensive Care unit with tubes stuck up various orifices of my body, barely staying alive.

"But I'm here, able to get around, though I don't see much of anything anymore. And yes, it hurts to get around, but at least *I can.* So, why should I fret when things *could* be a lot worse. *Don't sweat the small stuff*—just worry about things you have no control over, like 'acts of God' and epidemics. Everything else is bound to work itself out somehow sooner or later."

🌿 GRACEFUL AGING—TIP #4: YOU'RE NEVER TOO OLD TO LIVE

The Jablonskys are an interesting pair to study. They combine wit with wisdom to get them through their physical handicaps. Eugene, who was 83 in May of 1996, observed with sharp humor about his wife, Gloria, then 67 years old: "We met, fell in love, and got married in February [of the same year]. Now if that isn't a *blind* date, I'd like to know just what is!" Clearly, their vision impairments haven't handicapped their thoughts or emotions.

"The priest who married us in the Cathedral of the Madeleine [in Salt Lake City]," Eugene continued, "told my wife and I that we were one of the oldest couples he had ever married. He said he usually got them much younger, and that at our age, he was usually giving *last rites* to folks on their death beds. He was naturally concerned about our extreme ages, and wondered in private with us before the ceremony started, if the thing [our contemplated marriage] would last very long.

"But I reassured him, 'Look father—you just do the marrying and let us worry about the rest of the details. As far as Gloria and I are concerned, it's *never* too late to love, nor too old either. Age makes no difference when two people care about each other like we do. Our bodies may be falling apart in places, but our hearts and minds are as young as two teenagers in love for the first time. Our love is what keeps us going, when the rest of us wants to lag behind and rest a spell."

🦌 Graceful Aging—Tip #5: Be Happy all the Time

There we were, eight of us, packed like sardines into a big 1995 Lincoln Towne Car, merrily rolling down the highway to a free church luncheon and volunteer reading session that particular Friday in May of 1996. Scrunched somewhere in between us in the front seat was 85-year-old Lena Chipman. Next to her was Virginia Clegg, also 85. That left me hugging the left door of the driver's side and Leona Simmons, age 75, hugging the opposite door side.

"Hope we're not over the limit," Lena loudly remarked.

Someone else with better sight leaned forward and looked at my speedometer. "Oh, we're okay," came the reply. "The doc here is only going 45."

"No, that's not what I meant," Lena corrected the other. "I meant I hope we're not over the *age* limit of how many old folks you can sandwich into a car at once." She then went on to mention that just in the front seat alone (not counting the driver who was near 50 at the time) there were people totaling 245 years. Then in the back, she calculated there was represented about 300 years: Fredda Cohen at 69; Gloria Jablonsky at 67; Eugene Jablonsky at 83; and John Mativietch at 81.

Then, as an afterthought, she added in the same whimsical tone: "That's an awful lot of *accumulated* wisdom to be packing around in one car!" Everyone enjoyed the mirth of the moment.

As if on a roll with the dice in a Las Vegas craps game, Lena continued and kept the rest of us in stitches. "An Idaho farmer was spreading some fertilizer over his strawberry patches. A schoolboy walking down the road noticed what the man was doing and stopped to shout out, 'They go better with cream and sugar, mister.' The Devil and Saint Peter get into an argument about where the boundaries of Hell are supposed to be located.

There appears to be no end in sight to their contention. Finally, Peter hits on a brilliant idea. Say, Luce, why don't each of us get ourselves a set of attorneys, have them study the matter over, and then argue each of our positions before the Great High Judge and let Him decide the matter for us. Well, the old Devil he smiles a bit and remarks, 'It's a good idea, Pete, but I'm afraid it won't work.' 'And why not?' inquires the other. 'Because,' Satan says with a wide grin, 'I got all the lawyers down here with me.'"

Mrs. Chipman informed me, after we had arrived at our destination and was getting out of my vehicle with a little offered assistance, that she had made it a point "early in my life to always be happy and cheerful, even when things look bleak and glum. I *never* let myself get depressed or down. I'll think happy thoughts that cheer my soul and fill my spirit with light. That way, I don't feel so old and can cope better with my different problems."

GRACEFUL AGING—TIP #6: VARIETY IS THE SPICE OF LIFE

Paul Petzoldt never felt "younger in my life than I do right now," he told me in late May, 1996. I was curious what would motivate someone almost 89 years of age to make such a statement. How could anyone *that old* lay claim to renewed and youthful vigor? I mean, the guy's hair and bushy eye brows were extremely gray; his skin sagged in many places; the liver spots on the backs of both hands were the size of silver dollars; and, he walked with the assistance of a cane. Was I missing something here, by chance?

I met him and his wife of eight years at a private lecture he gave at the University of Utah in Salt Lake City. Although both have an official residence on Lake Sebago, Maine, they maintain "a humble [Indian] wicikiup" in Victor, Idaho, nearby the Grand Teton Mountains he loves so much.

"I broke the mold for being a social stereotype," he admitted with rough candor. "I would have been dead a long time ago if I had followed the system that other men have." He paused for a moment to give a faraway look as he pondered what conformity might have done to him. "The *sameness* of everything would have killed my spirit in a hurry," he continued somewhat soberly. "And eventually broke my health and body for sure."

"The only think that has kept me intact has been the *rich variety* of my intensely interesting life. I've gained international fame by scaling many of the world's highest peaks. I've become something of a legend in mountaineering, I must admit. I served honorably in World War II in the 10th Mountain Division ski troops, helping to fight the Germans in the Scandinavian countries by doing 'renegade runs' against them. Gad! Did that ever give us one great adrenaline rush, blowing up their petrol and ammunition dumps, and then skiing away in the dead of night.

"I've bummed rides on freight trains from Yuma [AZ] to Duluth [MN] after the war. I later worked for the mysterious Howard Hughes as a blackjack dealer at one of his casinos in Vegas. Later, I took to playing poker professionally, and won myself a few dollars to boot. I also was in the used-car racket for awhile, but eventually got out of it, because I didn't like having to lie all the time, especially to sweet, little old ladies. I even managed to trek to distant Kashmir, India, and spent a couple of months in a commune with an 'Ascended Master.'

"That probably did me the most good of all. Sort of cleared my conscience, I suppose, from my gambling and car selling days." Here he paused to evoke a throaty chuckle. "My guru told me to 'get some variety' to my life. He said that the problem with all Western men and women, was that they lived dull lives of mental and emotional deadness. He said that you're never any good if you go through life as a mere 'rock of a personality.' That's when I decided to become more adventuresome, and I'm glad I did. And I don't regret one minute of it either!'"

Petzoldt believed that "adventure is an integral part of growing up. It's like exercising the muscles of your body—the more *different* kinds you do, the stronger they'll become." Conversely, "the more varied experiences you have, the stronger your life is going to be." That, to him, is aging gracefully.

HEINERMAN'S ENCYCLOPEDIA OF ANTI-AGING REMEDIES **175**

But before we parted, he let me in on a little health secret of his. "Last Fall [October, 1995]," he began, "doctors at the University of Utah Medical Center bluntly told me in no uncertain terms that the peripheral vision in my left eye and tunnel vision in my right one would be gone in just a couple of months without risky surgery. They gave me these two options: guaranteed blindness without the operation, and possible blindness because of the surgical risks involved.

"Well, I must admit, it left me pretty rattled at first. I felt as if I'd been dumped off a cliff into a big snowbank and buried for good. But as I got to assessing the thing and looking at it from a gambler's point-of-view, I figured, 'What the heck—I'll lose for sure if I don't and, at least, increase my chances of winning if I get it.' So, I went ahead with the operation. And wouldn't you know, I won 'the luck of the draw' in this high-stakes poker game. My card hand was mighty good and surgery came out successful."

Paul told me in parting that his schedule remained just as hectic as ever. "I give lectures everywhere on using good judgment in mountaineering, on what constitutes appropriate behavior for expeditions, how to protect our environment, and just having plain fun in the outdoors." We shook hands and as I walked away I tried imagining what this man might look like sitting in a rocking chair back home watching television. Somehow, I just could *not* envision this ever happening, much as I tried to.

GRACEFUL AGING—TIP #7: STAY YOUNG WITH STINGING NETTLE SAYS FAMOUS TV DOCTOR

Anyone who is in the habit of watching "Good Morning, America" on ABC television will be immediately familiar with the name of Nancy L. Snyderman, M.D. Besides being the in-house medical correspondent for this program, she is also an associate clinical professor of otolaryngology (ear, nose, and throat branch of medicine) at the California Pacific Medical Center in San Francisco.

Not too long ago, she wrote an insightful column on the common weed stinging nettle for *Health Confidential* newsletter (Vol. 10, no. 4, p. 6, April 1995). She recommended it as an ideal treatment for allergies and related problems that might contribute to poor health and faster aging.

She declared "nettle [to be quite] safe even when taken over an extended period [of time]." While not giving any specific amounts to take, she encouraged her readers to "be sure to follow the dosage directions listed on the bottle." She mentioned that the herb is available both in capsule as well as tincture forms.

Her own introduction to this wonderful weed came while doing an interview on ABC's "Good Morning, America" show sometime in 1995 with alternative medical advocate Andrew Weil, M.D. He told her of his own clinical experiences with this herb and how much it has helped older people to feel *young* again. It is not know, though, by what mechanism the herb works to accomplish this.

GRACEFUL AGING—TIP #8: PEPPERMINT WILL KEEP YOU KICKING YOUR HEELS FOR YEARS TO COME

T. Upton Ramsey, a retired chef, thinks he may have found *the* miracle herb for reversing aging. This enthusiastic 75-year-old can't sing enough praises about one of nature's greatest herbs. "Peppermint is to the body of an old person what running may be to that of a college kid," he chimed. He feels that peppermint can *invigorate and revitalize* systems that are . . . well, to put it plainly, "over the hill and ready for recycling."

He adores peppermint tea. *"The* most exhilarating drink one can find," he purrs. To make the *perfect* pot of brew, simply bring one pint of water to a boil. Then add one-half cup of *fresh* peppermint leaves, cover, and set aside to steep for 15 minutes. Or, two tablespoons of the *dried* leaves may be substituted instead. Strain, sweeten with a little *pure* vanilla flavoring, and E-N-J-O-Y! And why the vanilla, instead of honey or sugar? "It gives it a truly distinctive flavor."

His mint vinegar makes an ideal dressing for tossed salads and will certainly add more years to your life.

Peppermint Vinegar

6 cups apple cider vinegar

3 lemons

¹/₂ cup honey

2 cups fresh peppermint, loosely packed

1 cup fresh peppermint sprigs

Heat the apple cider vinegar in a saucepan to 150° F. and set aside for awhile. Cut fine strips of lemon peel with a sharp paring knife. Then combine the peel, mint leaves, and honey together. Next, add the hot vinegar and stir with a wooden spoon, gently crushing the leaves. Cover and store for two weeks. Strain through a fine mesh strainer. Discard the peppermint. Pour the liquid into decorative bottles. Place a mint sprig into each bottle. Cork them and store in a cool, dark place for up to six months. Yields 6 cups, and makes a lovely gift for holidays or special occasions.

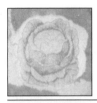

Handicap Helpers

"HOW A FAMOUS POLITICIAN AND VIOLINIST OVERCAME THEIR PHYSICAL CHALLENGES"

When Given a Lemon, Make Lemonade

As we get older life sometimes hands a few of us a lemon in the form of some type of physical handicap. This can be in the form of sight or hearing impairment or a limit on our efforts of mobility. Whatever it may be, such restrictions can work to our disadvantage if we let them. On the other hand, we can simply accept them for what they are and make the best out of a bad situation. In other words, turn something sour into pretty good lemonade.

THE POLITICIAN AND THE FIDDLER

Two men who come to mind who've managed to do this very thing are Senator Bob Dole (R-Kansas) and world-renowned violinist Itzhak Perlman. Both men, for very different reasons, sought to overcome potentially damaging handicaps early in their adult lives. And, in doing so, became a hope and inspiration for millions of others similarly handicapped in some way.

At age 19, Robert Dole quit school and joined the Army's Enlisted Reserve Corps. On April 14, 1945, on an erupting battlefield near Bologna, Italy, he felt a sharp sting in his upper right back, probably an exploding shell. His collarbone was crushed, his lung was punctured and his vertebrae were damaged. He was paralyzed from the neck down. He thought his arms were missing.

Itzhak Perlman was born in the same year that Dole was seriously injured—August 31, 1945 in Tel Aviv (then Palestine). He was somewhat of a child prodigy and began playing the violin at age 3, much to the delight and astonishment of his parents, other family members, and friends. Everyone had great hopes for this exceptionally talented child.

But then tragedy struck only a year later. At age 4 young Itzhak came down with polio. Everyone became very sad, imagining the worst for this *wunderkind*. It seemed like the musical gift in the child wanted so very much to come out, but his crippled little body just wouldn't let this talent be fully expressed the way he wanted it.

PATIENCE THROUGH STRUGGLE

Private Dole went home in a plaster cast from his ears to his hips. Over the next several years he somehow managed to survive fevers as high as 108° F. His right kidney was removed. He couldn't feed himself for months. His weight dropped from 194 to 122. He wondered if he would end up selling pencils on street corners.

The townspeople of Russell, Kansas, pitched in, though, with a "Bob Dole Get Well fund" to cover his medical expenses. Contributions ranged from 30¢ to $100 to a live mallard duck. When he returned to his hometown in 1976 as a vice presidential candidate, the good senator openly wept as he thanked folks for standing by him all these many years.

The disability Dole handles so effortlessly is a constant, occasionally painful presence. He keeps his limp right arm at an angle, his curled hand grasping a pen. His left hand, he told me back in the Fall of 1992, feels like it's in a glove. He was in Utah at that time to briefly campaign for then senator-elect Bob Bennett. I got a chance to interview him for a few minutes at the home of millionaire Joe Cannon in Provo, in my capacity as editor of *Utah Prime Times*, a monthly, free distributed newspaper for senior citizens. Dole noted that his left arm isn't strong enough to cut meat. It becomes even more of a challenge for him when he has to periodically struggle with milk cartons or childproof caps. And dressing himself every morning "takes a very long time," because he has to do it with a button hook.

Dole said that out of his physical disabilities, there grew within himself a "quiet patience" towards people and events. "In politics, you quickly learn," he said with a sober scowl, "that things don't always move in the direction you like them to. You have to be flexible and bend a little. Patience taught me how to compromise and get along with everybody . . . even with the Democrats," he chuckled after a momentary pause. "I believe if I hadn't been injured in the war, I might have ended up a lot more cantankerous and ornery than what I've sometimes been accused of being."

Clearly, Bob Dole's physical handicap tempered his impetuous and unruly nature in youth just enough to eventually make him into the strong political leader that he has become in the late 1990's. This same quality of mental toughness enabled him to withstand a rigorous and very combative political race against U.S. President Bill Clinton in the 1996 presidential campaign; he came out of it gracefully and with his dignity intact.

🌿 PLAYING SECOND FIDDLE TO NO ONE

Itzhak Perlman eventually recovered, in part, from his bout with polio. But it left him somewhat disabled, and it is today quite obvious whenever he gets up to walk. "I determined very early in my childhood," he said, "that I *would* continue to play the violin *in spite of* being crippled." Then, after a moment's reflection, added: "I believe much of my success for this could be attributed to my determination to *separate* my abilities from my disabilities." Looked at another way, he mentally dropped the negative prefix *dis-* from dis-ability and instead focused solely on the remaining word itself.

Remembering that he had been featured on the cover of an old *Newsweek* magazine sometime back in 1980 with the banner "Top Fiddle," I inquired somewhat mischievously: "Do famous violinists like yourself ever get riled up when someone calls you a fancy 'fiddler?'" He quickly shook his head and replied, "Oh no, not at all. In fact, violinists use the term all the time themselves. We might pay another colleague a compliment for the way he played a particular piece by saying to him, 'You're a pretty good fiddler.' Or, we might tell someone else, whose instrument we admire very much, 'That's a pretty fine fiddle you got there.'"

Perlman made his initial television appearance on the old *Ed Sullivan Show* way back in 1958. In 1964 he won the Leventritt Competition for young classical musicians. He gave his first solo performances with the Israel Philharmonic orchestra at its concerts in then Communist Poland and Hungary. In 1990 he was invited to Russia to give a solo violin performance at a concert held especially to celebrate the 150th anniversary of Tchaikovsky's birth. And in 1993 he did the haunting violin solos for the disturbing film *Schindler's List*, which depicted the stark brutality and terrific horrors of the Jewish Holocaust.

🦁 THE BEST AWARD IS SOMETIMES A HANDICAP

Since 1977 Perlman has won a total of 14 different Grammy Awards for his musical accomplishments. In 1986, then-President Ronald Reagan awarded him the Medal of Liberty. A TV documentary later on his tour of the Soviet Union with the Israel Philharmonic won him a prestigious Emmy Award.

And yet for all of the honors which the world has heaped upon this man, he still manages somehow to retain his humility, humor, and common sense. "I would have to say probably that my handicap in early childhood has awarded me more things than all of the plaques, trophies, medals, and certificates that I've received since then." He then went on to enumerate those attributes, he believes, life has given him on account of his apparent disability: courage, determination, faith, hope, perseverance, and persistence. Without these qualities Itzhak might have turned out to be a far different person than the one he is now. But it took a handicap to instill these wonderful virtues within him.

I noticed he had a pair of antique violins at least two centuries old. "What are these?" I asked out of curiosity. "This is my Stradivarius and this here is my Guarneri," he said with obvious pleasure. "I play one in the summer and the other one in the winter time. I like to change off every so often. It does me good and keeps my music sharp."

Healthy Bones

"HOW TO BONE UP FOR A MORE ERECT FIGURE"

🦁 EXERCISE AND DIET TIPS

Although bones may seem to be rigid and fixed, they are actually more like muscles, capable of growing or shrinking with use.

Each time a bone is moved, it bends ever so slightly, just enough in fact to trigger electrical and biochemical changes that stimulate bone formation. The more force, the greater the bending, and the greater the stimulus for new bone formation. A normal amount of movement keeps the density of bone constant, while additional bending—say, from a brisk walking routine—can cause bone mass to increase. Less frequent bending, on the other hand, signals to the body that it doesn't need so much bone mass. When a wrong message like this is sent out, the bones become thinner and more brittle.

Although the ability to increase bone mass is going to vary from person to person with age and gender, everyone can benefit from exercise and a balanced, calcium-rich diet. Here are some easy suggestions to follow for a healthier and more upright skeletal structure.

- Walk, jog, run, or dance. Any activity done in an upright position helps because muscles and bones work together against gravity to hold our frames erect. Swimming and biking, while great for the heart, don't do very much for the bones.

- Lift weights. The benefits of weight-bearing exercise can be enhanced by strengthening specific muscle/bone groups.

- Exercise moderately 3 to 5 times every week, for at least half an hour each time. Although there are no clear guidelines for maintaining bone mass, this amount of aerobic exercise is a good guide to follow.

- The public has been repeatedly encouraged by the American Dairy Council to drink more milk every day for stronger bones and teeth. But the adult human body lacks the necessary enzyme to properly digest milk. As a result, most of those who drink a lot of milk tend to have mucus accumulation problems in their upper respiratory systems. Much safer alternatives would be tofu milk, calcium-enriched soy milk, and goat milk. And unless a person has hypoglycemia, calcium-fortified orange juice is good. A juice mixture made from one cup each of kale and collards and $1^1/_2$ cups of pineapple juice, mixed together for two minutes in a Vita-Mix Whole Food Machine, is an outstanding drink for strengthening the bones in older people. (See Product Appendix for more information on the Vita-Mix.)

- Eat calcium-rich veggies. The calcium in bok choy, broccoli, Brussels sprouts, and kale is best absorbed.
- Consume plenty of leavened wheat bread. It does not contain much calcium, but what's there is readily absorbed.

(See also FRAILNESS PREVENTION.)

Healthy Head of Hair

"CAVALRY HERO OF FOUR WARS RODE WITH BUFFALO BILL AND LEARNED THE SECRETS TO A WELL-GROOMED MANE"

MOST OF HIS LIFE WAS A GALLOP

Sometime in 1980 I was in Riverside, California, visiting with a friend of mine. She took me over to meet a very remarkable gentleman by the name of Lieutenant Colonel Nelson Robert Moon, who was then about 86 years of age (he died a couple of years later at age 88). We spent an enjoyable four hours with him.

If every life is a book, his could fill the shelf. This man had fought in four major conflicts, ridden in Buffalo Bill's "Wild West Show," served as a judge in the 1932 Olympic Games and appeared in several cavalry movies.

Moon began honing his extraordinary horsemanship skills in 1901, when at the age of 8—he was born in Syracuse, New York, on March 2, 1893—he would vault onto his steed from the steps of a post office in upstate New York where he would pick up the mail for his foster dad.

When he first tried to enlist in the U.S. Cavalry, he was told he was too thin. But that didn't stop him. "I immediately found a job at a Woolworth department store luncheon counter," he recalled, "and there I consumed more than my share of food. I stuffed myself sick with bananas and milk to up my weight to Cavalry caliber."

After he joined in 1913, Moon was sent to help hunt Pancho Villa along the embattled Texas border, where about 200 American civilians were killed in attacks by Villa's army. Moon's Troop K was part of the Sixth Cavalry that later chased Villa until about 1917. In 1916 Moon was picked by General John "Blackjack" Pershing to go into Mexico alone and hunt Villa.

"We came within that far of capturing him," Moon told us, holding his thumb and forefinger about an inch apart. "It was early one morning when the military outpost we were encamped at near the American-Mexican border was suddenly attacked by Villa and his ragtag army of peasant rebels. All of us stumbled about dazed, clad only in nightshirts, sure prey for Villa's raiders. But I rallied the troops into quick action and we managed to get to our horses in the nick of time with weapons in hand, but not much more than that. Some of us didn't have much more than our longjohns on. But we mounted and fought hard against them, killing a number of them. They were badly organized and we gained the advantage over them in this respect. I came within 15 feet of Villa himself. He looked over in my direction and I gave chase. But he was suddenly surrounded by a band of loyal guard and managed to escape from our grasp. The fighting was fierce and there were casualties on both sides. That was my only brief encounter with this Mexican Robin Hood. But after that, he never again dared to conduct a raid on the American side of the border."

🌿 RODE WITH BUFFALO BILL

When Moon was about 20 years of age, he got a job as a stunt rider in William "Buffalo Bill" Cody's Wild West Show. He had to travel between Texas and Oklahoma quite frequently. He stayed in the Cavalry and drew his $25 a month pay.

I asked the Lieutenant Colonel what kind of horseriding tricks he did for Buffalo Bill's crowds. Moon stated that his forte was to ride standing up on the backs of two running fillies while they jumped over obstacles. "But the most daring and breath-taking part of my whole venture in those days," he said in a gravelly voice, "was to jump through huge fire hoops in a standing position on the backs of those horses. That was something to see! I almost got my face and hair singed a couple of times doing this daredevil stunt. Yes, I worked with the famous Buffalo Bill himself, who was then well into his 70s and with Annie Oakley, the best woman sharpshooter with a rifle I've ever seen."

🦎 HAIR TONIC SECRETS FROM THE AMERICAN INDIANS

Moon was the one who brought up the subject of natural hair care before I ever did. My lady friend had informed him in advance over the phone that my profession was studying and writing about folk medicine as a medical anthropologist. The old gent ran the fingers of his right hand through his thick shock of mostly black hair to get my attention.

"If you look carefully enough," he continued, "you'll notice that I have most of my *original* hair. And there isn't very much gray in it either. Not bad for an octogenarian?"

I had to admit to myself after focusing more thoroughly on his scalp that he was entirely correct in his statement. Now I'm not a professional hairdresser or barber by any means, and know very little about what would constitute a well-groomed set of hair on a man or woman. But two things were quite apparent with Mr. Moon. First of all, he wasn't bald; and secondly, he had very little gray in his mane.

But this cavalry hero from another period of time wasn't finished yet with showing me some beautiful hair in old age. He called his wife of some 35 years, Eloise Moon, into the living room from the kitchen where she had been working the daily crossword puzzle from the local newspaper. "Honey, tell Dr. Heinerman and his lady friend when was the last time you went to a hair dresser?"

Mrs. Moon momentarily demurred answering her husband's question, probably more out of shyness or embarrassment than anything else. "It's probably been *30 years,* dear," she replied.

My lady friend and I both blinked in astonishment as we looked at her head and then at each other. Before I could get my question out, my friend had asked one of her own already. "You mean to say, Mrs. Moon that you've *never* had a perm in all that time?"

"Well, yes. At least not the standard perm ladies get from their hairdressers periodically. I have a friend cut my hair sometimes when it starts getting a little longer than I want it to be. I don't like it down past my neck and have always worn it short this way."

Before I got a chance to slip another question into the conversation, our retired army host picked up the tempo again. "The reason our hair looks so great is because of the things we use and what we do. I learned from Buffalo Bill himself, who had the neatest hair of any fellow I've ever met in my life, what he did to keep it looking so nice and healthy. And he got these secrets from a number of different American Indians whom he had met earlier in his life while riding the Great Plains. Buffalo Bill and Annie Oakley always took great pride in how they looked and spent a lot of time fixing up their hair. It's the same things Eloise and I have been doing ourselves for many, many years."

BUFFALO BILL'S HEALTHY HAIR PROCEDURES

"Buffalo Bill told me when I was just a young man working for him, that the Indians always ate a lot of fish to keep their hair in great shape. And sometimes they'd even take to rubbing some of the fish oil into their scalps, believing it added luster and shine to their hair. Of course, they also used things like bear grease pretty regularly to rub into their scalps, but I think the fish probably did more for them than the other did."

The fish which the Indians always ate was haddock, cod, salmon, and mackerel. Most of these tribes lived near large bodies of water and subsisted primarily on fish, along with some other staples, of course. The great plainsman told Moon that these Native Americans always seemed to have the most vibrant and shiny hair, more so, in fact, than did those tribes which ate very little fish.

Moon claimed he tried rubbing fish oil into his hair for awhile, besides eating it often, but finally gave it up because "it stank too much and drew every cat to me from miles around." He said that a person could get just as good results by eating several helpings of any oily fish at least three times a week. "Eloise and I have eaten tuna, sardines, halibut, and swordfish. But the other fish, especially the *canned* mackerel or salmon seem to have done the most for adding luster to our hair and keeping the ends from splitting or going gray so fast."

I checked into some of my nutritional reference books when I returned home and discovered that all of these fish are extremely high in biotin. This important nutrient has been recommended for many years by veterinarians to farmers for keeping their animals' coats beautiful and their hooves stronger. This "hair-and-nails" supplement should be taken regularly; it is non-toxic to the body. Three milligrams a day is sufficient. It works better, though, when taken with 25 mg. of zinc.

A number of Indian braves would boil the bones of any slaughtered animal in an iron kettle suspended over a campfire. They wouldn't necessarily throw any vegetables in with them, but just boil the bones in plenty of water for several hours until about half the amount remained. This they drank copiously when cooled. Moon and his wife have done this for years. He said the mixture is rich in calcium, magnesium, potassium, silicon, and other minerals essential for healthy hair.

🦌 DEALING WITH DANDRUFF

Imagine yourself sitting perfectly still in a chair for awhile. You don't shift or move around; you don't twitch a muscle or even scratch an itch somewhere. You become almost like a mannequin, except you can still breathe and blink. As fantastic as it may seem, you will have shed more than a million flakes of skin in that hour of near perfect stillness. And when you scratch or undress or dry yourself off with a towel following a shower, that flurry becomes a veritable downpour. The flakes come off in tiny clusters too small to see as a general rule. On the scalp, however, where there is more shedding than anywhere else on the body, flakes can get trapped by hair and oil. They eventually fall in large, conspicuous clumps which everyone immediately notices. That's called dandruff.

Admittedly, it's not a major problem. Most of us would like to think that there are far more important things in life to worry about. But let's face the facts for a moment and do a reality check on ourselves—every single one of us is as concerned with the cosmetic as we are with the cosmic. That's the reason why we have mirrors all over our house, in our cars, and even on our persons.

Scientists have better things to do with their time than to investigate shedded flakes. No one has yet won a Nobel Prize for Medicine in dandruff that I know of. But awhile back I met a gentleman who is the world's expert on the subject. Back in 1988 Dr. Albert Kligman was then 71 years of age and still working at the University of Pennsylvania as a dermatologist.

I soon discovered that this guy was a regular Renaissance man in terms of minor medical maladies. He had authored numerous published papers on such unimpressive health topics as athlete's foot, body odor, diaper dermatitis, itchy earwax, and sticky nose snot. (Excuse the grossness, but the themes were very real that he had devoted a lifetime to studying.)

But most of all Dr. Kligman was considered to be without an equal in his field and then reigned as the undisputed "King of Dandruff." His classic 1976 paper entitled, "The Nature of Dandruff" drew rave reviews from other medical professionals not only because of its thorough research but also because of its singularity.

I visited with the good doctor in his home one evening while back in his home state giving some lectures on herbal folk medicine. He rattled off dandruff facts and figures the way a football or basketball fan might do with sports statistics. That night I learned:

- About 20% of the population has dandruff.
- This number is about the same for men and women, blacks and whites.

- Dandruff declines in the summer.
- By age 75 it's rare, and by 85 almost nonexistent.
- Some people are more prone to dandruff than others.
- Those with dandruff simply create and shed skin cells at a faster than average clip.

I asked Dr. Kligman the Number One question that dandruff sufferers all over America have probably been wondering about themselves for a very long time: "Just what *is* the most effective dandruff remover?" His straightforward answer took me completely by surprise, seeing as how it came from a dermatologist. "*NONE* of the medicated shampoos or other treatments on the market will do much good for someone who has dandruff. In my opinion," he continued, "they're pretty worthless."

So then, I inquired of the good doctor, "What do *you* recommend in their place?"

"I've studied the problem of dandruff for many years," he said with careful deliberation. "And found that there are really only just a few things which are effective in the removal and future prevention of dandruff." He then itemized what they were:

A. *Keep the scalp clean at all times.* "If you shed skin cells faster than the normal rate, and have greasy hair to go with it, then you'll need to wash and rinse your hair morning and evening," he advised.

B. *Think zinc for fair hair.* "Dandruff sufferers who've been placed on 50 to 75 mg. of zinc gluconate daily have had considerably less flaking," he noted.

C. *Clean with coal tar and rinse with aspirin.* Dr. Kligman stated that scalp preparations containing coal-tar were still the safest and most effective means of controlling and preventing future dandruff problems. Coal-tar products may be purchased at any drugstore. After washing the scalp with this kind of soap or shampoo, he advised giving it an initial rinse with cool water. Then the scalp was to be rinsed a *second* time with an aspirin solution. He explained how this could be made. Crush 6 to 8 Bayer aspirin tablets into a fine powder. Stir into one pint of *distilled* or *spring* water and mix or shake thoroughly before using.

Rinse with this solution and then dry the hair after that. The good doctor remarked that salicylic acid—the stuff of which aspirin is made—is "probably one of the best dandruff controllers around." "Maybe if the aspirin manufacturers knew about this," he observed with a certain wit to him, "they might be able to develop a product that could remove both your headache and dandruff with just one use."

To his recommendations I would like to add a few of my own. Oat bran or pine soap can be used in place of coal tar preparations if desired, though more will have to be used of the former than the latter. Also, rinsing the hair with boiled cabbage juice (strained, of course) seems to work just as well as the aspirin solution does. Also taking 200 micrograms of selenium three times weekly for the first month, two times weekly for the second month, and once a week for the third month, really helps to control dandruff buildup and recurrence.

🦎 CROW AND BLACKFOOT HAIR CARE SECRETS

One thing above all stood out in my mind in my visit with Lieutenant Colonel Nelson R. Moon some years ago at his home in Riverside, California, in company with a lady friend of mine. He told us that "if you want information about *good* hair care, *don't* look to any hairdresser for that; instead, look to Native American wisdom of the past to find useful things for the present." From a cultural perspective, I could see just how true that was. White men who visited Native American tribes throughout the U.S. and Canada in the last couple of centuries had always remarked on just how fond these people, especially the men, were of their hair. In fact, they usually considered their hair to be the most important part of their bodies, and would naturally lavish a lot of attention and care on it.

In 1970 I met an Indian couple named Adolph and Carol Hungry Wolf. At that time they resided near Glacier National Park in the top part of Montana. I never really learned their particular tribal affiliation, but have reason to believe it was either

Blackfoot or Crow. They provided me with some interesting information on personal hair care that might prove helpful to some readers of this book. It is passed along in that spirit.

"Combs were not known in the Old Days, but the hair was often brushed," Adolph told me. "A primitive brush consisted of a handful of flexible twigs, bound together with buckskin. The most common brush among our people then was made by inserting a stick of wood into a porcupine's tail. Our ancestors also cut off a handful of horse hair from the tail end, wound it tight and then doubled it over to make a soft hair brush. We still like to brush our hair with this."

His wife Carol, who had remained silent in the background for awhile, then spoke up with these comments. "Both my mother and grandmother would make hair tonics and washes from the different grasses that grew in abundance on the plains or in the meadows around us. Sweet grass and common bear grass were the two most often used. They would be boiled in water, cooled down, and then rubbed into the hair every day. Such grasses leave the hair smelling sweet, almost like clover. In fact, red or white clover tops may also be used for this. They would sometimes mix in cedar leaves for better aroma and medicinal effect. I've discovered in using it in my family, that it has kept our hair from falling out."

Along more disgusting lines, they talked about the use of bear grease, buffalo dung, and deer urine for the hair, that many braves in "the Old Times" were in the habit of using in their hair. "But now we are educated and know better," Adolph said. "We know that such things are not socially acceptable by the Whites. So we rely on plants instead."

One thing which Mr. Hungry Wolf emphasized, that is worth repeating here, is "to always brush or comb your hair every day," because that seems to "keep the hair from getting old and gray and falling out." I think what he meant to say was that as long as your scalp get plenty of exercise *every day* and blood circulation to it, your chances of going gray or bald will be drastically reduced.

Hearing Loss Solutions

"GOLFING LEGEND ARNOLD PALMER SOLVES HIS PROBLEM GRACIOUSLY"

🦎 THE '96 SENIOR SKINS GAME

There they were, four of golf's greatest players, all assembled on the 6,938-yard Mauna Lani Resort South Course in Kawaihae, Hawaii, to play the annual Senior Skins game. On the weekend of Saturday and Sunday, January 27 and 28, 1996, the greens on this oceanside course were softer than usual on account of the rains earlier that week. And there was barely a hint of wind anywhere, which made putting the ball a lot easier.

Arnold Palmer, Jack Nicklaus, Jim Colbert, and Ray Floyd battled it out among themselves to see who could get the most skins and win the most cash. On the first day of the tournament, Palmer was hampered by a balky putter and missed his first two putts. But Floyd edged ahead of him and won $60,000 for his first three holes or skins. He observed on camera that "I felt Arnold would make his putt on the first hole, since he had a much easier putt. I didn't really expect to make my shot from 20 feet away."

The next day Palmer blew an opportunity at the 10th hole. His first two shots were "right on schedule," he said, but reluctantly admitted that "I lost a lot of momentum after that. The 10th hole burst my bubble. That was a real downer. I did everything according to plan, but I just couldn't close for some reason. I really worked hard to get that ball on the green and was successful at doing that. But it turned out to be only a disappointing three-putt instead."

Floyd handily won his third consecutive Senior Skins that day by taking home eight skins worth $240,000 and, in the process, running his total winnings to $960,000. Colbert finished with seven skins worth $180,000. Palmer managed to come in third by picking up $80,000, and Jack Nicklaus rounded out the event with only $40,000, failing to win any skins in regulation.

🌱 PALMER'S SOLUTION TO HEARING LOSS

On September 10, 1995, Arnold Palmer turned 66. Exactly two months and nine days later, he teamed up with golfing pro Peter Jacobsen to play in the $1.1 million Shark Shootout. This tournament was played at the Lake Sherwood Golf Course in West Lake Village, near Thousand Oaks, California. It was hosted as usual by Greg Norman, who, ironically enough, has yet to win one of his own tournaments. While Palmer and his partner didn't win any of the big money at stake, for Arnold it was special for another reason.

"I shot a 66 during my 66th year," he told a television reporter during a break in the Senior Skins game in Hawaii. He described it as "a special moment in my long golfing career."

Palmer also shared something else with the reporter. "A few years ago I began to lose my hearing. At first it wasn't such a big thing, but as time went on hearing became increasingly difficult for me. I resisted wearing a hearing aid, thinking that I didn't want to be bothered with such a thing. I mean, with a device like that sticking out of your ear . . . it really tells everyone just how old you're getting. I was rather sensitive about wearing something that would let others know immediately this guy can't hear very well."

But something along the way eventually changed Palmer's mind about the matter. "Whenever my grandchildren would come to visit my wife and I, they would naturally want their grandpa to play with them," he said. "But in doing so, I discovered I couldn't hear very much of what they were chattering about. I felt like I was missing out on a lot of the good things that grandkids love to tell their grandparents. That's what it took to convince me that a hearing aid was a necessity, but not something to be ashamed of. Now I can hear everything they say crystal clear. It's almost like being young all over again."

Palmer currently appears in television ads for the hearing aid company, whose device he himself wears. His solution to the former problem was relatively simple, but not an easy thing to do until he finally managed to get a different perception of the thing in his mind. Once he was able to see it in a more positive light, then the obvious benefits became all the more apparent.

🌿 FENUGREEK TEA RESTORES HEARING

The following true story doesn't make claims to curing deafness. Nor does it suggest that this particular remedy is some kind of a "magic tonic" that will immediately restore someone's hearing loss. Rather, it is one woman's attempt to deal with a vexing health problem for which there were no real medical solutions.

Roberta Janeway is a 57-year-old computer operator for a large Midwestern corporation. She is happily married and the mother of six children. Until just a few years ago, she never imagined herself as having any kind of serious health problem. That is, until she started losing her hearing. "It came on quite suddenly, one day," she said in a letter to me awhile back. "At first I though that both of my ears were plugged up and attributed it to an allergy of some kind. I went to an allergist, who could find nothing wrong with me."

After this, she decided to visit an eye-ear-nose-and-throat specialist, who thoroughly examined her. He asked some pertinent questions during the diagnosis and learned from her that she had been down with a serious fever about four months prior to the onset of her hearing loss. He attributed this period of illness to that problem. A prescription was written out, but she never got it filled.

"I wasn't about to put strange medicine into my body," she said in her letter, "without first knowing what the risks and consequences were. Neither my doctor nor the pharmacist was willing to tell me the long-term side effects of this medication. So I simply tore up the prescription and started looking elsewhere for a much simpler solution."

It was about this time that she got an advertisement in the mail about one of my previous books. "I read," she continued in her letter, "about that woman from Eugene, Oregon, who drank fenugreek seed tea for the 'funny' noises in her ears. I figured, 'Hey, what the heck! If it worked for this lady, then it oughta do something for me.' So, I bought some of the seeds at a local health food store and made a tea just like the woman in your story did." (Leota Lane, the other person mentioned in that account, didn't cook the seeds, but instead let them soak overnight in cold water and strained off some of the liquid the next morning.)

Ms. Janeway followed this routine for about a week, but with no results. "I wasn't getting anywhere with the remedy," she stated in her correspondence. "At first I wondered if it was really valid. But then I decided to *boil* the seeds and see what that did." She boiled a pint of water and added one level teaspoon of fenugreek seeds. She covered the small saucepan with a lid and turned the heat down low and allowed the contents to simmer for about five minutes. Then she set the pot aside and let the tea steep further for 20 minutes. While it was still *lukewarm*, she strained a cup and drank it on an empty stomach.

"I did this faithfully day in and day out for almost two months," she concluded. "And I can testify to you Dr. Heinerman, that I was frankly amazed at just how well the thing worked. I mean, within the first week I could start hearing better again. I finally discontinued taking any more of it once most of my hearing returned. I probably now only have a 10 to 15% loss, but that's a lot better than the 55 to 65% I had before. The tea works great for something like this! Thanks a lot for recommending it. Keep up the good work." She signed herself, "Gratefully Yours, R. Janeway."

Hints for Hypertension

"DRUGLESS THERAPY FOR HIGH BLOOD PRESSURE"

 ### LAUGHTER RELIEVES THE HEADACHES

A prominent doctor once told me that humor always helped those of his patients suffering from hypertension. He said those who followed what he styled as his "yuk-yuk prescription" and learned to laugh more, always had blood pressure readings that were consistently *below* 140/90.

He thought that laughter helped to diminish stress. When this happened, he reasoned, then the force that the blood was exerting upon the walls of the arteries subsided, too. Overall, he felt that humor was a very relaxing form of therapy for hypertensive patients to regularly engage themselves in.

 ### GARLIC TO THE RESCUE

In keeping with my medical friend's recommendation, I wish to share with you something about garlic. Garlic, as most herbalists know, is outstanding for high blood pressure. But no one seems to understand exactly how it works within the body to accomplish this.

That is, until now. I've finally figured out how the stuff works so well for hypertension. Now high blood pressure, as everyone knows, is induced by stress. And stress, of course, is caused by people. Therefore, it stands to reason, that if you eat lots of garlic, it will make the people go away, which in turn relieves the stress. And when this sequence of events happens, then blood pressure returns to normal.

Levity aside, garlic is great stuff for hypertension. In all seriousness, it's probably one of the best herbs for treating this problem. Raw or prepared garlic can be used for this purpose. Some die-hard garlic lovers claim that by chewing one clove a day, they never have to worry about elevated blood pressure levels again. Of course, these are usually the same *single* guys who brag about how great their bachelor lives are.

I've used prepared forms of garlic for many years now. I've recommended Kyolic Garlic to thousands of people, because I know from research that it is the very best kind of manufactured garlic anywhere in the world. No other commercial preparation of garlic can hold a candle to it. The average intake per day will vary, of course, depending on individual metabolic rates and the age, weight, and sex gender of the user. But for the most part 3 capsules daily is adequate for maintaining blood pressure that's within normal bounds.

❦ ANTIOXIDANTS, AN OVERLOOKED FEATURE

Somewhere around 25 million Americans are currently taking high blood pressure drugs of some kind. These medications consist primarily of diuretics, beta-blockers, calcium antagonists, and ACE inhibitors. But they tend to produce some serious side-effects if taken for too long a time: elevated blood sugar, depression, high cholesterol, aggravated asthma, potassium deficiency, and cardiac arrhythmia.

An interesting report authored by M. Cohen, J. Josimovich, and P. J. Lefebvre appeared in the scientific journal *Clinical Science* (81:739–42) in 1991. It was entitled, "Anti-Oxidants Show an Anti-Hypertensive Effect in Diabetic and Hypertensive Subjects." It demonstrated that such substances substantially lower blood pressure levels when used with consistency.

Spices are one important class of antioxidants. Besides garlic and onion, there are rosemary, sage, thyme, marjoram, and oregano. When regularly used in cooking, they hold blood pressure within safe limits. Besides this, there is the obvious benefit of making things taste better. If I had to choose another spice to go with garlic and onion, I would have to pick turmeric. This is the basic ingredient in curry powder. It has a decided therapeutic advantage in the liver. The Sabinsa Corporation of Piscataway, New Jersey, market a product called Curcumin C-3 Complex, which is the only standardized turmeric extract of high quality currently available. Taking some of this everyday will help to bring stability to elevated blood pressure. (Call 1-800-248-7464 or write to Sabinsa Corp., 121 Ethel Road West, Unit #6, Piscataway, NJ 08854 for more information.)

Within each of our brains, resides a tiny organ known as the pineal gland. It is about the shape and size of a single kernel of corn. Some consider it to be one of the body's "master glands" responsible for performing many multiple functions. One of these is the production of the hormone melatonin, about which much has been written of late.

As we become older, a number of vital hormones begin declining: testosterone, estrogen, growth hormone, DHEA (dehydroepiandrosterone), and, of course, melatonin. At one time the slow loss of these hormones was seen as a *consequence* of old age, but now their losses could actually *contribute* to the aging process. Which means that replacing them might just extend our youthfulness a little longer.

A lady judge (aged 54) I know of, discovered her blood pressure was 167 over 115, making her case extremely bad. She went to a local health food store (New Frontiers Natural Foods Market & Deli) and informed a clerk of her problem. The clerk suggested she try some melatonin, which proved to be helpful for her honor. She took two 3-milligram tablets every day for two months. By then, another check of her blood pressure showed it had dropped to borderline levels: 141 over 105.

An Ounce of Prevention Is Worth a Pound of Cure

Other measures can be taken to avoid or hold in check hypertension. Weight levels should be kept within a healthy, normal range. Cigarettes and their second-hand smoke should be avoided. Alcohol intake needs to be restricted to no more than two small drinks a day.

Plan on doing at least 25 minutes of vigorous exercise every day. This could vary from day to day with jogging, biking, dancing, or swimming to help break up the monotonous routine of regular exercise.

And plan to limit your sodium intake. Many foods have hidden salt in them. Your daily intake should never exceed 1,500 milligrams of sodium. *Salt is bad for hypertension.*

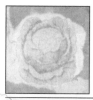

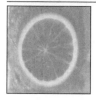

I

Immune System Buildups

"FOODS AND HERBS FOR RESISTING DISEASE AND FIGHTING INFECTION"

🌿 AN INTRODUCTION TO YOUR IMMUNE SYSTEM

Back when I was a kid the toy section in most department stores sold kaleidoscopes. These were cylindrical shaped tubes through which you could look at one end. At the opposite end were a few pieces of colored glass, that when turned could form an infinite number of geometric patterns.

In some ways, your own immune system is much like this apparatus that I enjoyed in my childhood. With only a limited number of weapons, it puts up an almost endless variety of defenses against diseases.

Personal immunity is threatened whenever there are antigens in the system. Antigens are viruses, bacteria, cancer cells, fungi, protozoa, particles and anything else that might challenge the integrity of personal immunity. In fact, antigens are the very reason that an immune defense exists at all.

The immune system employs different methods of fighting these antigens. One way is for some immune cells to "eat" antigens; these specialized white blood cells are called phagocytes. Another way is to cut a hole in the surface of the bacteria's cell. This then destroys the bacteria by permitting water, sodium, and other substances to leak in and out of the cell, upsetting its homeostasis or state of steadiness. Poison can be used to kill antigens. Or a cover can be slapped over that part of the antigen which does the damage (the toxic site).

There are different types of white blood cells, each with its own name, size, shape, and function. Besides a variety of phagocytes and leukocytes, there are also a number of different lymphocytes originating in the lymph glands of the body: T-cells, natural killer cells, helper cells, suppresser cells, and B-cells. But behind these immune troops is further backup in the form of the complement system, immunoglobulins, interferon, and interleukin. Everything that I've just mentioned forms your defense network. And as antigens float around in your system trying to form some pattern of disease, your immune system—like the kaleidoscope mentioned earlier—is forming endless arrangements to stop this process from ever happening.

🐉 STRENGTHENING YOUR OWN IMMUNITY

Before we can discuss what things will boost your immune defenses, you first of all need to know some of those things which tend to weaken it. Right off the bat, I'll tell you up front and personal that *any* food loaded with sugar or grease is going to pack a wallop and knock your immune system silly. Right after that comes *frequent and intense* stress: too much pressure for very long and your immunity is going to get knocked to the canvas in a big hurry. After this comes *prolonged* exposure to a lot of electrical devices such as microwaves, TV sets and radios, fluorescent lighting, electrical shavers, blow dryers for the hair, cellular phones, personal computers, and so forth. The electro-magnetic radiation they emit will deliver a one-two punch that will send your immune system into shock and unconsciousness. Breathing polluted air is another thing that's bound to "turn out the lights" on your immunity, if you're not careful.

So, obviously common sense dictates that you should avoid sweet and fried/deep-fried foods as much as possible; learn to relax more; divest yourself of some electrical gadgets or don't stay around them too long; and get out in nature enough to breathe good, clean air.

Another factor which I haven't discussed yet are bad thoughts and feelings. Negative emotions of any kind are like a ball-and-chain around the body's immunity and can really drag it down in more ways than one. Try to be of a more cheerful countenance, have hope, and think pleasant thoughts in order to enable your system to resist disease for a longer period of time.

Now for some of the things that will boost your own immunity. Seeds of all types are definite power foods that can really give things a lift. There are a class of compounds in all seeds, including beans and grains, called protease inhibitors (PIs). They limit the amount of nourishment that antigens can get. In other words, PIs help to literally "starve" these bad antigens out of existence. Munching on sunflower or pumpkin seeds, eating whole grain breads and cooked cereals, and dining on a variety of legume dishes will boost your body's immunity more than you may realize.

There are, of course, certain nutrients that are quite useful in strengthening natural immunity. They are vitamins A and C and sulphur. Dark leafy green vegetables are rich in both vitamins as well as red- or orange-colored fruits and vegetables. Many of these same items can be juiced: parsley, celery, spinach, apples, carrots, and oranges. I always recommend using a Vita-Mix Total Nutrition Center, which is the only machine on the market that gives you all of the food fiber with nothing wasted (see Product Appendix). Or, for greater convenience, you might want to mix some of these concentrated juice *powders* with water and take them that way. Pines International (see Product Appendix) makes a nice beet root juice blend and a 27-plant mixture called Mighty Greens.

The sulphur connection is found in a number of different Brassica foods: cabbage, kale, kohlrabi, Brussels sprouts, broccoli, and cauliflower. Other sulphur-rich foods include garlic, onion, figs, and dehydrated fruits. Most of these can be consumed either raw or else *lightly* cooked.

Grapes and wines, preferably the dark red types, are equally good for boosting body immunity. They have been tested in different laboratories around the world and proven to be very potent against common, ordinary virus antigens like influenza and herpes simplex.

We should not forget, of course, those medicinal herbs that have been traditionally recognized for a long time now as possessing definite antibiotic properties to them. Some of the more potent ones are listed below and the forms in which they best work: red clover (2 cups daily), echinacea (tincture, 15 drops twice daily); goldenseal (2 capsules twice daily); garlic (4 capsules Kyolic daily); feverfew (4 capsules daily); and ginseng (2 cups tea daily).

❧ Real People with Real Solutions

In my business I'm always running across new and different remedies for many of the common problems that cut our years short and cause us to age in hurry. Strange as it may seem, those diseases that seem to wear our immune systems out much sooner, aren't the major ones you read or hear about all the time. Granted that cancer, tuberculosis, or hepatitis may garner more press because of their extreme seriousness and expensiveness to treat. But, if the truth were fully known, common, everyday garden varieties of illnesses that plague us more frequently, actually are the real culprits for shaving time off our lives.

I'm speaking, of course, about the common cold, influenza, coughs, and similar respiratory disorders in general. These affect most of us more often than anything else seems to do. And they exert a heavy price in terms of work hours and productivity lost and potential income that could have been earned were we not home sick in bed with any of them.

In the pages that follow I present useful information that is going to be of great help to you the reader in coping with these things. Now, I'll admit at first glance, it may not seem like a common cold, influenza, cough, or lung problem belongs in an anti-aging book. But my own research shows otherwise. By following the simple solutions given in what follows, you will not only be feeling better, but actually *turning back* the hands of time on your own biological clock. For a *strong* immune system is one way to *cheat* the Grim Reaper and steal for ourselves many more years to live the "good life" and enjoy doing those things we've never quite got around to yet.

🌿 KITCHEN WISDOM

There is some medical validity to chicken soup as a tried and true age-old remedy for the common cold. The science behind it comes from work done by medical researchers at the Mount Sinai Medical Center in New York City. Hot chicken soup was credited with increasing mucus flow from the sinuses, back of the throat, and upper respiratory tract in patients suffering from nasty colds. Cups or bowls of hot chicken soup helped to relieve much of their congestion and miseries, but plain hot water did not.

However, the specific ingredients responsible for doing this job still remain a mystery. Scientists continue to speculate whether it is the smell or taste of the soup itself or perhaps the interaction of common spices with the fat from chicken parts when subjected to high temperatures that may be responsible. Whatever it is, though, is relatively unimportant just so long as the remedy continues to work in breaking up sinus and chest congestion.

🌿 AN EASY RECIPE FOR COLDS

Nearly everybody's grandma had her own special recipe for making a good, flavorful chicken soup, and I'm naturally partial to the one left by my own Grandmother Barbara Liebhardt

Heinerman. My father's mother emigrated to America with her husband and small child from Temesvara, Hungary (now part of Romania) in the early part of this century.

She lived long enough to help raise my brother Joseph and me to young childhood. I can still remember her wonderful chicken soup and present it here for readers to use whenever they get a bad cold. It is, first of all, quite tasty and, more important, effective food medication for what ails you. I encourage you to consume several bowls of the same over a 24 hour period. You will feel a lot better after having done so.

Grandma Heinerman's Ultimate Chicken Soup

1 chicken (3$^1/_2$ to 4 lbs. in weight), cut into 10 pieces (include the neck and gizzard)

1 medium onion, coarsely chopped

1 medium carrot, coarsely chopped

1 medium celery stalk (with leafy top), coarsely chopped

1 bouquet garni (see additional recipe below)

1 teaspoon salt

$^1/_2$ teaspoon Hungarian paprika

13 cups mineral water

$^1/_2$ cup rice

Bring all ingredients to simmer, skimming off the foam and fat as it rises to the surface. Continue to simmer until the chicken is tender, about 40 minutes. Remove and set chicken pieces aside. Add rice to broth and cook until tender. Return broken pieces of chicken meat to soup mix.

Set aside to cool at room temperature before refrigerating later on. When it comes time to reheat, *do not* remove any of the congealed fat on top; this is *essential* to making the soup work well as an effective cold remedy. Heat only what you need, but be sure to include the bouquet garni with whatever amount is desired, then return the muslin bag of spices to the remaining soup and refrigerate until next time. By including the bouquet garni *each time* a portion of soup is reheated, you are obtaining the full benefit of the spices in it. These help to contribute to the overall medicinal value of the soup itself.

You should consume several medium-sized bowls of this *nearly hot* soup within a 12- or 15-hour period. You may alternate between this hot soup and some hot apple cider flavored with a cinnamon stick. Both will help tremendously to break up congestion and make your body feel a whole lot better. In between I recommend short cat naps as rest is critical in order for the system to rebuild itself from its weakened condition.

Bouquet Garni

5 sprigs parsley, finely chopped

1 small sprig thyme, cut

1 small bay leaf, crumbled

1 garlic clove, peeled and finely cut

1 piece of dried orange peel, coarsely cut

1 sprig marjoram, cut

1 sprig basil, cut

$^1/_2$ small cinnamon stick, broken or crushed

Bouquet garni is the internationally used fancy French name for the common English "bundle (or faggot) of sweet herbs." Cut a square piece of clean muslin large enough to accommodate all of the foregoing ingredients. Then place everything into the center of it, drawing up the edges or sides afterwards. Tie a string or stout pieces of thread around the top, leaving a few inches for a tail to make lifting in and out of a pot easier to do. Include this spice bundle with the soup and with every *reheated* portion, too.

DON'T FORGET THE SUPPLEMENTS EITHER

A necessary part of common cold treatment are the nutrients vitamins A and C and zinc gluconate. They constitute the "healing triumvirate" for getting well, along with chicken soup, of course. Vitamin A is usually sold in 25,000 I.U. capsules; during a cold or flu you should be taking 4 such small capsules or up to 100,000 I.U. And with the recently discovered side effects to beta-carotene, you're better off choosing your source of vitamin A from fish oil.

As to the remaining pair of nutrients, this piece of information may prove interesting. The late Linus Pauling, Ph.D., the only person to ever win *two* Nobel Prizes, wrote a national health best-seller some years ago, *Vitamin C and the Common Cold* (Freeman and Company, 1970). In it he suggested that daily supplementation of vitamin C was absolutely essential to full recovery. He explained that vitamin C works so well because it is employed by the body to build many immune system factors, including the virus killer known as interferon. He also stated that vitamin C is necessary to repair cells damaged by stress, be it physically or emotionally induced.

Once a person has a cold, vitamin C can alleviate many of the symptoms because it is a natural antihistamine. It neutralizes histamine and its symptoms of puffiness, without excessively drying the delicate throat and nose tissues that are trying to wash away the virus. This nutrient, likewise, assists in reducing inflammation and, because it boosts immune functions, can lessen the body's need to create a high fever.

Dr. Pauling advised people to take anywhere from 3,500 to 5,000 milligrams of vitamin C daily during a bout with a cold or flu. After full recovery is imminent, then the daily dosage drops to around 500 mg.

The remaining nutrient to be given equal weight of importance here is zinc gluconate. Back in the mid-1980s William Halcomb, M.D. of Austin, Texas, conducted an interesting experiment with this vital trace element. He and his associates prepared two sets of lozenges—one containing 23 milligrams of zinc in the most useable form possible, namely as zinc gluconate. The other, a placebo, was nothing more than a blank look-alike tablet. During the study, volunteers with colds were asked to suck on two tablets of the test medicine every 2 hours during the daytime. The final, compiled results demonstrated that the volunteers who had been using zinc recovered from their colds an average of a week *sooner* than those who had been sucking on the fake lozenges.

There were only minimal side effects to this form of nutrition therapy reported. A few volunteers complained about the taste of the lozenges. And roughly one-fourth of the group tested with the real thing experienced mild digestive disturbances. Happily, though, this problem was solved when they later took the same lozenges with a meal.

In looking for a reliable zinc gluconate, make sure it *doesn't* have a Twin Labs or KAL label to it. Brands that I feel more comfortable with would include Richlife and Schiff. But even trickier than this is shopping for a really good, or should I say, a truly *honest* Vitamin C. Most of the brands out there in the health food market place aren't worth crossing the street for. I suggest a Super C with cayenne, ginger, and wheat and barley grasses from Native American Nutrition instead. (See Product Appendix under Pines International for more information.)

ELDERBERRY SYRUP FIGHTS RESPIRATORY INFECTION

In the early 1980s, an Algerian-born Israeli, Madeleine Mumcuoglu, traveled to Basel, Switzerland, to get her doctorate degree in virology. When it came time for her to choose a subject for her dissertation, she was advised to investigate the antibacterial/antiviral potential of one of Europe's oldest herbal folk remedies, namely elderberries.

The person responsible for pointing her in this direction was none other than Jean Linderman, the same scientist who discovered the body's own antiviral chemical, interferon.

Mumcuoglu discovered two particular chemicals in elderberry that prevent cold germs and flu viruses from ever invading throat cells. Either one must first seize control of throat cells in order to cause infection throughout the body. The chemicals in elderberry appeared as though they might protect people from either respiratory illness, both of which send tens of millions of Americans to bed with fever, joint aches, loose bowels, upset stomach, and other general miseries every single winter.

After earning her doctorate, Mumcuoglu returned to Israel. There she started developing an elderberry syrup containing the anti-cold/anti-flu compounds. Since elderberry's Latin binomial is *Sambucus nigra,* she decided to call her medicine Sambucol. She tested it several times whenever there were cold or influenza outbreaks at a kibbutz in southern Israel in 1992, where she was then residing.

ELDERBERRY BEATS OUT TYLENOL FOR RAPID RELIEF

At the first sign of a fever, half the residents were given four tablespoons of Sambucol a day. The other half received standard cold/flu therapies: Tylenol and cold formulas. After just three days, 90% of the Sambucol users felt well again. This was rapid recovery in a remarkably short period of time. But in the standard-care group, it took almost a week (about six days) for the rest to respond in a positive manner.

As a result of these and other clinical studies done in her country, Mumcuoglu's wonderful formula quickly became Israel's favorite cough-cold-flu medicine. It is currently being marketed throughout the rest of Europe, parts of Asia, and also in the United States.

MAKING YOUR OWN SAMBUCOL

In the event that you are unable to locate some Sambucol for your own health needs during cold-and-flu seasons, you can make some of it yourself by following the simple directions given hereafter. And instead of putting extra, unused syrup into bottles and canning them, you may wish to preserve it a couple of other ways. Freezing elderberry syrup helps to counteract the problem of fading color. Instead of using glass jars, pour any unused syrup into small plastic containers, leaving room at the top for expansion, then freeze. Ice-cube trays are another handy form for preserving it. Each cube will be sufficient to make one 1-cup drink. Freezing also solves the problem of sterilization for bottling, which is often a lengthy and cumbersome process.

Elderberry Syrup for Coughs-Colds-Flus

1. Using two quarts of elderberries, force them through a sieve to remove the seeds. If desired, add lemon juice to thin a bit.

2. Then strain the juice through another sieve lined with cheesecloth. Gather the corners of the cloth together and twist tightly to force out all the juice.

3. Add 2 cups of blackstrap molasses or thick, dark honey to every $1^1/_4$ cups of elderberry juice. Place over a low heat and stir to dissolve the molasses or honey, then slowly bring to a rolling boil. Less molasses or honey may be used, if desired, but it will reduce the time such syrup can be safely stored on a shelf in a glass jar. However, freezing won't be affected by less molasses or honey.

4. Lower the heat. With a spoon, skim off any scum. Dip a pastry brush in water and clean the sides of the pan to prevent burning. Cool before using.

5. Take 2 tablespoonfuls of this syrup every couple of hours throughout the day as necessary until the symptoms of the cold or flu are gone.

THE QUINTESSENTIAL COSMO GIRL DRANK HOT LIQUIDS

Way back in 1962 Helen Gurley Brown produced a book, *Sex and the Single Girl*, which made the *New York Times'* bestseller list. Three years later she took over as the editor of *Cosmopolitan* magazine. She changed Cosmo from a worn out magazine showing lackluster subscriptions (under 791,000 at the time) into America's leading women's magazine when circulation peaked at 3 million in the mid-1980s.

In her new administrative role, Brown issued a very clear command: sex was to be the prevailing theme around which nearly every major article or column would be wrapped. From this mandate there soon came sex and makeup, sex and career changes, sex and film stars, and even sex and winter apparel.

She literally plunged herself into her work. One staff member remembered that Brown literally "plunged herself into her editorial work," working many 12- to 14-hour days in the beginning, and "giving it her all." Such unswerving devotion to the task at hand, obviously led to occasional neglect of her health. Lack of sufficient sleep, inadequate meal consumption, and lowered immune resistance made her system more susceptible to flu.

But, according to her colleague, "Ms. Brown had her own methods for treating herself when sick" with the flu. These were undoubtedly developed through trial-and-error over a number of years. When Brown faithfully applied them, she "never failed to get better in a hurry." The main secret to such self treatments was "*hot* (or very warm) liquids." My informant noted that "Ms. Brown would restrict herself only to drinking *hot* teas, *hot* coffee, *hot* instant soup, *hot* chocolate, or other liquids, just so long as they were always *hot*."

The Cosmo staffer who shared these things with me sometime ago, gave as her opinion the idea that it wasn't so much *what* her editor-in-chief took when ill as it was the *temperature* of the *liquids* she drank copiously. This makes perfect sense when one considers the fact that heated fluids promote natural discharges of waste materials from different parts of the body. Hot liquids can quickly clear up mucus congestion in the sinuses, the back of the throat and in the lungs. They are able to raise body temperature just enough to promote perspiration, which brings some toxins through the skin. They also encourage more frequent urination and bowel movements.

But, most of all, hot (or extremely warm) liquids make it virtually impossible for disease-including bacteria or viruses to exist for very long in the system. Once heated fluids enter the body they begin isolating germs by flushing them out in the different ways just described. And the fact that such fluids are quite warm, actually encourages the immune system to begin producing more of its own antibiotic substances in order to fight influenza viruses better. Evidence for substantiating this logic can be seen in the *beneficial* effects of a *mild* fever upon the system: It actually is one of the body's own unique ways of recuperating. Therefore, the reasoning for drinking *hot* liquids (as Ms. Brown seems to have done for years) when respiratory problems due to infection prevail, doesn't seem so absurd after all.

In early January, 1996 Ms. Brown, still quite vivacious and energetic at 73, formally announced her resignation from the *Cosmopolitan* editorial board. When reporters inquired as to the reason for this decision, she queried them with a question of her own: "Just how long can you continue editing a magazine like this for a 23-year-old audience when you yourself are way, way, way *way* out of age range?" But she didn't plan to retire by any means. In 1997 she would become editor-in-chief of Cosmo's 27 international editions. "I plan to expand it to 50 editions around the globe by the start of the next century," she told reporters. "My work definitely is me," she continued. "And for me, work is [like] chloroform."

DON'T FORGET THE A & C

Two of the most important vitamins that anyone with a cold or flu should be taking in generous amounts are vitamins A and C. Due to the recent medical reports concerning the possible cancer-causing effects of *supplemented* beta-carotene, it is best to rely on fish-derived vitamin A in capsules. Generally, an average intake of 50,000 I.U. once or twice daily *only* during a bout with the flu, is recommended. (Taking this much every day for long periods of time can create adverse effects in the body, especially with the liver.) Vitamin A is sold in all health food stores in either 10,000 or 25,000 I.U.-strength capsules.

Vitamin C is probably the most studied and best known of all the vitamins. The late biochemist, Dr. Linus Pauling (the only scientist to ever win two Nobel Prizes) was its strongest advocate; he lived into his nineties and credited much of his own good health (including reversal of his prostate cancer) to this vital nutrient. Pauling himself took an average of 3,500 mg. every day; vitamin C usually comes in 500 or 1,000 mg. strength tablets. **The best time to take vitamin C is in the evening just before retiring to bed!**

Vitamin C is available in different forms. The chewable kind is handy to suck on and can be taken with you wrapped in some foil wherever you go. I always suggest that people buy the nonacidic kind, which doesn't upset the stomach like the cheaper ascorbic acid does.

Finally, and most importantly: remember to get plenty of rest (or Vitamin Z) and keep the bowels regular at all times when recovering from influenza.

Insomnia Nappers

"FORTY WINKS AND THEN SOME WITH THESE (Y-A-W-N) REMEDIES"

Get Your Z's with the Help of Melatonin

Melatonin (amply discussed under FREE RADICAL CELL AGING REVERSED) is a hormone produced by the pineal gland. Melatonin regulates the body's sleep-wake cycle. Blood levels of this hormone become elevated at night and drop dramatically by day; it reaches its peak in childhood and greatly subsides in old age. Melatonin is capable of helping people to fall asleep, and overcome jet lag and sleep problems associated with shift work.

If you decide to get melatonin don't buy the first product you encounter in a health food store. And don't be fooled by some of those melatonin preparations containing herbs and vitamins. You don't really need all that extra stuff packed in with it. Just get plain melatonin and *nothing* else included. Take one or two tablets in the evening about an hour before bedtime on an "as need" basis.

🌿 SNOOZE AWAY WITH DHEA

DHEA is an acronym for dehydroepiandrosterone. This natu-rally-occurring phospholipid is a steroid hormone produced by the adrenal glands. DHEA is produced in larger amounts than any other adrenal steroid hormone. It has sometimes been referred to as "the mother of hormones" because it is a precur-sor for the manufacture of many other hormones, 50 from the adrenal glands. These are responsible for the maintenance of numerous body functions including fat and mineral metabo-lism, controlling stress, maintaining male and female character-istics, and others.

Although DHEA is produced within the body and convert-ed on demand to these other hormones, extra supplementa-tion is sometimes still necessary. One biochemist conducted a somewhat novel experiment with DHEA on animal models. Wistar mice were given minute doses of this phospholipid in hopes it might show some signs of age reversal. While old mice did regain some of their youthful vigor and experience a return to their former sleek and glossy coats, quite a number of them also fell *asleep* within half an hour of taking DHEA.

This suggests a snooze pattern inherent with the consumption of DHEA. As to exactly how much humans would have to take for this, still remains a mystery. But, when coupled with the melatonin, DHEA might yet prove helpful for an insomniac get-ting a good night's rest.

🌿 COUNTING SHEEP WITH WARM CHAMOMILE

Are you one of those unfortunate people bothered with empty dreams at night? You see the lovely meadow or pasture separat-ed down the middle by a low-built wooden fence. But where are the sheep to jump over it? You toss and turn in the hopes they might appear, but never do. Disconcerting, isn't it?

Well, you'll rest a lot easier knowing that one cup of *warm* chamomile tea will do the trick every time. Just sip this wonderful herbal beverage, after it's been moderately heated and steeped for 7 minutes. Then fluff your pillow up again, lay back down, close your eyes, and dream woolly dreams for a change.

INSOMNIA INSPIRATION?

Some years ago a Hutterite minister named John Wipf from the Martinsdale Colony near the town of Martinsdale in Wheatland County, Montana, gave me a copy of this formula. He said that whenever he had difficulty sleeping, he would read it over several times and fall to sleep "almost instantly."

He claimed that the reason for its success was that it promoted "a happy heart and a peaceful disposition."

Happy Home Recipe

4 cups of love

2 cups of loyalty

4 quarts of faith

3 cups of forgiveness

2 spoons of tenderness

1 cup of friendship

5 spoons of hope

1 barrel of laughter

Take love and loyalty; mix together with faith. Blend with tenderness, kindness, and understanding. Fold in friendship and hope. Sprinkle last of all with laughter. Then bake with sunshine and much warmth. Serve daily in generous helpings.

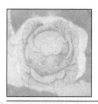
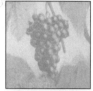
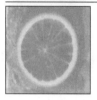

Loneliness Lifted

"WHAT TO DO FOR SPIRITUAL HEART DISEASE"

🌿 FRAGMENTATION OF SOCIETY CONTRIBUTES TO LONELINESS

Today in America more people die from coronary heart disease than any other single illness. Various reasons have been assigned to its causes: some say it's the bad air we're breathing, others the chemically-ladened food we're chucking down, and still others the tremendous amount of stress that we're all subjected to.

Well, they're all right to some extent. Foul air, crummy food, polluted water, and material stress do take some toll on the heart, that's for sure. But I've looked at the problem from an entirely different perspective. Actually, an anthropological one that involves culture. Ours has undergone unbelievable fragmentation. Because of this many people middle-aged and older are now experiencing a sense of loneliness, alienation, and isolation.

Half a century ago, many people still lived in the same neighborhood they were born and grew up in. They went to the same church, synagogue, cathedral, or temple to worship for a number of *decades*. Many men held down jobs that they had been at for 15 years or better. And many people back then had their extended families living within a one-hour driving radius of themselves.

That was *then*, but this is now. Few people in our population anymore can experience this kind of stability that our parents or grandparents knew in their lives. As a result people are feeling more disconnected with things and becoming lonelier.

🦎 A SHORTER LIFESPAN

Study after study has repeatedly shown that lonely and isolated folks run a three- to five-times greater risk of premature death as compared to those who have a sense of belonging and community spirit about themselves. As a result of this disconnection with family and society as a whole, many older individuals have turned to self-destructive behaviors such as smoking, gambling, overeating, drinking, or overusing prescription medications to fill the void in them. Such behaviors only tranquilize the disturbed soul, but fail to heal it.

🦎 OPEN YOUR HEART

Dean Ornish, M.D. is author of *Dr. Dean Ornish's Program for Reversing Heart Disease* (Random House) and *Eat More, Weigh Less* (Harper-Collins). He has also been an official physician to U.S. President Bill Clinton. For the past two decades he has devoted himself to understanding the lack of stability in our society as it relates to the health of the individual, especially the health of a person's heart.

Ornish offers a unique "Opening Your Heart" program as a means of combating the pain of loneliness and isolation. The program uses heart disease as a catalyst for changing unhealthy behavior as well as the conditions that cause them. Many people begin the program for medical reasons: they may want to unclog their arteries or develop better dietary habits. But the spiritual and emotional nourishment the program provides is at least as valuable as the physical benefits patients receive.

The doctor's program is an unusual type of open heart procedure. Rather than telling his patients to avoid the pain of loneliness, he encourages them to feel and understand it—to actually embrace in totality. He supports them in redirecting their emotions into an avenue for healing rather than harm and helps them manage the stresses in their lives rather than avoid them. To illustrate the difference between health and healing, Ornish recalled an occasion wherein his fictitious spiritual teacher Swami Satchidananda was asked, "What are you, a Hindu?" "No," he replied, "I'm an Undo. I'm trying to teach people how they can *undo* the patterns that cause damage to their minds and bodies so they can begin to heal."

Ornish's sweeping program draws its success from a low-fat, vegetarian diet; cessation of smoking; meditation and visualization; communication skills; safe and moderate exercise; and stress management techniques which are designed "to assist people to calm down their minds and bodies enough to experience more of an inner sense of peace, joy, and well-being." It teaches them to communicate with people in ways that don't invite judgment or attack.

He likes to encourage support groups that create a safe haven, "safe enough for people to talk about what's really going on in their own lives without fear or shame or rejection or criticism or abandonment," he carefully observed. "And, when we do that," he continued, "we find that people are more likely to change their lifestyles in self-enhancing rather than self-destructive ways." (The author is indebted to Lauren Mukamal-Camp of Santa Fe, New Mexico, for much of this data in the form it appeared.)

✿ THE HEALING POWER THAT COMES WITH DOING GOOD

Feeling a bit lonely or rejected these days? Feeling that the world or friends have turned their backs on you? Still feeling sorry for yourself again? Then maybe you need a change of pace—maybe, just maybe, you need to get up off your duff, out of those four home or apartment walls that you've made into a "prison" and look for someone to render assistance to. This will work better than you think, because, you see, new research suggests that by lending a hand to someone else in need, you're also helping yourself as well.

In 1987 a survey was sent to volunteer workers at more than twenty social-service organizations around the country. And from the 3,296 surveys returned by a broad range of volunteers—including helpers of AIDS patients, homeless families, shut-ins, crime victims, runaway youths, hospital patients, and others—the cause-and-effect relationships between helping and good health became abundantly clear.

According to the survey's findings, the dramatic health improvements produced by regularly helping strangers happen in a two-part process. The healthy-helper syndrome begins with a physical high, a rush of good feeling. Ninety-five percent of the survey's respondents reported experiencing this immediate physical sensation, which chased away not only their loneliness but also many of their aches and pains.

Some psychologists have termed this the "helper's high." The high has clear and definite components: Nine out of ten helpers felt one or more sensations from a characteristic set that includes a sudden warmth, increased energy, and a sense of euphoria. These sensations strongly indicate a sharp reduction in stress and the release of the body's natural pain-killers, namely the endorphins.

Phase two of the healthy-helping syndrome is a longer-lasting period of heightened emotional well-being, a sense of calm. In our survey, 57% of the volunteers said they experienced an increased sense of self worth, and 53% noted gains in such areas as happiness and optimism, as well as decreases in feelings of helplessness and depression.

Experiencing the full healthy-helping syndrome provides a powerful antidote to life's daily stresses. It also can be effective to some degree for virtually every sort of human ailment, besides just loneliness of the heart and abandonment of the soul. In the survey, volunteers who regularly helped others reported effects ranging from diminished pains of arthritis and lupus erythematosus to reduced frequency of asthmatic symptoms and migraine headaches, and of colds and bouts of influenza. Helping others can also mitigate against the stress and other conditions that eventually lead to strokes and heart attacks.

A combination of factors appear to be at work here: the strengthening of immune system activity; the diminishing of both the intensity and awareness of physical pain; the activation of emotions vital to the maintenance of good health; the reduction of the incidence of attitudes, such as chronic hostility and constant self-pity, that negatively arouse and damage the body; and the multiple benefits to the body's systems provided by stress relief.

Volunteers who reported health benefits in the survey tended to have at least one other thing in common as well: They *perceived* themselves to be in good health. Of the respondents who reported the helper's high, nine out of ten rated their health as better than others their age. This feeling of well-being is critically important. Studies have documented that raising a person's perceived health status leads to reductions in stress that help create actual health improvements. And in the survey, respondents frequently dated their perceived improvements in health to the beginning of their helping efforts.

Unlike regular exercise, which many engage in for healthy benefits, helping has a vaster potential. Not only does it benefit the health of individuals but also our entire tension-ridden society. According to the results of the previously cited study, once people involved in helping acts experience the strong good feelings they then become motivated to help that much more. Their empathy for others—especially strangers—increases as their own health does. And as awareness spreads of the potent sense of well-being and related health benefits, more folks are likely to try helping acts for themselves. Hopefully, this could eventually lead to a new level of daily altruism in our society. Whenever this happens, the healing power of doing good will have come full circle for once. (I am deeply grateful to Allan Luks and Peggy Payne for this important data and their kindness in permitting its use here.)

🐾 The Animal-Human Connection

The plain fact of the matter is that pets are good for you—good for you if you are lonely, depressed or physically challenged in some way. They're good if you're unlucky enough to be confined in a nursing home or psychiatric ward of a mental health facility.

Anybody who's ever loved an animal readily understands the value of owning pets. They give us something which psychologists claim we receive only from our mothers—*unconditional love*. Animals are the ultimate friends to have. They're nonjudgmental, entirely devoted, selfless, and possess a limitless supply of affection. It may not be too far off the mark of good reasoning to say here that animals express many of the same noble virtues found in the Creator Himself. How ironic then that the beasts, birds, and fish, which make all of our lives a great deal better, are capable of a much higher love than men and women are.

One study on the "socializing effects" of pets for the physically challenged showed that people in wheelchairs were more likely to get a positive reaction from passersby if they have a dog than if they do not. Dogs facilitate smiles, but handicapped people seldom do.

In 1991 I brought into the Anthropological Research Center located here in Salt Lake City, Utah, a small white kitty cat who was promptly named Jake by a former employee. Everybody took to him at once and he took to us, albeit rather clumsily and with some mischief at first. But eventually he settled in, grew into a big tabby cat, and had full run of our entire office until late June of 1996 when I gave him to a 16-year-old boy in Gunnison, Utah. Stephen Kjar and his mom, Mary Ann, now enjoy Jake's companionship even as I did.

But prior to his coming, we had nothing in the way of pets. Not even so much as a goldfish or parakeet, let alone something bigger. Jake came to us by happenstance, and we've never regretted it one minute. Before his arrival, I used to be more tense and nervous. But Jake's presence had a slow, melting effect on my irritable nature and soon much of my pent-up stress was released. Jake did, indeed, have a definite mellowing effect upon me, as well as the rest of our staff. His was a calming and reassuring presence, something with which we are intimately familiar and very comfortable having around. There can be no better friend in your life than a pet!

For those who reside in apartments or condominiums where rules preclude having a cat or dog, consider other options. Do as Joe Morgenstern, a writer based in Santa Monica, California, did back in 1989 sometime; he built a bird feeder outside his tenement window and soon enjoyed the delightful company of several scrub jays. There are also goldfish, finches, parakeets, and even turtles to consider as potential pets in the event you can't have a cat or dog on your premises. But, for heaven's sakes—get a pet of some kind and enjoy the wonderful therapy that they bring for very little investment into our chaotic lives.

Longevity Secrets

"WIT & WISDOM OF THE WORLD'S YOUNGEST AND OLDEST SENIORS"

"WHAT, ME WORRY AT AGE SIXTY?!!"

In 1989, author and playwright Larry L. King (no relation to the TV-radio talk show host of nearly the same name) celebrated the beginning of *his* old age at age sixty. He did so knowing that he was the proud father of two children, a girl Lindsay, 10 and a son, Blaine, 7. "I got started somewhat later than most," he teased.

He denounced the customary "giving up" which routinely comes with aging. "We have a clear choice in the matter—using our remaining time as best we can, or simply giving up on life all together." He then defined some of the ways by which people surrender: losing interest in work or the world and becoming a couch potato; becoming abnormally fearful of death; becoming embittered that one's life somehow hasn't attained earlier great expectations; attempting to flee reality. "Our decision to 'live' or 'die,'" he reasoned, "is really an individual one when you come right down to it."

"There should be a sense of urgency about accomplishing work one feels compelled to do—yes, a sense of limited time—but we should have no frenzy in it. There is no need hanging cloud raining dark thoughts of approaching infirmities or death. One simply knows what one wants to *do* with the remaining good years and plans the doing as efficiently as circumstances permit."

"However," he cautioned, "this drive to accomplish work left undone must be balanced against both the need and the wish to share and assist in important events and key moments in the lives of one's growing children. I don't want them to remember their father as one who was so preoccupied with his own creations that he had little time for those he helped to create. I want to leave them warm memories: bedtime romps; cheering together at football games; a Christmas weekend in New York City; popping popcorn in front of the fireplace on snowy winter nights. Good moments *shared* and not lost.

"I am gratified that life has taught even a slow learner [like myself] that it is far better to hang in there, mixing it up, than to quit on one's corner stool in the early or middle rounds of living."

He Bicycles at 70

Cecil Cripps turned 70 sometime in 1996. Now a retired journalist, he has been a racing cyclist for 58 years of his life. He has been a national amateur and pro champion, winning some of cycling's biggest events for seniors. He won two Gold Medals and one Bronze at the 1995 Huntsman World Senior Games held annually in St. George, Utah.

He contacted me by mail in early January, 1996, when I still served as editor of *Utah Prime Times* (a monthly newspaper for seniors; I resigned in April of that year after almost five years of editorship). Cecil offered up a little bit of what he called "me kangaroo philosophy 'bout life in the outback, mate."

He declared that some form of intense exercise—he opted for bicycling over say, hang-gliding off Mount Everest, to "work out me frustrations and boredom in a meaningful way." He said that anyone 60 and up, who started to feel "sorry for hisself" should attempt a sport that requires a lot of endurance, patience, and energy.

"The thinking here, mate, is that your mind is troubled with somethin' you can't rightly handle, then it's best that you work out these frustrations with 'kangaroo-intensity' exercises. And just like them kangaroos, always bouncin' around here and there and everywhere, you'll soon get yourself so bushwhacked that you won't be able to lift a little finger. But that's good, mate, 'cause then you'll be too exhausted to ever notice what was bothering you in the first place."

He Earned His College Degree at Age 70

I interviewed Marinus Palache on Monday, June 14, 1993 in my research center in Salt Lake City, for a story I was doing for the seniors newspaper *(Utah Prime Times)* I edited at the time.

Marinus was born September 28, 1915 in Poland and eventually emigrated to America sometime in 1947. He commenced working in the jewelry trade in Ogden, Utah, sometime after that. Later he hired on at the *Salt Lake Tribune* (a local newspaper) and worked there for 33 years as a typographer before finally retiring in 1980.

But it soon dawned on him that he just couldn't putter around his Rose Park home. "I thought, 'What am I going to do?

Rake the leaves? Cut the lawn? Walk the dog?'" That's when he decided to sign up for a state program that allowed students older than 62 to pay $10 a quarter to audit university classes.

Eventually, Mr. Palache enrolled for credit, slowly working toward his philosophy degree by taking two classes a quarter. He enjoyed talking with the young people, asking many questions and learning new things from them all the time.

"They kept me young, because of their youthfulness," I remember him saying. "Through them I learned to stay in touch with life." He swam a half-mile four times a week. Asked the reason for this, he replied: "If you don't you shrink up like an old prune."

Yet there were times when the septuagenarian definitely showed his age. Once in his "Human Sexuality" class, Mr. Palache was asked by the liberal professor to speak about how things were different when he was young. He modestly admitted that he and his late wife knew each other for six years before they ever got married.

"*Then*, and only then, came sex and three children," he explained to 117 astonished students. "But the girls in the class liked it very much, what I said, and wished it could be that way now for them."

On Friday, June 11, 1993, at age 77 he became the oldest student ever to receive his baccalaureate degree from the University of Utah. "It took me about ten years," he said with a grin. "But it was worth the wait and effort. Now, I got to go out and look for a job," he joked with obvious mischief in mind.

BRIDGE FOREVER, HOUSEWORK WHENEVER

As little girls, growing up in the same Ogden neighborhood, Marjorie Jennings, Phyllis A. Chatwin, Helen "Pat" McCraley and Marion Reese knew each other fairly well. They would frequently walk together to Madison Elementary, Central Junior, and then old Ogden High schools.

The four, who now live in the Salt Lake City area, even knew each other's parents. There were the usual sleepovers at each other's homes when mere girls. And occasional "post office" games with "rowdy" boys. None of them really cared for the "Special Delivery" or "Air *Male*" suggestions proposed by the boys. "We always ended up giving them the 'Return to Sender' signal," said one of their number. "That's because they had 'Insufficient Postage,'" joined in another.

They graduated together from high school—three had special parts on the program—and were the workhorses for a recent 60th high-school class reunion. The women—Marj, Phyl, Pat, and Marion—all turned 80 during 1996. For each birthday, they went out to lunch.

But the birthday celebrations had to be scheduled carefully. There is never *any* excuse for interrupting their favorite foursome pastime—bridge—every other Monday at 1:30 P.M.

This is a *really* dedicated bridge group as I was soon to find out. Their bridge napkins said it best when I was visiting at one of their homes: "Bridge Forever, Housework Whenever!"

I asked them why they've played this game faithfully for so many years. Their reply was that the game gets them together. "Playing bridge gives us something to do with our hands while we talk," Marj observed.

"Getting together is social first," Phyl chimed in, "while bridge is second." All agreed that it was probably the best form of therapy for them. No shrink, no analyst's couch here—just loving hearts and understanding minds since grade school to hear each other's bi-weekly woes and fourteen-day joys. The ups and downs of daily living and everything and anyone with whom they interact is fair game for discussion at a typical bridge session.

"We're more like sisters than friends," another noted. "Our feelings and affections for one another go deeper than the roots of that big tree standing out there in the front yard."

Bridge has helped them to survive and *stay alive*. Without these regular get-togethers, each woman would have to shoulder her own frustrations and unhappiness alone. But bridge allows them the vehicle by which they can unite to communicate and inform each other of where their individual hearts, heads, and lives are presently at.

"Bridge," said Pat with some thought, "may not always keep us young, but it certainly has kept us *sane*." It's a tough road for the elderly to hoe by themselves. But coming together by a common interest in a popular card game has kept these four gals a-going for a long time now in spite of some physical limitations due to the infirmities that come with old age.

"AND NOW ABIDETH FAITH, HOPE, AND CHARITY" (I CORINTHIANS 13:13)

In the Spring of 1994 I happened to be in Texas fulfilling some speaking engagements when someone told me about the famous Cardwell triplets. I decided to travel to Sweetwater, Texas, and visit them at the Holiday Retirement Center. They were born on their parents' cotton farm north of Waco way back on May 18, 1899. The doctor who barely arrived in time to deliver the last one suggested they be named Lillie, Lola, and Lula. But their parents, Elza and Eliza, didn't much take to those names—or, for that matter, to any others suggested by well-intentioned folks.

For six months, the babies went nameless. Word of their parents' dilemma got into the newspapers and finally reached the ear of Frances Cleveland, wife of President Grover Cleveland. She recommended that the babies be called Faith, Hope, and Charity—and so, in order of birth, they were.

At the time of my visit with them, these three 95-year-old sisters had outlived 18 American Presidents and a total of six husbands. The 1992 *Guinness Book of Records* proclaimed them to be the world's oldest triplets.

Charity, who did most of the talking for the trio, chuckled as she quoted me her favorite scripture from I Corinthians 13:13 that goes, "And now abideth faith, hope, charity . . ." She paused ever so briefly and then completed the verse with her usual flourish, "but the greatest of these is charity."

Charity attributed their remarkable longevity to several things. "We was always working hard in the fields, picking cotton. Faith here ran a family-style diner later on. As for myself, I kept myself busy at my beauty parlor. Hope helped both of us out when we needed it. We never strayed very far from our hard-scrabble roots down here. We stayed close to the land and worked our fingers to the bone in whatever we decided to tackle."

One of the attendants on staff told me in private later on, that each of the sisters still has her own room. "They still fight," she said softly, "just like sisters will do."

Hope started to speak, but Charity quickly interrupted and continued on with the conversation. "It's a good life for us. We play dominoes. We play every kind of game you think of, old-fashioned games." I challenged her to a checker game, so the attendant brought a game board and playing pieces for us. I set it up and went one-on-one with Charity. We played six straight games in rapid succession and, I'm sorry to say, that feisty and outspoken lady skunked me all six times. To be beaten is bad enough, but to have it done that many times by someone old enough to be your great-grandmother was too much for my pride and self-esteem to bear.

On May 16, 1996, I placed a call to the Holiday Retirement Center in Sweetwater. With the assistance of a head attendant, I was able to carry on a very brief conversation with a partially deaf Hope Brock, who was in her 97th year of life. I learned that her sisters, Faith and Charity, had passed on a year before. Mustering enough strength in her wheelchair to laugh, she wise-cracked in a feeble voice: "Faith faileth, and Charity passeth away; but Hope continues on." At least the old gal still had her sense of humor fairly well intact, though other parts of her body were definitely not operating very well.

I could clearly overhear the attendant shouting my ques-tions, very slowly and carefully into Hope's one good left ear. Hope mumbled something that escaped my notice until repeated by the attendant a moment later. "She said that her two sisters are still with her in spirit form. She can see them plain as day, and talks to them all the time. She said they never leave her side. She said that Charity still does most of the yakking, just as she did in real life. Some things never change, do they?"

I thanked the attendant for her kind assistance and asked her to convey my gratitude to Hope for speaking with me a little.

🦁 LAUGHTER MADE THEM KINGS OF LONGEVITY

The barrel-chested and very robust Hal Roach (January 14, 1892–November 2, 1992) and the diminutive, soft-spoken George Burns (January 20, 1896–March 9, 1996) couldn't have been more different from each other in terms of physical appearance, stature, and achievements. But for what they lacked in differences, they easily made up for in a shared trait: they loved to laugh and enjoyed making others laugh as well. It has been said of them that "laughter made them the kings of longevity" in a ruthless and highly competitive place (Hollywood) not known for having too many centenarians around.

Both loved good cigars, enjoyed playing an occasional round of golf, liked sipping martinis, and ate whatever they wanted. When asked individually about their gregarious appetites, each man responded in his own unique way. Roach: "Health food is what you can eat anytime in big enough quantities that won't kill you." Burns: "I've always been on the see-food diet, myself— I see this and I eat it; I see that and I eat it. Works out pretty good for me, though."

In 1912 the Titanic sank, vitamin A was discovered and Hal Roach got his first job in the movies—for a dollar a day, carfare, two sandwiches, and a banana. He got good use out of that one and many more bananas besides. "We must have had somebody slip on a banana peel 50 different times," he remarked. He put comedian Harold Lloyd and Oliver Hardy through their banana pratfalls without much difficulty, although a chiropractor may have been sorely needed on many of those occasions.

"Our Gang" comedy shorts was another Roach original. The series began in 1922 and became immensely popular with the advent of sound. When they later appeared on television in the 1950s, the name was changed to "The Little Rascals."

"Roach had that most mysterious of Hollywood talents," wrote Stephen Hunter of *The Baltimore Sun*, "the most difficult to pin down and dissect. He directed but he wasn't really a director. He wrote screenplays but he wasn't truly a screenwriter. He acted but he wasn't an actor, not really. He thought up gags but he wasn't a gag man. He was fundamentally a producer, which is the key job in the industry and is almost the industry itself. He produced. It means he recognized talent, not only in and of itself but was able to project it and imagine how it might fit with other talent and from the sparks could be created something exquisite. He was the prime mover, and his Hal Roach Studios was a font of creativity for 30 years. . ."

On March 31, 1992 the movie thriller "The Silence of the Lambs" garnered the lion's share of Oscars at the annual Academy Awards show. Hosted by Billy Crystal, that evening's first standing ovation went to Hal Roach. When he tried to offer a brief speech, there was no microphone near. Ever the quick wit himself, Crystal dryly observed that it was appropriate since Roach began his own career in *silent* films instead of the "talkies." He was then presented with an honorary Academy Award "in recognition of his unparalleled record of distinguished contributions to the motion picture art form." His two previous Oscars were less pompous.

Well into his nineties, Roach still did his own bookkeeping. "My mother took care of her own finances until she was 95," he said. "Most of the money I have to live on now is money I gave her and she turned into good investments." Roach died of pneumonia at his home in Bel-Air, California, on Monday, November 2, 1992.

George Burns was born as Nathan Birnbaum in a slum tenement on the Lower East Side of the New York borough of Manhattan in 1896. He had seven sisters and four brothers. Until his teenage years, his family lived in near abject poverty. By the time he was 15, George knew he wanted to be a vaudeville actor. At 16, he began smoking cigars to look like an actor— and never gave them up. At one time he was puffing his way through 20 El Productos a day, but eventually cut down to five.

One day, as a booking agent came looking for a monologist named George Burns, he jumped up and said, "I'm George Burns." That got him a job at the Myrtle Theater in Brooklyn; three days for $15—big money in those times! But he was called offstage and promptly fired after his first raunchy joke.

He soon met Gracie Allen, a jobless, 17-year-old Irish-American dramatic actress who had been thinking about becoming a secretary. They performed together one time and discovered that the audience liked them as a team. They married in 1926 and thus began a lengthy stage, radio, TV, and film career that lasted almost four decades. She died in August of 1964 at the age of 58; her passing devastated Burns and it took him a full year to come out of his depressive slump.

He slowly went back to work in television and doing occasional nightclub shows. Then, quite suddenly, he became a movie star at 79 in the hit movie, "Oh God!," won an Oscar for it at 80, and went on to make seven more pictures as an accomplished actor throughout the rest of his 80s and into his early 90s.

Humor was clearly one of the major keys to his longevity success. When asked by curious reporters what he attributed his long life and good health to, he gave them the standard reply. "Drink three martinis a day, get very little sleep, eat fried foods, make love at least four times a week, and smoke cigars. I smoke about 15 a day myself. Three doctors told me to stop the cigars years ago. Of these three, two are already dead—and the third one has been coughing a lot lately."

The other secret to his longevity was to keep himself busily occupied with those things that he enjoyed doing the most. "The older I get, the more I seem to want to do," he said on one occasion. "The main thing is to get a job and love what you do. That keeps you young. I was old at 27, because I wasn't working. But now I'm young, because I'm busy. Idleness will get you old in a hurry."

Two American Presidents honored him. President Ronald Reagan helped him to celebrate his 90th birthday in January 1986. And when Burns died of heart failure one Saturday morning, President Bill Clinton read a statement heralding him "as one of the great entertainers of all time," adding: "George Burns' sense of timing and captivating smile touched the hearts and funny bones of more than three generations. He enables us to see humor in the toughest of times and laugh together as a nation."

For many years prior to his death, Burns had always insisted in a gravelly monotone: "I don't believe in dying . . . It's already been done for me by someone else." He may have been guilty for smoking cheap cigars, but certainly deserves our respect for having lived a rich and varied life.

✿ OLD ENOUGH TO HAVE BEEN GEORGE BURNS' MOTHER!

Meet Jeanne Calment, the world's *certified* oldest woman *and* rap singer. She was 121 as of 1996. Up until January of that year before he died, she was old enough to have been the mom of comedian George Burns (who himself was 100 years old at the time). She has lived through the administration of 18 French presidents and once met artist Vincent Van Gogh, whom she described as being "ugly as sin" and "ill tempered as the Devil himself!"

This incredible woman is something like the Energizer battery bunny seen on these cleverly cute TV ads all the time: she just keeps going and going and going, never seeming to stop. At least that's what banker Andre-Francois Raffray's family learned, much to their own regret.

Andre thought he had the deal of a lifetime in 1965: He would pay a 90-year-old woman $500 a month until she died, then move into her spacious and grand apartment in Arles, located northwest of Marseilles in the south of France.

But on December 25, 1995, Raffray and *not* Jeanne Calment, died at age 77, having forked over a whopping $184,000 for an apartment he never even got to live in one day of his life. On that same Christmas day, Jeanne dined on *foie gras* (goose liver), duck thighs, cheese, and chocolate cake at her nursing home, not far from this much sought-after apartment.

She doesn't need to worry about losing any income just because Raffray passed away before she did. Although the amount he already paid is nearly three times the apartment's current market value, his widow is obligated to keep sending that monthly check of $500 anyway. And if Jeanne manages to somehow outlive Mrs. Raffray, who was reported to have been in somewhat ill health herself, then the Raffray children *and* grandchildren will be forced to continue with these monthly payments.

When asked to comment on this strange twist of circumstances, Jeanne replied, "In life, one sometimes makes bad deals. And this was a bad one for Monsieur Raffray." The apartment currently is unoccupied. Buying apartments *en viager*—or "for life"—is common throughout France. The elderly owner gets to enjoy a monthly income from the buyer, who gambles on getting a real estate bargain—*provided* the owner drops dead in due time. Then, upon the owner's death, the buyer inherits the apartment, regardless of how much was paid for it. Jeanne Calment has proven to be the worst nightmare of all those who have bought real estate *en viager.*

Pity the poor Raffrays and cheer Miss Calment who got the deal of a lifetime from a (supposedly) shrewd French investment banker.

At the time of her 121st birthday on Wednesday, February 21, 1996, a slew of reporters gathered about her, clamoring for interviews and photo ops of the world's oldest person in modern times whose date of birth could be authenticated.

"Madame Calment, why have you lived so long?" shouted one journalist (she is partially deaf).

"Because I've been forgotten by a good God," came the humorous reply.

"Miss Calment," another yelled. "What is your vision of the future."

She gave a mischievous grin and replied: "Very brief."

"Oh, Miss Calment," another screamed from some distance away. "What healthy lifestyle have you followed to live to such an incredible age?"

Without missing a beat, she mumbled: "Eating anything that is delicious. Nibbling on chocolates has been one vice. Smoking two cigarettes a day for 103 years is another." (Nursing home authorities and her own doctor forced her to give them up, however, sometime in 1995.) She finished answering this last reporter with a final thought: *I have a single glass of port [wine] before every meal."*

That, more than anything else, may pretty much sum up *why* she has lived so long, unless, of course, you include her sharp-edged humor along with it. It's being called the "French Paradox" and seems to have given Miss Calment a long lease on life, besides the one she already has on her apartment with the very unhappy Raffray family.

The Paradox may be explained this way. When international surveys in the 1980s showed substantially lower rates of coronary heart disease in France than in other industrialized countries, scientists were puzzled beyond belief. How on earth could such a thing be true in the land of *pâté de foie gras* and Gauloises, burgundy, and béarnaise sauce? Such a contradiction has been labeled the French Paradox.

Medical researchers have suspected for some time now that wine, which the French drink in legendary quantities, might just explain why a diet relatively high in saturated fat and cholesterol was producing only half as much coronary disease as it would among Americans.

Scientists had several reasons for zeroing in on wine. Several prospective studies, including one done at Harvard Medical School, showed that consuming two alcoholic drinks a day for six weeks increased levels of "good" cholesterol, that's HDL (high-density lipoprotein), by 17%. This rise translates into an almost 40% reduction in the risk of heart disease. Additionally, other medical evidence gathered worldwide indicated that moderate drinkers usually have healthier hearts than people who don't drink at all or those who drink in excess.

At the 1994 American Heart Association Scientific Sessions, held in Atlanta, presentations on the French Paradox drew crowds of cardiologists and reporters. Participants already knew that people who want to protect themselves against cardiovascular disease should cut down on fats, eat their vegetables, and exercise regularly. But should they also, for their heart's sake be consuming one or two alcoholic drinks a day?

The experts who spoke at this particular AHA meeting (that I attended with a cardiologist friend of mine from Salt Lake City), were in general agreement that *limited*, regular consumption of alcohol appears to safely reduce the risk of heart disease for many adults. They were quick to point out, though, that this wasn't an across-the-board recommendation by any means. They emphasized that such advice should only come from an individual practitioner and should be directed to an individual patient. They drew the crowd's attention to the fact that heavy drinking is bad. What they hoped they got out was that *very small* intakes of alcohol every day would seem to do the heart some good.

The mechanism by which *red wine in particular* accomplishes this was discovered by a researcher at the Israel Institute of Technology in the city of Haifa in 1995. Michael Aviram attributed red wine's benefits to polyphenols found in grape skins. In a study bearing his name and published in the March, 1995 issue of the *American Journal of Clinical Nutrition*, he noted that by mixing red wine with "bad" cholesterol (LDLs or low-density lipoproteins), his team observed a 70% reduction in LDL oxidation, which greatly contributes to arteriosclerosis.

Next, they studied blood samples from two groups of people who had consumed two glasses of either red or white wine each day for 2 weeks. In the group drinking red wine, polyphenols were detected in the blood stream, where researchers said they bind with LDLs and prevent them from adhering to arterial walls. The same effect wasn't detected in white wine drinkers. In fact, just the opposite occurred: white wine was found to *increase* this negative oxidation. Grape skins are removed during white wine production, leaving few, if any, polyphenols.

Here then is the best medical explanation given as to why Jeanne Calment reigned undisputed as the world's oldest, living person in 1996.

Her sharp wit has also been studied by others for its positive health benefits. The late Norman Cousins devoted an entire chapter to it in his book, *Head First: The Biology of Hope* (New York: E.P. Dutton, 1989). "Just in psychological terms," he wrote, "laughter can confer benefits . . . Laughter has also been shown to be helpful in reducing discomfort . . . Laughter can improve one's perspective on life and on pain . . . It might [even] be helpful in combating unusual stress . . . Laughter produces . . . changes in blood pressure . . ." He quoted Dr. Harvin E. Herring of New Jersey's School of Osteopathic Medicine as saying that "the diaphragm, thorax, abdomen, heart, lungs, and even the liver are given a massage during a hearty laugh." The expression, though, which Cousins preferred in his first best-seller, *Anatomy of an Illness* was "internal jogging." The best thing you can do for a hospitalized friend or relative, he asserted, is not to give flowers, candy, or cards. But "consider sending the patient a funny novel, a book of jokes, a silly toy, a humorous audio tape, or a video recorder to show a funny movie on." This will do that person more good than just about anything else, he emphasized.

So You Want to Live to be 100?

Having reviewed the wit and wisdom of some of the world's youngest and oldest seniors, it is now time to summarize the highlights of what this very interesting section contains:

Larry L. King, age 60: "Don't give up; don't surrender."

Cecil Cripps,. age 70: "Exercise to distract your frustration."

Marinus Palache, age 70: "Educate the mind when you retire."

The bridge ladies over 80: "Talk things over with friends you trust."

The Texas triplets, age 95: "Work hard to stay young and live long."

Hal Roach and George Burns, age 100: "Enjoy a good cigar, eat what you want, like the things you do, and laugh a lot!"

Joseph Anderson, age 100: "Be prudent in your eating habits, swim and walk a lot, don't eat pork, and be active in religious matters."

John Carpenter, age 108: "Consume lots of vegetables (especially onions and garlic), live close to the earth, practice moderation in everything you do, have plenty of patience and tolerance for others, and be at peace with yourself at all times."

Jeanne Calment, age 121: "Choose good investments, don't always worry about good nutrition, keep a good sense of humor at all times, and be sure to have a glass of red wine *before* every meal.

While the foregoing information doesn't necessarily represent the direct quotes of every individual cited, the data does define quite concisely those factors most responsible for extended and healthy lifespans. Obviously not everything listed here will work for everyone. But many of these features will add *quality* years to your own present existence, so you can stay around long enough to get the most out of what life has to offer you!

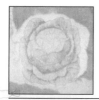

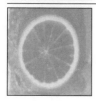

Memory Revitalization

"AT AGE 88 THE MIND OF JAMES A. MICHENER IS AS
STRONG AS EVER"

❧ His Specialty Is Historical Novels

In his 40 different books, James A. Michener has taken his fans
on an incredible tour of the literary universe: from the South
Pacific to the Chesapeake Bay, from Poland to Alaska, from the
sunny Caribbean to the vast blackness of outer space. So, in his
88th year, I wanted to know if there were any parts of the world
he hadn't yet explored?

"There are only about 30 left that I know of," he said in a long-
distance telephone interview in mid-December, 1995 from his
home in Austin, Texas. "I still receive about half a dozen letters
every month from fans suggesting areas of the planet that I

haven't covered yet. And all of them make sense. If I could turn back the clock to the time when I was a young man, full of energy and stamina, I would love to tackle every one of them."

Even my Beehive State, Michener believed, would make a rich subject for the sweeping historical novels that have become his recognized specialty. "It has all the right elements. It's a truly classic American story and a very unique one at that. I don't think I have that many years left to tackle something on this grand a scale. But I'm confident that somebody of equal talent will someday want to do a mighty saga of your people and their noble religion."

No Fading Memory Here

The thing which intrigued me most with this prolific writer was the excellent state of his mind. No fading memory here that I could tell. So, how were his mental capabilities anyhow, I wondered aloud. "Never better," he said matter-of-factly. But, at his age, I reasoned, many people are either faced with the unhappy prospect of failing memories or else have already become candidates for some degree of Alzheimer's disease. "How have you been able to avoid this from happening?" I asked point-blank.

Michener reminded me that he was a great novelist and not a great medical doctor. He couldn't think of anything offhand in his diet that might account for his strong mental powers. Nor did he take any of the known herbal or food supplements that are purported to invigorate the mind in later years and make near geniuses out of some older folks. "Maybe it's the exercise I get," he thoughtfully speculated.

But not just any ordinary kind of exercise, I might add. Michener stated with certainty that "I love to read books. I've read them all my life. I believe that when you store your mind with a host of good things, it doesn't shrivel up or waste away." After all, the brain is *a muscle* just like other muscles of the body found in our arms, legs, back, and abdomen which need to be regularly exercised so they don't go flabby or become atrophied. It is said that the *gray* matter inside our brains is where all of our thought processes take place. If this is the case, then Michener's gray matter, like that of Albert Einstein's, must be thicker than that of the average person.

Use It or Lose It

Smart people Michener's age, who are less famous and that I've had the pleasure of interviewing through the years, have all *actively* utilized their minds in a variety of ways. A few have been thinkers, others were creative souls, some liked to read, a fair number enjoyed the arts, and many more have contented themselves with doing crafts of various sorts. But all of them have kept themselves busily occupied in one way or another.

Television has been blamed by many educators for "wasting" the minds of America's young people. Numerous articles have pointed to the fact that young children and teenagers don't have to exercise much mental activity when watching the "boob tube." What's true for kids is equally so for senior citizens. In the many nursing homes, retirement centers, and hospitals that I've visited over the last couple of decades, the majority of the elderly I've met in such places have usually been glued to TV sets for many hours of the day. And even in many private homes, where older folks are still able to get around and take care of themselves, the TV set is frequently on and has a major focus of their attention.

Michener himself watches very little television. He thinks it's a complete waste of time and brain power. In his opinion, TV can stifle whatever creative talents a person may have. He claims that "by not watching TV, I've been able to produce those 1,000 page novels I'm so famous for, that would make other writers exhausted." Reading tends to *stimulate* the mind, providing it with a cultural excitement and literary exhilaration. Some of his best friends have been favorite books; but he can't say the same for TV programs. The mind *slowly vegetates* with excessive TV viewing, while it continually contracts and expands through reading good literature. If older people read more often and watched TV a lot less, they wouldn't find their mental powers failing so fast.

242 HEINERMAN'S ENCYCLOPEDIA OF ANTI-AGING REMEDIES

In fact, there is now some hard science to prove this very point. So listen up all of you television viewers and consider switching to book reading instead. A group of professors at the University of California, Berkeley, has a lesson to impart about overcoming the memory losses that often accompany aging. Psychologist Arthur P. Shimamura and his fellow coworkers administered a battery of memory and cognitive tests to 72 professors recruited from a wide spectrum of disciplines on the Berkeley campus. Volunteers fell into three age groups of about the same size: young professors, age 30 to 44; middle-aged professors, ranging from 45 to 59 years old; and senior professors, age 60 to 71.

To the astonishment of researchers, senior professors held their own quite well on two memory tests submitted to all three groups that required mental planning, organization, and problem solving. Scores on these tasks typically decline sharply in the elderly, Shimamura and company noted. But in senior professors, where TV watching was most *minimal*, their aged brains were still able to perform some difficult memory chores equal to younger counterparts. It is believed that *without* television, older brains subjected to increased reading, are somehow able to overcome a few of the biological glitches that come with aging, by devising innovative memory strategies. A full report of Dr. Shimamura's team research appeared in the September, 1995 issue of *Psychological Science.*

"It's Been a Good Life, Indeed"

Michener attributes much of his good fortune to the talents which a loving and divine Providence has so graciously bestowed upon him. His books have sold into the tens of millions of copies and been reprinted in some 38 languages. He has won a Pulitzer Prize, the Presidential Medal of Freedom and the devotion of history teachers everywhere for his novels, which often spur readers to study the culture and history of the places he writes about.

Reflecting back over his long writing career, Michener sounded almost adverse to appraising his large body of work. He said there is no one favorite book of his. It would be like asking a father to choose which of his many children he loves the most. "There is *no* favorite one, " he emphasized. Then, speaking more candidly with me, he added, "Truthfully, when I've completed a long manuscript, I feel like getting down on my knees and just thanking the Almighty that I was able to finish it. I believe in giving credit where credit's due!"

🌿 OTHER THINGS THAT SHOULD SHARPEN YOUR MEMORY

A high-potency B complex vitamin is always practical to take when the memory begins to slightly wane. Two tablets each day with the noon meal are recommended. But there is one member of this particular vitamin group which seems to do a very good job in memory improvement. This is choline, and along with inositol (another B vitamin), they make up the basic constituents of lecithin. Choline assists the body in manufacturing more acetylcholine, which is the message carrier of the brain. Average daily intake of choline is about 200 milligrams.

The next most important thing for increasing one's mental powers is to make sure that the brain is receiving adequate blood flow. Poor circulation can deny the brain the necessary oxygen it needs in order to function properly. In my many years of experience, I've found five things that seem to work very well together in making the mind razor-sharp. My simple supplement program for this is given below.

Memory Sharpening Program

2 capsules daily gotu kola herb

2 capsules daily Ginkgo Biloba Plus from Wakunaga

1 capsule daily cayenne pepper

50 mg. niacinamide (vitamin B-3)

1 capsule alfalfa leaf

1 capsule Korean ginseng root

Menopausal Assistance

"'CATCHER IN THE RYE': SALINGER WOULD HAVE DEARLY LOVED THIS REMEDY"

🌱 "DR. MARK'S HEALTH BREAD"

Not too long ago, I read a fascinating article in my international edition of *The Jerusalem Post* for the week ending February 10, 1996. The story by Esther Hecht concerned a Russian Jewish couple, Dr. Mark Shteintsig and his wife Vera, who operate a special kind of bakery in the new section of the Beit Shemesh industrial zone.

For Mark, age 50, baking bread is not so much a business as an extension of a philosophy: Good living requires good nutrition. "I just can't understand how people who claim they love their children can give them poison," he mentioned, referring first to cola beverages, then to artificial additives, highly spiced foods, and pesticides on fresh produce.

And as for bread? "Well, when Vera and I arrived in Israel from Minsk in September 1990, there was *no* bread!" He spits these words out disdainfully. According to him—in an overseas telephone conversation I had with the couple—"What passes for the 'staff of life' here isn't even fit for the pigs to eat!"

Mark received his training at the Minsk Medical Institute and the Minsk Institute of Physical Culture in the former Soviet Union. He specialized in Internal Medicine and Cardiology, before heading a rehabilitation department. But when he became seriously ill, his own conventional medicine was incapable of helping him get well. So, he undertook to cure himself, and did so in less than half a year with a combination of correct nutrition (vegetarian and whole foods), fasting and exercise. He claimed this program is "enough to be healthy if you want to be ."

For 20 years he worked in alternative medicine; 15 of those years were devoted to helping top athletes prepare for the Olympics, with special emphasis on their diet. Meanwhile, he gave courses in nutrition. And, along with his wife Vera, the top chef at a sports complex, held demonstrations and tastings of healthful cooking. He even had a monthly hour-long TV show back then.

Together they developed a very unique bread that has become the talk of Jerusalem and surrounding cities; they also bake rolls and cookies. "Rye flour is very capricious to work with," Vera told me by phone. "Think of it as a little child and you will then, perhaps, better understand just what I mean by that. You have to lovingly cradle it with your hands to reassure it, but not too much or else it becomes spoiled. Texture is everything here. You wouldn't believe the amount of dough that passes through my hands—about a thousand loaves every day, five days a week."

"EAT TWO SLICES AND CALL ME TOMORROW"

Many doctors like to prescribe drugs for their patients' different ailments—it's quick, easy, and profitable for the pharmacist. But some like Mark, prefer doing things the old-fashioned way: they like to prescribe *foods as medicines.* And this is exactly where "Dr. Mark's Bread" comes in.

He first noticed it with his wife, who started passing through menopause in a rough way. "I remember her getting lots of hot flashes and doing a great amount of sweating," he recalled for my benefit. "She became nervous, depressed, and had a hard time sleeping. Things were very difficult for her during this phase of her life."

Mark said that one day as she was munching on some of their special rye bread, Vera casually remarked to him, "I don't know what it is, but whenever I eat this bread I feel pretty good afterwards." There then followed a clinical discussion of this phenomenon. As it turned out later, *something* in the rye bread greatly relieved her menopausal symptoms.

Dr. Shteintsig decided to give some of their bread to other Israeli women they knew in their forties, who were going through the same thing. Imagine his surprise and delight to discover that they too experienced freedom from the pain and discomforts which often accompany menopause. Mark took this one step further and had some of his acquaintances living elsewhere in Europe, who were also going through their own menopauses, try some dark pumpernickel for a change. Again, reports came back on how much easier things went for them.

Nothing is ever put on the bread, Mark informed me. "I tell them to eat it plain, to take small bites and to chew it v-e-r-y slowly." Recently, he started having some of menopausal women drink cups of *warm* fenugreek tea with their bread. An amazing thing happened: The symptoms were more quickly relieved than with just the bread alone. The standard recommendation is two slices of rye or pumpernickel bread with a cup of the tea.

"I know it sounds strange," he finally admitted. "But I tell you in all truthfulness, *it does work!* I don't know exactly how the dark bread and tea interact, but they do in a way that brings relief to suffering women everywhere. It is nothing short of a miracle, I tell you."

 ## TRACE MINERALS FOR RELIEF

Several women locally here in the Salt Lake Valley have reported good results to me from using a couple of health products for their menopausal symptoms. They said that the Trascend for Women and Stress-X from Trace Minerals Research of Ogden, Utah, gave them much satisfaction for what had been troubling them. (See Product Appendix for more information.)

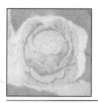

Natural Prozac Substitutes for Nervousness

"LONDON'S LORD MAYOR HAS PRESCRIPTIONS THAT
WORK"

🌿 BUSINESS AS USUAL SINCE 1189 A.D.

Decked out in a fur-trimmed scarlet gown and a black tricorn
hat with ostrich feathers, London's Lord Mayor Dr. John
Chalstrey waved to the crowds as he was paraded down Fleet
Street in an opulent horse-drawn carriage sometime in early
January, 1996.

To look at him adorned in all of his finery, one would hardly
suspect that he was the leader of one of the world's most important financial centers. But John Chalstrey, M.D., a surgeon by
training, is the highest-ranking public official in London's financial district, a one-square-mile area simply known as "the City."

When he isn't hopping from pageant to banquet, he overseas a 4,700-person bureaucracy that handles everything from street cleaning to tax collection. Other than the invention of paved roads and cars to pull floats on the parade routes, little of the ritual involved in the job has changed since the first lord mayor was elected in 1189 A.D. As some of the locals there put it, "It's been 'business as usual' with his lordship's position for well over 8 centuries now."

❦ RESEMBLANCE TO A MONTY PYTHON SKETCH

According to Tim Wright, a London-based vice president at the consulting firm Booz-Allen & Hamilton International Ltd., "the whole bloody system is right out of a Monty Python sketch." (For the uninformed, Monty Python was a very popular TV wit some years ago; his comedy troupe performed some of the most outrageous and ludicrous acts that kept millions of Brits laughing and faithfully glued to their "tellys" for many years (until they retired).

"The worshipful bottle washers wearing their big, funny hats," Mr. Wright went on to explain, "don't have anything to do with the serious things happening in London business. It's an anachronism for sure." Indeed, much of the lord mayor's one-year term is spent wearing medieval costumes while entertaining Lord and Lady So-and-So and assorted movers and shakers at an extravagant government-owned mansion. A black-and-gold robe is for banquets; a crimson velvet robe with an ermine cape is for receiving royalty. Sometimes, the lord mayor tops it all off with a scarlet hood called "the cap of dignity." (As his lordship explained to me by an overseas telephone call in early March, 1996, "I don't draw a salary, and must pay for nearly all of this regalia with my own funds.")

The work is also heavy on ritual. At a "silent ceremony" for the lord mayor's swearing-in, the incumbent passes a mace and sword to his successor in an intricate ceremony that involves "a lot of sitting, standing, and taking an assortment of hats on and off again." At some dinners, guests share the "Loving Cup," a huge glass of wine that is passed up and down long tables. One person drinks from the cup while another faces him and a third protects him from—get this—"being stabbed in the back" of all things!

🦎 "Good Health" to You

Upon assuming his office at the beginning of the year, Dr. Chalstrey decided it would be fitting to choose the theme of "Good Health" for his welcoming parade. "I urged the people not to labor so hard or for so many hours at a time," he told me by telephone. "Instead I encouraged them to learn how to relax more. I gave them some prescriptions for doing this, just as I've done with many of my patients over the years."

Here is a short list of Dr. Chalstrey's favorite methods of combating nervousness and stress. He said if they are faithfully followed, a person will feel less irritated and be able to enjoy life more.

R_x #1: SIP A WARM HERBAL TEA. Peppermint is the lord mayor's favorite tea, "brewed to perfection, and sipped with affection," as he good-naturedly put it. Other teas helpful for this are chamomile and lavender. "But they should always be taken *warm* in order to work," he emphasized.

R_x #2: DON'T FRET OVER LITTLE THINGS. "Learn to let the little things slide," he advised. "Otherwise, a person is in danger of wearing himself out over nothing." And as for the big things? "Well, they somehow always have a way of resolving themselves, don't they?" he reasoned aloud.

R_x #3: MIND THE MIND. "Take better care of your mind, or else it is apt to snap like a rubber band stretched too far," the good doctor noted. "Listen to quiet music. Read a good book. Stroll in the meadow. Or take a nap. But get your mind off of its anxiety. And stop worrying yourself to death, for heaven's sakes!"

R_x #4: KEEP THE SPIRIT IN SHAPE. Inside everyone of us, his lordship believes, there is an essence of spirit that needs to be nourished with religious things. "Keep the faith and hope of your spirit strong," he admonished, "and everything else will go along pretty well after that."

Nice Nails

"GIMME THAT OLD-TIME RELIGION AND GREAT-LOOKING NAILS"

❧ HER HUSBAND PASTORED SIX CHURCHES AT ONE TIME

Thelma Williams likes to tell folks that she's from "the *deep* South." "It's so deep, in fact, honey," she told me in a 1992 visit made at her home outside of Savannah, Georgia, "that you gotta use wading boots sometimes to get out here to visit us."

Her husband Isaac was fresh out of a Chicago seminary in the Spring of 1942, when he accepted a call to Georgia, where he pastored *six* churches *simultaneously*. "You heard right," Thelma reminded me, at the same time holding up half a dozen fingers as further proof. In order to cover his "parish" of churches, she continued, he followed a monthly schedule. Every Sunday morning, he attended Sunday School and conducted the service at a local church in one nearby community. Then he divided Sunday evenings between the two largest open country churches.

"On Sunday afternoons," she said, "my Isaac held one service per month at each of the other three churches. And whenever a fifth Sunday would pop up somewhere on the calendar, it was supposed to be his day off. But he usually found himself at one of the churches that needed some bolstering."

❧ GOOD NAILS ARE EVERYTHING

Even though her husband had a lot of responsibilities between these six churches, his income wasn't that great. So, Thelma went out to get some part-time work and ended up eventually becoming a professional manicurist. But beyond just trimming, filing, sandpapering, and polishing nails, she also became something of a "nail nutritionist" (a designation she invented to describe better what she did for a living).

"In my line of work, honey," she continued, "nails are everything. A woman may have the best looking outfit on in church, but if she has lousy nails, everyone will forget the dress and instead focus more on her fingernails." But in her self-appointed role this Georgia woman freely dispenses nutritional advice to her customers while caring for their cuticles.

"You want healthy nails?" she asked in a mocking tone. "Then you'd better eat high-protein foods." She listed egg yolks "from hens that have the pleasure of a rooster around them" as being one of the very best sources. "I tell my customers all the time to mix two tablespoons of a powdered protein mix with one glass of goat's milk and then to crack open 2 or 3 eggs and include their yolks in with it. Mix everything good by running it through a food blender and drink it for breakfast. Your nails will always look great with this healthy combo."

Thelma believes that "food is where it's at" when it comes to beautiful-looking nails. "I tell anyone who will listen to me," she continued, "to eat a bowl of cooked oatmeal for breakfast several times a week. Or have themselves a few slices of multi-grain bread in the form of regular toast or even French toast. Heck, a short stack of buckwheat pancakes will do the trick. Grains are good for the nails."

She discovered some years ago that two of the best food sources for *naturally* shiny nails were nuts and seeds. "Now them cashews, pecans, and walnuts not only make for good eating," she raved, "but have enough oils to give nails a natural kind of shine." When questioned in regard to certain nut butters, she momentarily hesitated before responding, then gave as her opinion that "as long as they're still nuts, they're probably okay to use that way." Munching on sunflower seeds helps to promote bright nails, too. And taking a teaspoon of sunflower or sesame seed oil for brief periods (2 weeks every month) would be of definite benefit.

🌱 SUPPLEMENT SECRETS

"Now that you've gotten all that down," my informant remarked off-handedly as I took notes of what she said, "let me give you something that *I know* works for a fact!" Thelma then told me about her three favorite supplements which, when taken *together*—"and *that's* the secret," she emphasized—virtually guarantee to give anyone "healthy new nails in a matter of months."

BREWER'S YEAST: 1 tsp. stirred into a glass of milk (goat's or soybean). "Has just about everything you need," she commented.

GELATIN: 1 tsp. Knox unflavored gelatin mixed in with the milk. "This is really the foundation where good nail care begins," she advised.

HORSETAIL: Empty the contents of 3 capsules of powdered horsetail herb into the milk with the other ingredients. "This is what 'cements' everything else together to make for terrific looking nails," she stated.

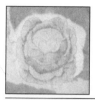

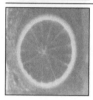

Old-Age Eyes Reversed

"NEW YORK BALLERINA KEEPS AGE FROM HER EYES"

✤ CRINKLES AROUND THE WRINKLES

Take wafer thin onion-skin paper, such as the kind frequently used in law and business for important documents, and crinkle a sheet of it several hundred times. You will eventually end up with something that's been pretty well used.

That's about the same thing that happens every time you open and close your eyes; this happens an estimated 30 times in a single minute, because I timed my own blinks to find out for sure. In a 16-hour waking day that's about 28,800 eyelids movements. Little wonder then that the paper-thin skin around the eyes becomes so crinkly and wrinkly after awhile.

❧ The Sun Her Worst Enemy

Natasha Oreznekov is a 50+ ballerina residing in New York City, who still manages to execute some beautiful moves on stage in spite of her age. "I may not do *Swan Lake* quite like I did 20 years ago," she said with a laugh, "but I definitely haven't lost my touch."

One day, about 15 years ago when looking in the mirror, she noticed crinkles starting to form around her eyes. At first she didn't give this much thought, until two months later she happened to focus again on the same area in the mirror. "It was then," she said, "that I realized for the very first time just how old I seemed to be getting."

She consulted with a licensed dermatologist in Manhattan, who told her that it was the sun that was doing this to her skin. "He said that lengthy exposure to sunlight in a big city was worse for me than if I was exposed to the same thing out in the country," she continued. "He maintained that because of air pollutants in the smog, more ultra-violet rays were getting through the ozone layers over large cities than they were in rural areas." And with her skin unprotected like it was, an "old age look" was setting in a lot faster than it usually took.

Her dermatologist recommended a particular brand of chemical-free sunscreen that was especially designed for the eye area; it had an SPF (sunscreen protection factor) of 15. He mentioned to her that products intended for this area of the face should be thick enough so that they don't run into the eyes following application. He suggested an additional safety factor: she was to give herself a no-sunscreen/no-moisturizer zone of about a quarter inch around the eyelashes themselves. This no-lotion zone around her eyelashes was soon protected with dark, polarizing, wraparound sunglasses.

After following these few simple procedures for a couple of months, she carefully reexamined herself in the mirror again, and was overjoyed to find that no additional crinkles had formed.

🎋 RUBBING YOUR EYES WILL MAKE YOU LOOK OLDER

One of Natasha's friends, a woman 59 years of age, had a long-standing eye allergy. She went to the dermatologist that this ballerina recommended. He informed her that she had to quit the habit of constantly rubbing her eyes. He informed her that the more she rubbed her eyes, the thicker would the skin become and the wrinkles would multiply.

Natasha's friend read in an herb book that parsley leaves were good for the eyes. So she procured for herself a bunch of parsley from one of the many Korean groceries dotting the five boroughs that make up greater New York City. She snipped two springs of fresh parsley with a pair of scissors into two cups boiling water, covered the small saucepan with a lid, and let the contents steep for 20 minutes. Then she strained the liquid out and allowed it to cool. Using an eyedropper, she dropped a tiny amount into each eye and rolled her eyeballs around to evenly distribute this weak parsley tea over their surfaces. She repeated this procedure every few hours or whenever her eyes felt itchy and she wanted to rub them.

This symptomatic relief caused her to discontinue her old habit of eye rubbing. Within a couple of months, she told Natasha that the skin around her eyes became less crinkly than before. She said people told her that she looked *five years younger* on account of this.

🎋 PUT IT ON TO TAKE OFF YEARS

Natasha also discovered an amazing thing, quite by accident."I found that by changing some of my makeup techniques, I was able to, literally, take off years from my face," she stated. "I now replace my mascaras every $2^1/_2$ months, because as they age, bacteria seems to grow more easily in them. And this buildup of germs always left my eyelids red and itchy, but now they aren't that way anymore."

When they did become inflamed, however, Natasha resorted to the application of cool milk compresses to them. "I would take several cotton balls and soak them in a little cool milk, then gently squeeze out the excess liquid, and put them over my closed eyelids for 10 minutes twice or three times a day. I noticed that whenever I did this the irritation would simply go away."

The dermatologist also pointed out to Natasha that with each passing year, she should shift her color palette and application method a little bit. Older eyes tend to look best when a woman stays with taupes and browns for the lid and a pale neutral under the brow bone. "The purpose of my eye color," Natasha told me, "is that as I get older it tends to add shape and definition rather than color alone." She now tends to avoid heavy frosts that could accentuate the crepey look of older eyelids.

Whenever she wants a little more definition, Natasha simply takes a deeper shade of brown and uses it on the outer corners of her eyes in the crease areas. "I just use a soft wash of color," she explained, as heavy shadowing closes the appearance of her eyes.

And for the smoothest application on slightly dry skin, an older woman should first prime the undereye area with moisturizer and concealer. The concealer should be used over the entire eyelid, however, as age tends to darken the pigment around the eyes.

Natasha laughed as she showed me, in detail, what she now does to her eyes to make herself look 5 to 7 years younger. "You'll know a lot more about eye makeup than you did before you came to my apartment," she said. "But it's doubtful you'll be able to use any of this information for yourself."

"I can use it in one of my books for my readers, though," I thoughtfully added.

Lining the eye becomes more difficult with the passing years, she declared. And it had nothing to do with dexterity either. It's just that applied incorrectly, eyeliner can accentuate bags or circles. "And that's the last thing a woman wants to show up," she mused. "The best thing I like to do is to dot the liner around my eyes and then smudge it a little. I use a pencil for its softer, smudgier look," she advised.

As the attractive ballerina that she still is, Natasha Oreznekov is a firm believer in the eye-popping, head-turning, lip whistling powers of mascara. But she applies this material only to her upper lashes. When she "put on her face" for my benefit, I noticed that she went a little heavier on the outer lashes. And for a little extra "opening tease" (as she playfully called it), Natasha curled her eyelashes, but didn't add any more mascara after doing this.

"My reasons for doing things this way," she concluded, "are very simple. I want to define and highlight my natural beauty, not to get a 'made up' look that hides it. This way, I'm actually giving the appearance of looking younger by keeping the appearances of old age from my eyes as long as I can."

Old Age "Fountain of Youth"

"WHAT SOME OF AMERICA'S FAMOUS OLD FOLKS ARE DOING TO STAY YOUNG"

"ON THE WRONG SIDE OF 30"

The great English satirist Jonathan Swift (1667-1745) is best remembered for his most famous work, *Gulliver's Travels* (1726), which was a keen satire upon cant and sham of courts, parties, and statesmen. In the last seven years of his life, he was increasingly lonely and haunted by a dread of insanity. From 1738 until his death he produced trivial, bitter, sometimes indecent works.

Among them was *Polite Conversation* in which he made an observation about a woman that doesn't seem very polite, even by the standards of his day. "I swear she's no chicken," wrote the acid-tongue cleric. "She's on the wrong side of 30, if she be a day."

One wonders just what he would think of Carol Channing, back on Broadway for the 1996 season starring in "Hello, Dolly!" at age 74. Or how would Swift view Julie Andrews, who had just turned twice the wrong side of 30 in 1995 and, night after night, as the star of "Victor Victoria," sung with stunning power and performed daring, athletic dances a year later.

HOW ON EARTH DID THEY DO IT?

Both Ms. Channing and Ms. Andrews are able to keep such rigorous performing schedules that demand a lot of physical energy, because they learned some years ago to take better care of their bodies. Both women watch their diets very carefully. They tend to eat more fruits, salads, whole grains, and prefer fish and chicken to beef or pork. Both avoid colas and soft drinks and opt for fruit and vegetable juices instead, some of which they make fresh every day and others they buy canned, bottled or packaged.

Exercise is very important for these ladies. Channing has been an advocate of hatha yoga for many years, and strongly believes that the stretching involved has kept her muscle tone in great shape. Furthermore, the meditation aspect of yoga tends to bring an inner peace to the soul and gentle calmness to the mind. This is important she says for maintaining a nice balance between your thoughts and feelings. Meditation every day helps to remove the cobwebs and gives the mind more clarity; it is the edge these ladies need late in life to carry out such demanding roles that ordinarily would go to other women on "the right side of 30."

OURS IS AN AGELESS AGE

The Dublin born Swift also once wrote: "Every man desires to live long, but no man would be old." But the 17th-century satirist would be astonished to find that nowadays no man or woman is old or need worry about admitting it.

Ours seems to be an ageless age. What proof for this? Consider the following several examples of men well past their prime, who still manage to carry out their different duties in capable ways.

At age 89, architect Philip Johnson has designed New York's most controversial skyscraper, "Gold Donald," a hotel and condo complex for Donald Trump on Central Park. At 92, theater caricaturist Al Hirschfeld attends every Broadway opening, puts in seven days a week at his drawing board and, since the death of his wife, has begun dating again. Poet Stanley Kunitz won the 1995 National Book Award at age 90 for *Passing Through*.

And what common secret do each of them share for still being so productive in the advanced years of life? You'll probably be surprised when I tell you. Each of these men pretty much gave the same answer when this very question was put to them. Architect Johnson noted that "I'm still able to do what I love doing the most." Artist Hirschfeld was of the opinion that "when I can't draw no more is when I die." And Poet Kunitz is grateful to the Almighty that his mind hasn't been debilitated yet by senility or Alzheimer's. "My greatest joy is poetry and the fact I can still write it is, I believe, what keeps me going."

In other words they're still able to do what they enjoy the most. Their bodies and minds allow them to perform to the maximum limit without serious restrictions on what they want to do. Their mortal vehicles work well enough to let them fulfill the creative desires of their inner spirits. But once something starts to give out and they're no longer able to do as well, then they think the end will have finally come for them. But until that moment does arrive, they intend to "seize the moment," and make every precious minute count with the wonderful opportunities still remaining for them.

THE POLITICIAN AND THE BOXER: WHAT DO THEY HAVE IN COMMON?

Anyone of a conservative mold will likely cheer this next fellow's name, while those of a more liberal bent might tend to send a few boos and hisses his way. I'm speaking, of course, about U.S. Senator Strom Thurmond (R-S.C.), who turned 94 in 1996 and announced that he would run for public office *again* for the umpteenth time. This becomes even more amazing when we consider that 13 of his much younger colleagues—such as Sam Nunn, Nancy Kassebaum, Alan Simpson, Bill Bradley, and Mark Hatfield—stated to the media in 1995 their intentions of giving up the legislative grind when their terms ended the following year. Thurmond is probably most remembered for his efforts to get abortion outlawed in America and to have homosexuality declared a criminal offense.

Boxer George Foreman, on the other hand, celebrated his 48th birthday in 1996. He is almost *half* of Thurmond's age, but considered by everyone in the boxing world to be "an old man" as he edges towards mid-century. But he set this sport on its ear the year before by regaining the heavyweight championship of the world, more than 20 years after he lost it. More incredible is the fact that just about all of his sparring partners these days weren't even born when he won the heavyweight gold medal at the 1968 Olympics in Mexico City.

Some 46 years separate Thurmond and Foreman. Their lifestyles are completely different as day and night. The senator is ultraconservative, while the boxer is somewhat more liberal in his views. One is very intolerant, while the other exhibits greater tolerance for others. One is close-minded, but Mr. Foreman is quite open-minded, even on some things he may not always agree with. The former is a crusty curmudgeon and has earned a reputation for orneriness; the latter, however, is quite good-natured, something of a practical joker at times, and fun to be around.

So with all of these stark differences, just exactly what do they have in common with each other? In a word, it is their *unshakeable* faith. Both enjoy reading their bibles, are devout churchmen, and engage themselves in prayer quite often. They're also strong family men and take the high road of moral virtues. Each of them has been interviewed on separate occasions by various reporters, who've probed into their religious sides. And both of them have stated in no uncertain terms, but in different ways, that they owe much of their present successes late in their careers to the *spiritual strength* within them. It is impossible, they argued, to get very far along in life, with everything pretty much still intact, and not have some kind of reasonable spirituality about you. They insisted that life cannot go on for very long without the spiritual dimension being present in some form. They felt that being active in some kind of religion helps to take the edge off of life in general, and renews not only the spirit but also the body just enough in order to keep carrying on.

🌿 WHY DO SOME MEDIA PEOPLE RARELY SEEM ANY OLDER?

Faces we are used to seeing and voices we frequently hear week after week on the broadcast waves seldom ever seem any older. It's almost as if they were frozen in time. They've been with us for so long now that it sometimes appears we've aged faster while they've remained younger.

In 1996, David Brinkley and Hugh Downs each turned 75, while Mike Wallace, Paul Harvey, and Andy Rooney hit 78. And Barbara Walters still looked pretty darned good at 65.

What I'm about to tell you could very well surprise you. In fact, it may even astound you! These half dozen media personalities have managed, either purposefully or unwittingly, to actually *slow down* the aging process. Is it some liquid elixir they gulp down or some miracle cream they rub on their skin every night, which has brought this about? Certainly not!

The "secrets" (if they can be called that) to their remarkable and resilient youthfulness lie in their diets. But they're still not what you think they might be. Oh sure, some of them eat healthy and organic most of the time; but a few of them indulge their appetites in things that wouldn't be considered exactly nutritious by those of us concerned about good health habits.

What it is they do right, however, is to eat *more frequently* throughout the day. Thus, their regular "meals" become more like snacks and are spaced apart about every 3 hours. The other thing they do is to have a *minimal* intake of fried and deep-fried foods. Scientists now know that one of the big factors which strongly influences the aging process is free radicals. These are scavenger molecules freely circulating throughout our systems, causing biological havoc and cellular deterioration wherever they roam. And foods that are fried or deep-fried happen to have *the most* free radicals in them, because of how they are cooked.

A third and final element with these six people is that they enjoy using spices a lot in whatever they prepare or have prepared for them. Spices are great antioxidants and, as such, sharply curtail the activity of free radicals within the body. The most preferred spices these broadcasters seem to lean towards are garlic, onion, rosemary, sage, thyme, basil, and tarragon.

THE DAY IS FAST APPROACHING WHEN MIDDLE-AGE WILL BE 70 OR 80

One of our nation's most famous documents, the Declaration of Independence, was formally adopted by representatives of the Thirteen Colonies in North America on July 4, 1776. But unfortunately, while our forefathers were declaring their freedom from Great Britain, they weren't living very long to enjoy the glorious fruits of their patriotic labors. You see, back then, life expectancy in the newly declared republic was a mere 35 years at most! During the Civil War over 80 years later, it had only nudged up to 40.

Today, however, things present a much different picture so far as what age can be achieved by each of us. The National Institute on Aging notes that people over 85 constitute the nation's fastest-growing age group.

Men and women "of an age," as the novelist Henry James delicately referred to the more mature members of his stratified society in the 19th century, no longer quietly fade away. More than any other age group, people over 50 spend more in the supermarket, watch more television, listen to more radio, read magazines and newspapers more , and wrote more letters to the editor and congressional representatives. They also tend to buy more luxury automobiles, gamble more in Las Vegas or Atlantic City, and certainly dominate the cruise and upscale vacation markets.

The cosmetics and fashion industries are pushing trendy new lines for older customers. Banks welcome their loans and mortgages. Hotels and resorts woo them with generous discounts. And politicians have learned to listen more carefully to them.

"Youth," noted the Irish poet and wit Oscar Fingal O'Flahertie Wills Wilde (better known as Oscar Wilde, 1854–1900), "is America's oldest tradition." But these days old age is starting to become more of America's newest myth instead. More of us are viewing old age as something that happened to people long ago, but not anymore. In just a few years from now, middle-age will start being for those in their 70s and 80s, rather than in their 50s and 60s as it still is at present.

 ## SOME WAYS TO SLOW DOWN YOUR BIOLOGICAL CLOCK

I might not be able to literally "turn back the clock" and give you any of the younger years you've lost, but I certainly can *slow* things down a great deal so that whatever time remains doesn't tick away so fast anymore. A summary of the things learned in this section will provide you with some valuable guidelines in what to do so you don't grow old so quickly.

The following list follows a somewhat unusual numerical order. Instead of the usual 1 through 7 count, I've reversed things. And also added a bunch of zeroes behind these numbers to reflect an *actual countdown* in the years that remain for you. So, that by my calculations, if you follow what is given here, you will probably feel and act with the wonderful exuberance that belongs to a kid of ten, when you've hit *middle-age at about seventy!*

TURNING BACK YOUR BIOLOGICAL CLOCK
FROM AGE 70 TO 10

Reverse Aging Down to 70: CONSUME MORE LEAFY STUFF, FRUITS, AND CEREAL GRAINS, AND EAT *LESS* MEAT.

Reverse Aging Down to 60: EXERCISE BY STRETCHING. AND PUT THE MIND IN HIATUS WITH SOME DAILY MEDITATION.

Reverse Aging Down to 50: CONTINUE DOING WHAT YOU ENJOY DOING THE MOST. AND KEEP YOURSELF REASONABLY FIT SO YOU CAN DO IT.

Reverse Aging Down to 40: MAINTAIN BALANCE IN YOUR LIFE WITH SUFFICIENT ATTENTION BEING GIVEN TO THE SPIRITUAL DIMENSION. A BELIEF IN DIVINE PROVIDENCE AND ACTIVELY STUDYING HOLY WRIT SEEM TO HELP MANY OF THE VERY ELDERLY LIVE LONGER.

Reverse Aging Down to 30: EAT SMALLER MEALS MORE FREQUENTLY THROUGHOUT THE DAY. AND LEARN TO SNACK MORE OFTEN ON HEALTHY *RAW* FOODS.

Reverse Aging Down to 20: MINIMIZE YOUR INTAKE OF FRIED AND DEEP-FRIED FOODS. LEARN TO COOK THEM BY BOILING, BAKING, STEAMING, OR POACHING WHATEVER YOU EAT.

Reverse Aging Down to 10:   ROUTINELY SEASON YOUR FOOD WITH HEALTH-GIV-ING AND FLAVORFUL HERBS. NOT ONLY WILL THEY MAKE THINGS TASTE A LOT BET-TER, BUT THEY WILL ALSO ADD MORE SPICE TO YOUR LIFE.

My Own Daily Supplement Program for Youth Restoration

During the weekend of March 15–17, 1996 I was in Anaheim, California attending the annual Natural Products West Expo being held in part of the sprawling Anaheim Convention Center. During that time I must have had half a dozen or more health food retailers—all of them women by the way—who compli-mented me on how "young" my skin looked. They concluded that I had some of the best-looking skin they had ever seen on a man. I mention this fact in passing, not out of vanity, but as a basis for the information to be given here.

Each of these ladies, ranging in age from the early twenties to the late sixties, wanted to know what I took in order to have such fantastic skin tone and texture. (Lest the reader think that all of me looks like a kid at age 50, I must hasten to insert here the fact that I have *a lot* of gray hair, am balding in the middle of my head, and have worn glasses ever since I became a teenag-er. But aside from these "aging" drawbacks, I *do* indeed enjoy very youthful skin.) Here's what I told them of *how* I've man-aged to accomplish this.

First of all, I *stay out of the sun* or else wear protective head and eye gear and the appropriate clothing (no shorts) to keep my skin from getting baked and tanned like leather. Believe it or not, I *don't* put much faith in sunscreen products and seldom ever use them. Instead, I take on a regular basis one tablespoon of extra virgin olive oil or Rex's Wheat Germ Oil. (This last product can be ordered for $65 from Anthropological Research Center, P.O. Box 11471, Salt Lake City, UT 84147.) When I travel to foreign climes where the weather is incessantly hot, I always bring some of this oil with me and take it faithfully.

It has been my experience that this oil, when taken *internally*, not only keeps my skin supple and resilient, but somehow manages to keep the sun's ultraviolet rays from damaging its surface. Thus, after some two decades of time spent in many countries encompassing the equator, I am still pretty much wrinkle-free and have skin as soft as that of a baby's.

Second, I *do not* use any kind of toiletries on my skin except for simple shaving cream or lathered soap. I discovered early on in my adulthood that aftershave lotions, colognes, and even underarm deodorants take a toll on the skin's health, that can eventually lead to roughness and dryness. I am also not one to use shampoos on my hair, but instead wash it with ordinary soap. I take a good shower every day, which nicely eliminates the problem of any body odor. I also try to watch what I eat so as to hold any odor to a minimum.

Third, I attribute my healthy skin to a simple diet, at least so far as breakfast and dinner are concerned. Those meals are pretty predictable and uneventful; some might even describe them as very boring. I have eaten a large bowl of cooked oatmeal with milk for breakfast every morning for the last 40 years or more. And in the late evening, say around 9 P.M., I have relied upon a bowl of dried cereal and milk to suffice for my dinner. I mix together shredded wheat and a little granola for crunchiness and pour over this mixture some raw, whole milk (when I can find it). Otherwise, I use regular, store-bought milk or sometimes opt for goat's milk.

My big meal of the day is always lunch, which I take anywhere from 12 noon to 2 P.M. It varies from day to day what I eat, but usually includes some kind of meat, except chicken or turkey which I believe greatly contributes to the cause of cancer. (See my article "The Case Against Chickens: People Who Live in Cultures That Do Not Eat Them, Don't Get Cancer!" in the Spring 1993 issue of *Folk Medicine Journal* for more information on the reasons for abstaining from poultry. You can order a reprint of this by sending $10 to: Anthropological Research Center, P.O. Box 11471, Salt Lake City, UT 84147. Be sure to specify that you want the "chicken article" when you order.)

The final part of my own "old age" prevention program for younger looking skin and more youthful feeling, is a simple supplement program that I devised myself and which has worked for hundreds of others to whom it has been recommended. Below is a list of the things I take every day without fail. These and maintaining a happy heart and care-free spirit have given me, what I believe to be, a restored youthfulness in every sense of the word.

Dr. Heinerman's Personal Anti-Aging Supplement Program

12-16 tablets of Pines Wheat Grass Juice

3 capsules Kyolic EPA Garlic (Wakunaga)

3 capsules Ginkgo Biloba Plus (Wakunaga)

3 capsules Kyo-Ginseng (Wakunaga)

2 tablets multiple vitamin (Native American Nutrition)

2 tablets multiple mineral (Native American Nutrition)

2 tablets Super C (Native American Nutrition)

(Consult the Product Appendix for more information on where to obtain these fine products.)

The other part of my Personal Anti-Aging Program consists of a simple vegetable drink that I take 3 to 5 times a week. I make it up in my office and it requires a Vita-Mix blender (call 1-800-VITAMIX or see the Product Appendix for more information on this superior juicer).

Youth Restoration Beverage

1 tablespoon liquid Kyolic Aged Garlic Extract

1 cup chilled tomato juice

2 tablespoons Pines Mighty Greens drink powder

1 teaspoon Pines Beet Root Juice powder

1 cup peppermint tea, cold

¹/₂ cup fresh spinach leaves, finely cut

1 cup ice cubes

Place all ingredients in a blender container in their given order. Secure the lid. Blend on HIGH speed until smooth. Drink immediately. Yield: 2¹/₂ cups.

Looking at Old Age with Good Humor

In my two-decade-long study of people who've lived to be 100 years or older, I've found that most of them had a pretty good sense of humor. I honestly think that when the heart is light and the spirit happy, the body tends to last a lot longer than it would where anxiety, depression, or stress constantly exist.

The following two items are both from unknown authors. But they do help us to look at old age in a rather jocular way, so that when the inevitable does arrive for each of us we don't take it too seriously.

I'm Fine in Spite of Myself

There is nothing the matter with me.
I'm just as healthy as can be.
I have arthritis in my knees;
And when I talk, I talk with a wheeze.

My pulse is weak and my blood is thin,
But I'm awfully well for the shape I'm in.

My teeth will eventually have to come out;
And my diet, I have to think about.
I'm overweight and I can't get thin,
But I'm awfully well for the shape I'm in.

Arch supporters I have for my feet,
Or I wouldn't be able to walk on the street.
Sleep is denied me night after night,
And every morning, I'm a fright.
My memory's failing, my head's in a spin,
I'm practically living on aspirin,
But I'm awfully well for the shape I'm in.

How do I know my youth has been spent?
'Cause my get-up-and-go has got-up-and-went.
But in spite of all this I'm able to grin
When I think where my get-up-and-go has been.

Old Age is Golden, I've heard it said,
But sometimes I wonder, as I go to bed . . .
My ears in a drawer, my teeth in a cup,
My eyes on a shelf, until I get up.
As sleep dries my eyes, I say to myself,
"Is there anything else I should put on the shelf?

When I was young, my slippers were red,
I could kick my heels clear over my head;
When I grew older my slippers were blue,
But I still could dance the whole night through.
Now I'm old and my slippers are black,
I walk to the corner and puff myself back.
The reason I know my youth has been spent,
My get-up-and-go has got-up-and-went.

I get up in the morning, and dust off my wits,
Pick up the "Amsterdam"* and read the obits;
If my name is missing, I know I'm not dead,
So I eat a good breakfast and go back to bed.

*Generic name for any daily newspaper.

THE WORTH OF THE ELDERLY AND THEIR FRIENDS

Remember, old folks are worth a small fortune. They have *silver* in their hair, *gold* in their teeth, *stones* in their kidneys, *lead* in their feet, and *gas* in their stomachs.

I have become a little older since I saw you last. A few changes have come into my life since then.

Frankly, I have become quite a famous old gal. I am seeing five gentlemen every day. As soon as I wake up *Will Power* helps me get out of bed. Then I go see *John* first thing. Awhile later *Charlie Horse* comes along; when he is here he takes a lot of my time and attention. After he leaves, *Arthur Ritis* shows up and stays all day. But he doesn't like to remain in one place for very long, so he takes me from joint to joint. After such a busy day, I'm usually quite exhausted and retire to bed with *Ben Gay*. What an exciting life I lead!

Oh, by the way. The preacher came by yesterday and said that at my age, I should be thinking about the Hereafter. I told him, "Why, reverend, I do that all the time, no matter where I'm at. If I'm in the parlor or upstairs, in the kitchen or even down in the basement, I'm constantly asking myself: 'What am I here after?'"

Optimism for Osteoporosis

"DIET AS A FIRST LINE OF DEFENSE, PREVENTION, AND TREATMENT"

 SOME ALTERNATIVE APPROACHES

Virginia M. Soffa is Director of the Breast Cancer Action Group in Burlington, Vermont. She is also the author of *The Journey Beyond Breast Cancer.* During 1996 she was working on her doctorate in human science at Saybrook Institute.

She provided some practical information on osteoporosis which my readers and I are indebted to her for. She uses a logical approach in assuming that it isn't so much what you *have* to take that matters, but what you probably *shouldn't* be taking that counts the most! In her view meat is the real culprit when it comes to loss of bone mass in menopausal women. She cited a study from Susan M. Lark's book, *The Estrogen Decision: A Self-Help Program* (Los Altos, Calif: Westchester Publishing, 1994; p. 140) that compared the incidence of osteoporosis in meat-eating women with that in vegetarians. The difference in bone density after age 60 was dramatic. Vegetarian women lost 18% of their bone mass, while meat-eating women lost 35%.

❧ CALCIUM AND VITAMIN D

A diet rich in calcium and vitamin D definitely protects against osteoporosis. Ms. Soffa cites seaweed as being "one of the richest sources of calcium." Seaweed such as kelp or dulse "is full of minerals that help to create and maintain bone mass" and "has the ability to bind high reactive biological compounds, called free radicals." Seaweed can be consumed regularly in the form of a salad, a vegetable side-dish, condiment, or seasoning, she insisted.

Not one to forget land-based vegetation, she mentioned "dark green, leafy vegetables such as kale, collards, beet greens, cabbage, brussels sprouts, and broccoli" as being especially high in calcium. Other sources besides these, she continued, "include artichoke, eggplant, and most kinds of beans, fish, berries, raisins, and some grains." And while dairy products may admittedly be high in calcium, they also contain protein and saturated fat, which she thinks could aggravate existing osteoporosis.

Vitamin D can be obtained from food, vitamin supplements, and activation of the provitamin 7-dehydrocholesterol in the skin. Egg yolk, organ meats like liver, and bone meal are common sources for small and variable amounts of this nutrient. Fish and fish oils are even better sources for it: salmon, mackerel, tuna, and sardines (all canned) can yield anywhere from 300 to 500 I.U. of vitamin D.

Exposure to sunshine or ultraviolet irradiation will cause the provitamin 7-dehydrocholesterol, which occurs in the skin and in the blood, to be transformed into vitamin D. The amount that can be synthesized by this method remains unknown. Atmospheric smoke and fog, window glass, clothing, and skin pigmentation limit the skin's exposure to ultraviolet light. In the

United States, exposure varies with the season; sunlight reaches its greatest intensity in the summer and is least in December.

 ## Estrogen Replacement Therapy

Estrogen should be started by a woman soon after her menopause ends, since bone loss usually accelerates at that time. There are certain herbs that, when used together at *different times* throughout a 24-hour period, can be just as effective as regular estrogen therapy. I've compiled a list of my favorites in the following table and give the best times, forms, and amounts for taking them.

Phytoestrogenic Herbs

Plants	Forms	Times
Alfalfa	Capsule (4–6)	Morning
	Tea (1–2 cups)	Morning
Black Cohosh	Tincture (15 drops)	Evening
	Capsule (2–3)	Late Morning
Chaste Tree	Tea (1 cup)	Afternoon
Dong-Quai/Tang Kuei	Capsule (4)	Mid-Morning
	Tea (1 cup)	Late Afternoon
Fenugreek	Tea (1 cup)	Afternoon
	Capsule (3)	Evening
Ginseng	Tea (1 cup)	Evening
	Tincture (20 drops)	Evening
	Capsule (4)	Any Time
Pomegranate	Fruit	Mid-Afternoon
Red Clover	Tea (1–2 cups)	Morning
	Capsule (5)	Morning
Stinging Nettle	Tea (2 cups)	Mid-Morning
	Capsule (4)	Afternoon
Wild Yam	Capsule (4)	Forenoon
	Tea (1 cup)	Forenoon
	Tincture (15 drops)	Forenoon

🌿 MODERATE EXERCISE

Leisure walking for 25 minutes twice a day can help to diminish loss of bone mass. *At all times* remember to take a magnesium:calcium ratio that is 2:1—the ideal would be 1200 mg. of magnesium to 600 mg. calcium. Also, take 4 tablets daily of a product called Arth-X Plus from Trace Minerals Research. It really helps to prevent the depletion of minerals from the body that are critical to bone formation (phosphorus and particularly calcium). (See Product Appendix for more data.)

(See also FRAILNESS PREVENTION and HEALTHY BONES.)

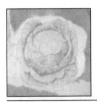

Physical Inactivity Corrections

"93-YEAR-OLD GRANNY GETS FUN OUT OF LIFE SITTING IN A (SKI LIFT) CHAIR"

🌺 Is This Granny Off Her Rocker or What?

At an age when most of her contemporaries are sitting at home somewhere quietly knitting or watching TV, 93-year-old Luella Seeholzer of Logan, Utah is having loads of fun sitting in another kind of chair. When winter comes to Logan Canyon each year, dumping its fluffy white stuff in great abundance on the nearby peaks, this feisty little lady takes off for Beaver Mountain to have some fun.

"I especially love riding up and down these slopes in the chair lifts," she told me one wintry afternoon in mid-January 1996. Her family has owned the ski resort there since 1937, making it the oldest ski area in America continuously operated by the same people. Her late husband, Harold, started the resort with the help of some friends and Logan City.

"Our very first cable lift," she noted, "was driven on a water wheel by a drive-train salvaged from a junked 1936 Buick. Because there wasn't any spur road off the Logan Canyon highway in those times, skiers needed to hike from the road up here."

These days, though, three lifts with a capacity of 2,600 skiers per hour serve the growing numbers of Cache Valley skiers. Skiers are now able to utilize 22 runs, eight of which are rated as for beginners, 12 as expert, and two as intermediate.

In an era of huge, sprawling resorts, skiing Beaver Mountain is like stepping back to the old days when family-run ski areas like Snowbasin, Brighton, and Alta (other Utah ski facilities) consisted of a few simple lifts and a day lodge. Frills were few and prices exceptionally low. With a $20 all-day pass, Beaver Mountain still ranks as one of the least expensive ski areas in the nation. The bargain carries through to the day lodge, where hamburgers cost less than $2.

"I try to get up here once a week to check on things," Ms. Seeholzer said in her typical matter-of-fact way. "Many of these younger skiers tend to give me long stares, wondering what on earth I'm doing up here anyhow," she said with a throaty cackle. "They think I'm nuts for being out here. But, do you know what I tell 'em? I tell 'em I wouldn't have it any other way."

This incredible granny loves the slopes like you wouldn't believe. "Downhill is the only way to go, once you've reached the top," she chuckles. "How else are you going to get down?" She said that skiing "keeps me fit, keeps my bones limber, and my muscles in shape. It is the most exhilarating feeling you could ever experience. I don't feel old when I'm up here, doing what I love most. But when I'm down in the city at my home or around some of my friends near my age, then's when I start feeling old again. Age is a state of being; it's all in your mind and just how you see yourself," she shouted, as she pushed off on her skis to check out some newly fallen powder.

How One 78-Year-Old Grandpa Manages to Keep Up with His Grandkids

I've known Robert "Bob" E. Crandall for almost 8 years now. He is a prominent Utah businessman and owns a historic land-mark—the Crandall Building—in downtown Salt Lake City. On Tuesday, January 30, 1996, I sat down with my friend, who was born in 1918, to find out what his "secrets" were for staying so physically active in the advanced years of life.

"My forefathers on my mother's side of the family," he began, "lived into their late 80s and 90s. My grandfather died at age 93 and had good health until just two years prior to his own demise. My grandmother died at age 89. My father's sister lived to be over 100 years old. So I guess you might say that 'good genes' run in our family.

"None of my forebearers, father or mother, ever used tobacco or drank alcoholic drinks of any kind. I have never used tobacco products or used alcohol myself. And I've been very careful about working in areas where tobacco smoke used to be present.

"I have generally been physically active all of my life. In high school I loved to swim, play tennis, go hiking in the mountains, and snow and water ski. I have always maintained a healthy interest in boating, tennis, golf, and walking. I also routinely do exercises at home. I average about 40 pushups every morning and spend 20 minutes or so on my Health Rider (a mechanical exercise unit) four times a week. I love gardening and working in the yard, be it spring, summer, fall or winter.

"I've always tried to maintain prudent eating habits. I always try and eat three balanced meals every day. For breakfast I usu-ally have a small glass of orange juice, half of a grapefruit, cooked cereal such as oatmeal, six grain cereal, or cream of wheat, two slices of whole wheat stoneground toast (delicious bread which my wife bakes every week for us), and a glass of 1% milk.

"For lunch I usually have a stoneground whole wheat sand-wich with tuna fish or cheese, a banana and an apple or some other type of fruit. I try not to overeat at midday, unless some-one comes along (looking over in my direction) who himself likes to eat and takes me out to a big lunch somewhere. Then I

get stuffed, which I don't think is good for someone my age."
Here he paused momentarily in his narrative and asked this curious question: "John, are you going to be truthful and identify yourself in your book as the one being guilty of causing me to overeat sometimes?" I gave no reply; we both enjoyed a good laugh, and he continued with the interview.

"At dinner I eat a cooked meat with a salad. This is about 2 or 3 ounces of lean meat, cooked vegetables, baked or mashed potatoes, and a non-fattening dessert. The meat my wife Evelyn fixes can be either a small [New York] strip or T-bone steak, a small pot roast or nice roast chicken sometimes. We periodically eat fish, but not that often. Evelyn will vary our vegetables—sometimes they may be frozen (corn, peas, beans, mixed vegetables), at other times fresh (broccoli, asparagus spears), or even in season (succotash and various squashes). Desserts are always simple: whole-wheat raisin cookies or some kind of Betty Crocker cake.

"I regularly eat three meals a day, but generally try to restrict my calories to not more than 2,000. My serum cholesterol has always stayed near 196 milligrams, which is pretty good my doctor tells me.

"Although I have had periods of stress in my life, I have always been optimistic as a rule. I've tried to look for the best in others and have been contented with my lot in life. I've never tried to want more than what was necessary to have in order to be comfortable. I've always lived within my means and have never incurred short- or long-term debts beyond my ability to repay them. I think that has kept me from having a lot of financial worries.

"And during the few crises that I have had in my life, I've been able to handle such reverses fairly well. I had almost back-to-back tragedies within a little over a year of each other. In January, 1962 my first son suddenly died at the precious age of 6. Then in March of the following year, this entire building sustained major water damage due to the top of the roof burning off. But my optimism held firm and carried me through both ordeals with very little anxiety. It's hard to describe what I mean by this, John. But I think what I'm trying to say is my contentment with life and hopeful outlook on things has always sustained me, even in trying circumstances like these.

"Being with my family has always been central to my contentment. I take two or three short vacations a year with Evelyn and some of our kids. We try and include as many of the grandkids as we can on any of them. And we always have the grandkids over for birthdays, holidays, and other special occasions. They know me as the 'fun grandpa,' because I will participate in many of the things that they like to do. Some of the older ones have wondered how their grandpa manages to keep up with them. I believe it's all in the way you live your life."

Bob Crandall has been in the insurance business for many years, being associated with The Lincoln National Life Insurance Co. of Ft. Wayne, Indiana since September 1947. He is a graduate of Harvard Business School and a licensed CLU and ChFc in insurance. He and his wife reside in a modest home on the east bench of Salt Lake City and live very frugally.

Prostate Potentials

"FOR MEN ONLY: VALUABLE TIPS ON HAVING A HEALTHY PROSTATE"

A 'HUSHED UP' AILMENT

Former U.S. President Ronald Reagan had two of them. But 1996 U.S. Republican Presidential contender Senator Robert Dole only had one of them. What did both of these fellows have in common that is shared by some 135,000 other men in America every year? It is some type of prostate difficulty that invariably strikes many men, sooner or late, past the age of forty.

But, because men (and their male doctors) simply don't want to talk about it in public, this remains one of the least known of our national health problems. Yet, the facts beg for it to be given greater attention: prostate disorders affect 60% of adult males over the age of 50, with prostate cancer being the number one cancer killer of American men throughout the 1990s.

I talked to one psychologist specializing in the psychic traumas induced by major health problems within the system, as to why it wasn't being discussed more often. He was of the firm opinion that prostate troubles bring most men to the sudden and unhappy realization that they are simply getting older. And most men just don't like to face up to this reality check and admit that it is so. Hence, they choose the easy way out and avoid mentioning it altogether. Another factor, which he felt went right along with this was what he termed the "sexual dimension." "Look," he observed, "the prostate gland produces liquid semen and, therefore, is readily identifiable with sexuality. So, if you tell a guy there's something wrong with his tool down there, he might suddenly suffer a severe drop in his macho self-esteem. He will either want to push it out of his mind or maybe punch out the lights of the doctor who just informed him of a problem down there in that area."

❧ WHAT TO DO FOR PROSTATITIS

Prostatitis is merely an inflammation of the prostate. Attending symptoms include low back pain, fever, pain on defecation and cloudy urine. Three specific types of prostatitis include:

1. The acute bacterial type, which is an infection that often originates in the urinary tract.

2. The chronic bacterial kind, which is a symptom frequently denoted by recurrent bladder infection.

3. The chronic nonbacterial form (and prostatodynia), which are two very similar problems with a cause that's not easy to find, thereby making it hard to treat.

Over the years through much trial-and-error, I've had ample opportunities to develop a fairly reasonable supplement program for treating prostatitis. Much of it involves the use of reliable botanicals, which have never yet failed to clear the condition up eventually. The length of time it takes to do this and the success rate depend largely upon the age of the man, his diet, mating habits, work pattern, and so forth, and will obviously vary from man to man as the case may be.

But, generally speaking, the nutrition program I've managed to test on hundreds of men, who've inquired of me through the years what herbs to take for this condition, has proven to be extremely successful with only a small number (probably no more than 15%) of failures ever reported. The list below represents a concise form of it and may be used to good advantage for as long as is necessary.

Nutrition Program for the Prostate

DAILY MAINTENANCE SCHEDULE

1 tablespoon of Pines Mighty Greens superfood blend. It is *the single best* product for the health of a man's prostate that I know of. It contains 27 different botanicals, vegetables, and other natural substances. It was introduced by Pines International at the Natural Products Expo West convention in Anaheim in March, 1996 and became an instant, runaway hit with the health food industry. It is best mixed with 8 oz. of purified water or juice and can be taken alone or with a meal. (See Product Appendix for more information.)

1 teaspoon of Wakunaga's liquid Kyolic Garlic Extract. There is no finer garlic preparation in the world than the one manufactured by Wakunaga Pharmaceutical Company of Hiroshima, Japan and distributed by Wakunaga of America Co., Ltd. Just add it to the Mighty Greens drink blend and stir thoroughly. (See Product Appendix for more information.)

7 drops of ConcenTrace from Trace Minerals Research. This is the most potent way to obtain life-giving trace elements from Utah's own inland sea, namely the Great Salt Lake. Add the drops to the Mighty Greens blend and stir before drinking. (See Product Appendix for more information.)

About 50,000 I.U. Vitamin A (fish-oil derived). There occurred early on in my research for the "perfect" prostate nutrition program, a fact that I don't believe other medical researchers have looked at very much. In my worldwide wanderings and travels for little known or as yet undiscovered health secrets, I began noticing that men in traditional fishing cultures (such as the Eskimo) or who worked on fishing trawlers and consumed an inordinate amount of fish were hardly ever bothered with prostate problems. This set me to wondering if the vitamin A in fish oil might have something to do with this. Further research turned up the evidence I was looking for, but not exactly in the way I had hoped to find it. Vitamin A from fish *does* work to keep the prostate in a healthy condition, but not so good if taken in capsules. Rather, the vitamin A must be obtained *directly* from the fish oil itself to do any good. So, while I mentioned a suggested daily intake for it, a man is much better off taking some kind of *fish oil* daily. *One-half teaspoon is adequate.* Fish oils that would be the most readily available for this are: cod liver oil (remember that stuff from our childhood days? yecchh!); salmon or tuna oils (both drained from the cans they're packed in); and, believe it or not, *sardine* oil from the same source!

One tablespoon of Rex's Wheat Germ Oil. Still the best source around for all of your vitamin E needs. And the most potent by far! The can label says that it's only for animal consumption, but don't worry about that. I've been taking the stuff myself for many years now, along with my father and brother and hundreds of other men to whom it has been recommended, and we're all still alive and kicking without any side effects. Because it is exceedingly difficult to find, you may want to order a quart from our research center, which carries it only as a convenience to readers of my different books in which it is always recommended. Send $65 to: Anthropological Research Center, P.O. Box 11471, Salt Lake City, UT 84147.

3,500 mg. Vitamin C. Yeh, yeh, I know—you're probably thinking I'm recommending any brand from your local health food store. But were the full truth of the matter known, nearly all of the vitamin C products on the market today aren't worth crossing the street for, let alone to be taking. There are only a couple of brand exceptions to this rule. One of the best out there in the market place, with natural ingredients you can trust, is a vitamin C product made by Native American Nutrition (a subsidiary of Pines International (see

Product Appendix for further details). You're better off getting your daily vitamin C rations from *fresh* citrus juices, *fresh* berries and berry juices, and chlorophyll-rich vegetable juices. The Vita-Mix Corporation, which offers the public an outstanding juice machine, includes a large recipe book with many creative ideas for making delicious juices that are high in this very important nutrient. (See Product Appendix for details.)

Other Supplements. Through the years German urologists have routinely prescribed for their many prostate patients saw palmetto and echinacea (two capsules each a day) with relatively good results. Other useful botanicals include hops tea (1 cup) or capsules (3) and kava kava capsules (2) from Nature's Way.

The foregoing program is well suited for any type of prostate disorder, but has been especially adapted to the needs of those suffering from prostatitis. Above all else, a man thus afflicted should remember to implore His Creator for divine assistance in the healing process. That's precisely what the gift of faith is for!

🌿 Assistance for an Enlarged Prostate

In healthy men, the prostate is a small glandular organ located at the point of transition from the bladder to the urethra. But as men approach sixty, many of them tend to experience a strange enlargement of it. The fancy medical terminology for such a problem is benign prostatic hypertrophy (BPH) or adenoma of the prostate.

It is a progressive thing and may even halt sometimes at any point in its slow development. In other cases, however, it usually proceeds along at snail's pace for several decades before the problem finally becomes evident. The most likely symptom to be noticed is an inability to pass urine. At this point, urologists generally recommend surgery. But there are better ways to address the matter, than subjecting a poor fellow to an operation of such serious consequences. In fact, doctors are often too knife happy to suit me—better to trust in some of the botanical creations of the Almighty.

Conservative herbal treatment might begin with saw palmetto, for which there is documented evidence that it works good for BPH. A randomized, double-blind, placebo-controlled study of 30 male volunteers experiencing BPH, were treated with an herbal extract or given a look-a-like placebo. Those receiving the saw palmetto had diminished enlargement, while the control group did not. It is suggested that up to four capsules a day of this herb be taken for this problem.

Pumpkin seeds are also quite useful for BPH. They can be purchased whole and thoroughly and slowly chewed before swallowing. An easier method, of course, is to take the encapsulated form (3 capsules twice daily). But the careful mastication of two tablespoons of pumpkin seeds is the preferred way to go for something like this. A popular herbal prostate medicine sold in German apothecaries under the name of Prostamed (from Klein Pharmaceuticals) contains not only pumpkin seed in the form of pumpkin globulin in pumpkin seed flour, but also has fluid extracts of goldenrod and aspen leaves in it.

Because pumpkin seeds are rich in the trace mineral zinc, they are able to benefit the prostate a lot. Zinc by itself is very helpful, too, when it comes to problems affecting this glandular organ of the body. James F. Balch, M.D., a nationally recognized urologist and co-author of the health best-seller, *Prescription for Nutritional Healing* (Garden City Park, NY: Avery Publishing Group, Inc., 1990; p. 272) proclaimed it as the *first and most essential* nutrient for all prostate disorders. He prescribed 80 mg. daily.

An excellent herbal combination of stinging nettle, couch or quack grass, and hyssop works good for BPH, too. Add one tablespoon each of the above herbs to one-half quart of boiling water. Stir, cover with lid, set aside and steep for 30 minutes. Drink 2–3 cups a day in between meals.

"DESIGNER FOODS" THERAPY IN THE TREATMENT OF PROSTATIC CANCER

I am indebted to Dr. Robert Buist of Manly, New South Wales, Australia for sharing with me the following case study sometime in 1992. He is a licensed osteopath and chiropractor and has treated numerous cases of prostate cancer with natural food therapy, believing that it is the best approach to a problem so severe as this.

"Ray, 67 years of age, had a history of prostate operations during 1984 after a biopsy revealed precancerous cells. Following surgery (and radiation during the first weeks of 1985) the PSA (prostate specific antigen) remained below 10 ng/ml (nanograms per milliliter) until April 4, 1990 when a routine check revealed an elevated PSA of 75 ng/ml. A whole body bone scan, taken on June 8 indicated extensive metastic involvement of the bone. This was largely confined to the axial skeleton, although there was one area of metastic disease involving the right femoral trochanter.

"After a lecture that I had given several months previously, Ray had noted that I suggested raw foods and the PriMale Energy formula (6 tablets daily) from Trace Minerals Research of Utah, U.S.A. [See Product Appendix for further information.] As he was dropping [in] weight, he incorporated the foods I had prescribed into his diet (this started on June 14, 1990). One week later he had an orchidectomy [excision of one or both testes], followed by a nine-day course of estrogen while still maintaining a raw fruit and vegetable diet.

"On July 13, his PSA had dropped to 3.1 ng/ml and at this stage he stayed at a health farm in Queensland for several weeks while still maintaining my prescribed diet of raw fruit and vegetables. In addition, I had him drink some wheatgrass juice from Pines of Lawrence, Kansas, USA [see Product Appendix]. He also had enemas. He noticed that his weight had dropped from 71 kg [kilograms] to 61 kg and that there was a noticeable loss of muscle strength.

"When Ray came to my consulting rooms on August 8, I modified his daily nutritional support. I had him combine two parts [two tablespoons] of Pines organic beet root juice powder with five parts of Pines wheat grass juice powder. I also suggested that a pinch of Pines rhubarb juice powder be added with each mixture as well. I held his PriMale Energy at their previous intake levels. But I added calcium orotate at 400 mg. twice daily. I also put him on pancreatic enzymes, an animal glandular supplement sold down here under the name of Bioglan Panazyme [but any brand will suffice]. He took four of these tablets each day. I then added four papaya tablets to help improve his digestion so he could start regaining some of his lost muscle weight.

"Ray's PSA had dropped to 0.1 ng/ml by September 12, 1990 and was down to 0 by December 7th, where it has remained ever since.

"During a nutritional checkup at my clinic in May 1991, he had gained weight and muscle strength. The PSA still remained at 0. His PAP (prostatic acid phosphatase) was 1.5 ng/ml, which was well within the normal range of up to 3.5 ng/ml for cancer cases like this. A report accompanying his total body scan May 29, 1991, in part, read as follows: ' . . . The study is normal. There is no [further] scan evidence of metastic disease.' This was certainly a very excellent result in view of the previous June 8, 1990 scan which indicated 'extensive metastic involvement of bone.'

"Following the successful outcome with Ray's 'designer foods' therapy, I put other older male patients suffering from similar prostatic cancers on the same rigid program. They, too, experienced noticeable and significant improvements just as my first patient had done." Dr. Buist included a more complete list of Ray's diet, other than those things which have already been cited and have no need of being repeated again.

Ray's Diet

NOTE: This excludes the items which have been previously mentioned.

1. *Breakfast:*

        Watermelon (one large dinner plate piled high)

        Cantaloupe (rock melon)

        Honey dew melon

2. *Lunch* (varies with the season):

Two Bananas	One Orange
One Mango	One Peach
One Apple	One Pear

A soup plate of fruit salad containing pineapple, kiwi fruit, strawberries, passion fruit (varies with the season).

3. *Dinner:*

        One heaped plate of salad, consisting of:

        Mixed vegetables (cabbage, cauliflower, corn, onion, garlic, etc) in a marinade.

        Tomatoes

        Cucumbers

        Green peppers

        Pumpkin, grated

        Snow peas

        Carrots, grated

        Lettuce

        Celery

        Spinach

        Sprouts, home grown (alfalfa, mung beans, fenugreek)

        Nut Sauces

        Tabbouleh, homemade

        Avocado sauce

        Kelp powder

To this salad he later added the following cooked items (**cooked food eaten after raw food**):

Lightly steamed potatoes and asparagus, cooked beetroot in cider vinegar, lavash flat bread (unleavened), spread with tahini, steamed fish in lemon juice and poached eggs.

4. *Extras between meals:*

Boiled brown rice

Mixture of barley, rice, millet flakes and buckwheat kernels soaked in water overnight and eaten an hour after breakfast with orange juice.

Acidophilus yogurt

Organic eggs eaten raw in orange juice—two per week.

Fish fillets, eaten raw after soaking in lemon juice—two per week.

One teaspoon of black molasses per day (because he felt like it).

Peppermint tea

Dr. Buist's remarkable nutrition program appeared in an expanded version in an issue of a scientific publication that I once edited and our research center published on a quarterly basis. (See "'Designer Foods' Therapy in the Treatment of Prostatic Cancer: Three Cases Studies" in *Folk Medicine Journal*/Summer 1993 (1:3:181–85). His article was a followup to a report I had already done in a previous issue. See "For Men Only: Your Prostate and Your Health" in *Folk Medicine Journal*/Winter 1993 (1:1:10–21). To order photocopies of both articles, send a check for $10 specifying exactly what you want to: Anthropological Research Center, P.O. Box 11471, Salt Lake City, UT 84147.)

🐉 MENTAL IMAGERY AS PART OF THE HEALING PROCESS

One final item which Dr. Buist sent along is worthy of inclusion here. He asked his first patient to record some of his own thoughts and observations regarding the healing process itself. I include them here just as they appeared in our journal article. The reader may benefit from what the fellow had to say.

RAY'S PERSONAL NOTES
ON USING THE MIND

Affirmation

Believe to the point of certainty that you are getting well. "I have everything to live for and have no intention of dying. Many others have beaten cancer and so will I."

Visualization

I concentrate my mind on the cancer areas so that I feel them being attacked, eaten, wiped out, carried away by the white blood cells . . . or their more easily visualized equivalents. I imagine Pacman eating the cancer cells or a high pressure jet blasting the cancer cells away. However my preference is to visualize cancer-eating ants crawling over the cancer and attacking it fiercely.

I concentrate on the prostate site, then on virtually each individual vertebra in turn. This produces a highly localized feeling which is so strong that it reaches the threshold of pain. It is a mixture of ache, tingle, and pressure. It takes enormous concentration (which often lapses) and it takes at least thirty minutes to "do" my prostate and spine.

My control is such that I can focus first on the front and then on the back of each vertebra. I do this twice a day; first on waking and then following a short rest after lunch. I need to lie on my back in a quiet darkened room.

Meditation and relaxation

I also practice meditation and relaxation but tend to fall asleep. I avoid, as far as possible, any mental stress—no deadlines, no frustrations, jobs can wait.

Possible causative factors

- The loss of a son in Vietnam.
- The tensions and frustrations associated with my job.
- Early exposure to many chemicals during university days and later in teaching science.

- Exposure to herbicides, pesticides, and diesel exhaust gases when we ran a cattle property from '71 to '86.

Side effects of the new lifestyle

- Dilatations are no longer necessary. The flow remains excellent. This might be coincidental.
- I seem to need less sleep and I am fully alert on waking.
- Bowel movements are always easy and complete.
- I no longer wear glasses when driving and a chronic tinea problem has disappeared. These changes might also be coincidental.

5

Senility Savers

"STOP FRETTING OVER FORGETTING WITH SOME
SIMPLE TIPS AND A LITTLE EFFORT"

🦃 MEMORY LOSS NATURAL FOR OLD AGE

Senility is pretty much synonymous with aging—the older you
become, the more likely you're apt to forget things. Doctors
define this condition as the physical and mental deterioration
usually associated with the advancement of years.

Can't remember your new neighbor's first name? Or your
wedding anniversary anymore? Or where you parked the car?
Or what you went back upstairs to get?

Don't fret about it. Just relax and accept it as part of growing
old. Scientists who study this phenomenon say it's as natural as
the turning of colors in tree leaves during the early autumn.

Periodic forgetfulness doesn't mean you're becoming a candidate for early Alzheimer's; it's more likely you're getting Oldtimers' instead.

I spoke awhile back by phone with Anneliese Pontius, a psychiatrist at Harvard Medical School in Boston. "Senility is just a part of the normal memory system," she noted. "It's nature's defense against too much information. People would go crazy if they didn't blot out all but a tiny fraction of the sights, sounds, and impressions constantly bombarding their brains every single day."

In a new book by Barry Gordon, who runs the Memory Disorders Clinic at Johns Hopkins University in Baltimore, he offers reassurance to Americans who are worried about their leaky memories. According to *Memory: Remembering and Forgetting in Everyday Life*, Gordon writes: "Most complaints of memory loss are not due to Alzheimer's disease. Many people with memory complaints will simply be experiencing normal memory loss due to aging."

Adults remember little, if anything, that happened to them before the tender age of 5. By the time they're thirty-something, they typically begin to experience a drop in memory ability, Dr. Pontius and Gordon both observed. A steeper decline begins in the 60s and gets worse in the 70s and 80s.

There is, of course, a much nicer term for the common condition of senility. Doctors who are sensitive to older patients' needs, now prefer to use the more politically correct term of "Age Associated Memory Impairment" instead. In a 1993 survey by the Dana Foundation of New York, close to 70% of the adults interviewed claimed they experienced varying forms of memory loss. Forgetting whether you locked the door, fed the cat, turned off the stove or made sure the fridge door was closed, were some of the most common complaints.

🦎 WHY PEOPLE FORGET THINGS

Researchers give a variety of reasons for memory impairment in healthy seniors: loss of aging nerve cells, interference from more recent memories, and sheer information overload. Alan Parkin, chairman of the psychology department at the University of Sussex in Great Britain, said old folks have fewer neurons in the front part of their brains, where intellectual functions are concentrated, than younger adults do. "With advancing age, the frontal cortex declines more rapidly than many other parts of the brain," he noted, "and this decline may be responsible for at least some of the memory deficits we observe."

Furthermore, physical and mental functions naturally tend to slow down after years of wear and tear. "With age, our neural mechanisms may not be functioning so well," Gordon wrote in his book. "It could even be a little slower, a little noisier than when you were young." On the other hand, while older folks respond more slowly, their judgment in matters may actually improve. John Blass, a neurologist at the Burke Medical Research Institute in White Plains, New York, told me in a recent telephone conversation that it is "the wisdom which goes with age. Our grandparents respond more slowly these days, but they sure got a lot of common sense to them."

The most significant explanation from such experts is that our memory systems can only hold so much. Because of the massive amount of information they are subjected to on a daily basis, brain cells tend to be used over and over again to carry newer, different memories. As Gordon writes in his book: "The memories that result may well be torn, shredded, stretched, pounded, modified, mixed with other memories, and often changed beyond recognition. Your memories may not get erased, but they may get overwritten and interfered with."

Some memories, however, are best forgotten. These are the ones that carry with them a lot of grief, pain, and personal unhappiness. Also, the differing interests of men and women explain, in part, why they remember things differently. Researchers find that women tend to be better at remembering names, faces, dress, and appearance. Men are better with cars, gadgets, and the position of things in space.

🌿 Use It or Lose It

Just as with muscles, the nerve connections that are the basis of memory grow stronger with use and weaker with disuse. Everytime a person exercises his or her memory in some way, it's comparable to an electrician heavying up the wiring in someone's house. Therefore, say the experts, it's far better to play bridge or work a crossword puzzle than to slump in front of a television set all day. Elderly people in nursing homes do worse on memory tests than those living at home, simply because they're parked in front of turned-on TV sets and left there by attendants, who busy themselves with other things.

Dr. Parkin of Sussex, England, noted that "the brain retains a degree of functional growth and a repair capacity throughout the lifespan that can be induced by stimulating activity. So, be sure to encourage Gramps or Granny to do their crosswords often." Brain cells do not renew themselves as other parts of the body, such as the liver, can do. But to the extent that we use our brains, we can preserve our mental abilities for a much longer period of time.

Many of us have a problem with remembering the names of people we meet. A few simple suggestions can greatly assist us in remembering them better. Having a genuine interest in the person helps; we seldom forget those we like or who impress us in some way. Become better acquainted with the individual upon meeting him or her. Ask the person to repeat his or her name, several times if necessary. Use it in conversation with that person. Upon bidding the individual good-bye, call that person by his or her given name.

Another helpful way is by association. If you can put the person's name into a mental image of some kind, you'll be less likely to forget it. For example, remembering the name of Mary can be hard for some, because it is so common. So by associating it with the first line of a Mother Goose nursery rhyme, "Mary, Mary, quite contrary . . .", you'll be able to recall it better by bringing to mind the "quite contrary" part and then knowing that it rhymes with Mary. Or, how about Tom or Bill? Associate them with a small-headed drum commonly beaten with the hands (called a *tom*-tom) or *bills* that come due the end of the month.

This technique has always worked for Harry Lorayne, author of the book *How to Develop a Super-Power Memory*. With many names that have no meaning to you, you may need to substitute a word that resembles the name (as in "contrary" with "Mary"). It doesn't even matter if your substitute word doesn't exactly match the sound of the name. Your own memory will be better able to recall the name from the association. And when you make up your own words and pictures, the impression is much stronger. For example, you have just been introduced to a Mrs. Bettina Auchincloss. You might substitute *button organgloss*. Then visualize a button bouncing back and forth over the keys of an organ. By practicing such techniques diligently for awhile, you'll be amazed at just how well they work for you.

Memorizing lists is quite another matter, though. A simple method you can employ is called the link system. Here is basically how it works: You form a visual image for each item in the list and then associate the image for the first item with the image for the second item, then do the same for the second and third items, and so forth. For instance, you have to get five items at the supermarket: milk, bread, a light bulb, onions, and ice cream. Start by linking milk to bread. Imagine yourself pouring some warm milk over broken pieces of white bread in a bowl. Following this association, continue on with the next items. Associate the light bulb with any idea that occurs in your brain. This is usually what cartoonists do when any of their various comic strip characters come up with a brilliant idea; they will draw the outline of a light bulb above their character in a balloon space and then connect that with the head of the same character. Think of an idea like a light bulb going on in the mind somewhere; by carrying this mental cartoon image with you to the store you'll remember to buy that item when you get there.

Branching off from the light bulb, then imagine that same bulb becoming rounder and more squat in shape. Picture yourself crying over this kind of bulb, and you immediately have the mental image of an onion *bulb* before you. This *morphing* or transformation of a light bulb into an onion bulb is easy and stays with you. Finally, the ice cream is simple to remember: just imagine *yourself* (I) *screaming* (scream) at the top of your lungs: This "I scream!" image won't let you forget to pick up some ice cream, too.

You can use this same method to form lists of your own. Make them as long as you like. Bear in mind, though, that to make the association more memorable, you should inject some humor or outlandish comparisons. Putting a little action into some of those pictures, helps too. Now some may object to this method taking longer than by simply memorizing the list. But it usually takes more time to explain than to use. Once you've practiced this enough, you'll be forming similar associations with many different things quite easily. By doing so, your own recall, as well as speed of learning, will have greatly improved, especially if you've done this *with* a coherent system of some kind. When 15 people were asked to remember a list of 15 random items without the benefit of a system, their average score was 8.5. But by using a system of linking visual associations on another list, the same group averaged 14.3. Of course, if you remember to take a *written* list of these same items when you go shopping, that will give you a score of 15 or 100%!

🦌 HERBS TO THE RESCUE

Finally, two herbs which will greatly assist in sharpening your mental skills as you grow older, are ginkgo biloba and gotu kola. Ever since I've been taking them for the past several years, I've been astonished at just how much more I've been able to remember and how more quickly my mental recall has become.

Both are quite safe and available at all health food stores or herb shops. I prefer to take the product called Ginkgo Biloba Plus from Wakunaga (makers of Kyolic Garlic), since it seems to work better for me than any similar product I've ever tried. I usually take 2 or 3 capsules every morning with water. This permits more blood to circulate through my brain, thereby providing better nourishment for my tired brain cells. I'm never without it. (See Product Appendix for more information.)

The other herb is a weed common throughout Southeast Asia. This is gotu kola. In one of my other books, *Heinerman's Encyclopedia of Healing Herbs and Spices* (Englewood Cliffs, NJ: Prentice Hall, 1996), I cite clinical evidence from India (pages 266–67) to show that gotu kola greatly enhanced the learning abilities of mentally impaired children. To quote from the medical report I cited there: [Gotu kola] "increased [their] powers of concentration and attention" [span]. Again, it seems to work on the circulatory system to accomplish this, but in a slightly different way than ginkgo biloba does. I also take two capsules of this herb along with Wakunaga's Gingko Biloba Plus.

It's a smart thing to do. And, I believe, will greatly enhance your mental powers of concentration and remembering. These are two wonderful botanical products that can rescue your worn out brain cells from the senility that accompanies old age.

Sexual Vitality

"SOME SECRETS TO ANTHONY QUINN'S LOVE MAKING SUCCESS AT AGE 81"

 ### DANCING WITH HIS OWN DEMONS

For decades, famed silver screen actor Anthony Quinn carried secrets. But recently he found some relief in being able to discuss them freely in public for the first time. The man who is best remembered for his starring role in the classic motion picture *Zorba the Greek* turned 81 in 1996. He admitted to having a dozen kids by five women. He claimed his children were scattered all over the world.

Quinn dubs his three sons—two by the same woman in Germany, and one by a *"mademoiselle* of some distinction" in

France (as he coyly phrased it)—"my biological accidents." In his soul-baring book, he went on to say: "I imagine there's a lot of guys who have similar biological accidents and won't own up to it because it might hurt their careers. A lot of people in Hollywood—Orson Welles, John Houston—lived these extracurricular lives. But at least I own up to mine."

Quinn put much of the blame on Hollywood for his wayward ways with women. "How was I able to resist falling in love with every beautiful leading lady they brought me, when I had to pretend I was loving them in front of the camera?" he asked a reporter with a puzzled look.

His straight-forward autobiography which appeared in mid-1995 was called *One Man Tango* New York: HarperCollins, 1995). In it the actor recounted his life from dirt-poor beginnings in Mexico through two marriages to the July, 1993 birth of his young daughter Antonia with then-current love interest Kathy Benvin, 32, who was once his secretary.

🎇 How Did He Do It at 78?

The reporter who interviewed Anthony Quinn wondered how on earth this man was able to father his last child at the remarkable age of 78? Okay, so admittedly the guy still had enough of what it takes to sire posterity well into his advanced years. But the more deeply probing question is "How did he manage to make love with such physical gusto?" After all, most guys his age are usually impotent by then and suffering from low self-esteem, not to mention a quashed sexual ego.

"Tony" (as he likes to be called) got serious during this part of the interview and shared with the reporter from an Italian tabloid some of his own health "secrets" for preventing and overcoming repressed sexual activity, especially in the areas of maintaining an erection, halting premature ejaculation, and ejaculating at the appropriate moment.

Quinn is gung-ho when it comes to natural foods, supplements, and herbs. He insisted that *boiled* beef tongue or *baked* beef liver were just the ticket for "getting in the right mood" and being able to "perform on cue" as Nature intended it to happen when people of the opposite sex were intimately attracted to each other. The beef tongue, after being boiled for a couple of hours, was plunged into cold water to cool, and then had the tough outer membrane peeled away with a sharp knife. After being refrigerated for some hours, it was ready to slice. Tony claimed it made "terrific sandwiches," which made for even greater "conquests in the bedroom." The beef liver, on the other hand, "should always be eaten warm, straight out of the oven." "None of this fried crap," he told the reporter. And, oh yes, "always be sure to season the liver lightly with delicate herbs like basil or tarragon, which brings out its flavorful essence." Onions can be thinly sliced and arranged over the liver before it's baked; but he attributed "judicious use" of the other two spices to making this organ meat "real he-man food."

Tony Quinn isn't that big on vitamins or minerals, although he thought (at the time of the interview) that "some vitamin E and a little zinc each day is going to help get things perking," while at the same time flashing a "thumbs-up" sign with one hand to his interviewer. No specific amounts were mentioned in the article that later appeared in one of Rome's major newspapers, *Republica*. But if I were to hazard some sort of a guess for optimal but safe intake, I would probably lean towards 55 I.U. of vitamin E and 50 mg. of zinc every day. The former would be taken in a gelatin capsule, while the latter should be sucked on as a lozenge, instead of being directly swallowed; this way more of it can get into the system.

This actor has always been a big fan of orange juice. "Never can get enough of the *freshly squeezed* kind," he said. "I usually have a nice big glass of it just before I . . " There he trailed off, leaving his interviewer to guess the rest of what he had in mind.

While there is no scientific proof that *fresh* orange juice is going to make you any sexier, nutritionists have told us before that several thousand milligrams of vitamin C every day will keep the sperm from clumping and make it more motile.

🌿 DADDY AT 80

Quinn entered 1995 as an octogenarian grandfather *and daddy* to "my little cutey" two-year-old daughter. "Imagine, at my age," he chuckled, "being both a grandfather and a father all at the same time." He told the reporter he didn't intend giving up making films . . . nor more babies for that matter. "If God wants me to be a father again . . . (thoughtful pause here) . . . Well, I've proven it already, haven't I?" he stated with an enormous grin.

Several other things which will help older men suffering from some form of "crippled sexuality" are as follows:

L-arginine, an amino acid that dramatically increases male sperm count and may prevent premature ejaculation. It is available in health food stores in 500 mg. capsules. Double or triple this amount may be necessary for desired effects.

Ginseng is one of the most popular herbs of all times. It is used extensively throughout the Orient by millions of men for increasing their sexual prowess. The best kind typically sold in most health food stores goes under the brand name of Ginsana. 2–3 capsules an hour before love-making begins is advisable. Also, sipping 1 or 2 cups of *hot* ginseng tea minutes before intercourse will often encourage penile erections in older men.

Certain products from the beehive may be efficacious, too. Two capsules of bee pollen and an equal amount of royal jelly have helped some men and women with their impotency and frigidity problems.

Slenderizing Middle-Aged Spread

"EXCITING SOLUTIONS THAT REALLY WORK"

 ### Not a Myth Anymore

Middle-age spread isn't just another health myth as some would like to believe. As statistics indicate, American women, on average, gain weight with age, and begin to do so even in their 20s and 30s. After menopause the extra pounds tend to roost around their midsections. Moreover, even those who don't put on pounds could eventually witness their waistlines expanding, seemingly for no reason at all.

In early times, this fact of life was met with resignation and a trip to the "matron's" racks at the dress shop. In the last few years, however, health authorities have told women that as their waistlines increase so do their health risks. (Burgeoning buttocks don't seem to have the same effect, though, for some unexplained reason.) If you divide your waist measurement by your hip circumference and come up with a number greater than .8, you're at elevated risk for heart disease and stroke.

Why Women Get Fatter As They Age

Some experts cite evidence that the change in women's bodies is due to a change in their behavior. They invoke evidence that women become more sedentary with increasing age. As a result, not only do they burn fewer calories by exercising, but their resting metabolic rates fall as well.

Others refer to research that implicates menopause more directly. As women might already have guessed, just going through the menstrual cycle consumes extra calories. By some estimates the metabolic rise in the last two weeks of each menstrual cycle accounts for 15,000–20,000 calories a year. Several studies have also determined that postmenopausal women tend to have more fat and less lean tissue than younger women do. Because fat requires fewer calories to maintain, female metabolic rates decline as their fat-to-lean ratios increase.

🌺 EVER WONDER WHY YOUR WAISTLINE SWELLS AS YOU BECOME OLDER?

In a 1991 randomized controlled European trial, a group of post-menopausal women who were assigned to receive hormone-replacement therapy (HRT) tended to develop less abdominal fat than a similar group who drew placebo treatments.

A few investigations have suggested why this may be. One group of European scientists discovered that the enzyme lipoprotein lipase, which is responsible for the growth of fat cells, becomes more active in abdominal cells than in other regions of the body as women pass through menopause and estrogen levels fall. Thus fat is preferentially deposited around the middle.

Another study determined that levels of sex-hormone binding globulin (SHBG) drop after menopause. SHBG is a molecule that attaches to testosterone—the "male" hormone, which is also produced in small quantities in women's ovaries and adrenal glands. With fewer SHBG molecules to take testosterone out of commission, circulating levels may increase—a factor that appears to be associated with the accumulation of upper-body fat in women, much as it is in men.

🌺 THINGS A WOMAN CAN DO

Unfortunately, as women get older they usually have to work harder to hold their ground. The best defenses against the middle-age spread are (yup! you guessed it!) exercise and diet.

EXERCISE. Weight-bearing exercise, a term encompassing almost any activity requiring weights or performed standing up, builds both muscles and bone mass. Aerobic exercise raises metabolic rates. Although you may have to exercise longer to get the same results you did a decade ago, you can be assured that exercise does make a difference. For instance, a 1992 study determined that among sedentary women, those who were postmenopausal had, on average, 26.8 lbs. more fat than premenopausal women who were similarly fit.

While an increase in the ratio of fat to lean tissue appears to be an unavoidable consequence of aging, there is evidence that it remains lower in postmenopausal women who exercise regularly than in sedentary women the same age.

DIET. Although a woman shouldn't be increasing her intake in midlife, restricting calories isn't as important as distributing them properly. The dietary guidelines put forward by the National Research Council offer a reasonable prescription—no more than 30% of calories from fat (including 10% of the total from saturated fat), and copious amounts of fruits, vegetables, and grains.

There is also the important role which spices can play in the diet to help a woman lose some of her middle-age spread. Besides flavoring a wide variety of culinary dishes, spices also help to "reset" a person's "fat thermostat" by nudging up a few degrees higher the internal combustion by which the body chemically "burns" off excess fat. Spices which are helpful for doing this include rosemary, sage, thyme, garlic, onion, marjoram, and turmeric. Another herb (actually a seaweed) kelp would be used, too. It is high in natural iodine, which is important for the regulation of the thyroid gland, which helps the body's metabolism function more smoothly. Kelp may be purchased from supermarkets or health food stores in granules or tablets. Food should be regularly seasoned with it in lieu of using salt or pepper; when this isn't always feasible to do, then two kelp tablets should be taken with a meal.

ESTROGEN. In the Postmenopausal Estrogen/Progestins Interventions (PEPI) Trial, women who took HRT (estrogen alone, estrogen and cyclic or continuous progestin, or estrogen and micronized progesterone) gained significantly *less* weight over three years (an average of just 1.5 lbs.) than those on placebo (3 lbs.). Some doctors interpret this to mean that HRT might actually help to *prevent* middle-age spread.

Herbal sources for estrogenic-like compounds include alfalfa, blach cohosh, red clover, St. Johnswort, and sarsaparilla. These are herbs which have proven to be a definite asset in helping quite a number of women keep their weight down. All of them are readily available from any health food store or herb shop. The simple table below lists the forms and given amounts in which they seem to work best for this.

ALFALFA	Capsules: 8 per day.
BLACK COHOSH	Tincture: 15 drops daily. Capsules: 3 per day.
	Tea: 1 cup every day.
RED CLOVER	Tea: 2 cups daily.
ST. JOHNSWORT	Tincture: 8–10 drops twice daily. Tea: 1 cup every day.
SARSAPARILLA	Capsules: 2–3 daily. Tea: 1 cup daily.

ACCEPTANCE. If you don't have a condition such as diabetes or hypertension, then don't worry. And if you aren't more than 10% over your recommended weight, then stop fretting. If your waist/hip ratio isn't above .8, cease the anxiety. And if maintaining your youthful proportions isn't your top priority, then you may just want to let out your waistband, kick back, and treat yourself to a piece of chocolate cake for a change!

🦁 LOSING 50 POUNDS THE HONEST WAY WITH JOAN LUNDEN

Good Morning America has consistently been the nation's Number One morning variety talk show for a number of years now. It is hosted by the pleasant and easy-going Charlie Gibson and the friendly, effervescent Joan Lunden; they are joined by the dignified news anchor Morton Dean and the witty weatherman Spencer Christian.

For years Ms. Lunden has seen her weight yo-yo up and down by as much as 30 pounds or more. In her new book, *Joan Lunden's Healthy Cooking* (Boston: Little, Brown and Company, Inc., 1996) she recalled early efforts in her "Battle of the Bulge":

For many years, food was my friend *and* my enemy. When I woke up in the morning, one of the first things I thought about was how I would stick to my diet-of-the-week. I went on the Atkins, Scarsdale, grapefruit, high protein, and the one that makes your breath smell bad. I tried every stupid, idiotic diet there ever was. And I'd have a little bit of success. But a diet is a false state of living you can't maintain. I'd lose five pounds and gain back seven. Then I'd find another diet, and start the cycle of frustration once again.

After so much of this seesawing between defeat and victory, Joan decided to take matters into her own hands. With input from program colleagues and friends, plus some of her own research, she came up with a program that helped her lose 50 pounds without proving to be an ordeal in the process.

🦎 TRUTH THAT HURTS ALSO MOTIVATES

As Ms. Lunden tells it, some of her greatest weight gains came after each of three daughters—Jamie, 15, Lindsay, 13, and Sarah, 8—were born. These added pounds ranged from 50 to 70 and, worst of all, didn't drop that significantly after the birth of each child. In her mind, she had figured that she might only gain 20 to 30 pounds, have a 7- or 8-pound baby, then lose an additional 5 to 10 pounds as a result of giving birth, and end up with only a modest 10 or 12 pounds more to shed. But was she ever in for the shock of her life!

Instead of things going the way she had imagined they would, they went in reverse. Following the birth of each daughter, she actually put on far more weight than originally anticipated. After her first daughter, Joan was getting desperate to hide all of her extra weight. So she approached *Good Morning America's* wardrobe consultant, Ellie Dell, and implored her to come up with clothing that would "creatively" hide these unwanted pounds. "I became an expert camouflage dresser," she admitted in her new book.

But this rug of deception got yanked out from under her in a most unexpected and confrontational way. She returned to work three weeks after delivering her second kid and encountered an

ABC Television executive, who wasted no time in getting to his reason for wanting to see her. He told her, quite blatantly, that she looked way too fat and needed to get in shape in a hurry.

Joan reacted instantly on the spot. "I exploded. How dare he say this! Here I was, busting my butt to come back three weeks after having a baby, and he was telling me I should weigh less? I was incredibly defensive because I knew he was right."

The next reality check for her came about in another unanticipated and somewhat embarrassing way. Sometime in 1988 the show's crew went to the Virgin Islands to do two broadcasts from there. After finishing up the second day's show on St. Thomas, everybody had to board a seaplane for the trip back to St. Croix. One of the requirements for boarding, though, was that everyone had to be weighed.

Joan made different excuses to not be first and let the rest of the crew go ahead of her and get on the scales. Even after this, she still fudged until a government official told her , "I'm sorry, Ma'am, but it's a regulation. You *must* get on those scales. There is no other way around this." She did so very reluctantly and must have felt considerable inward shame at having others know what her true weight was.

Following their Caribbean trip, the cast and crew headed for the 1988 Democratic Convention in Atlanta, Georgia. While struggling with a lot of extra luggage for the umpteenth time, Joan remarked to fellow cast member and friend, Spencer Christian, that she really needed to lose some weight. He took the bold and daring step to tell her face-to-face, "Stop talking so much about it and do something for a change!" She agreed then and there to take his advice, and this became the turning point for her in serious weight loss efforts.

🦎 SLOW BUT SURE

She began by choosing all the low-fat items from the hotel room's service menu. Next, she started working out in the hotel gym each day with Spencer after the show was done. The first day was the most discouraging of all for her. "I tried the exercise bike," she wrote, and ended up hating every moment of it. "Let's face it," she admitted, "after not working out for some 20 years, anything would have been hard" at this point. But Spencer stuck by her, offering lots of encouragement and hope. She somehow managed to press forward and stayed with these initial workouts during the entire week of the political convention. Upon returning home, she weighed herself on her bathroom scales and was shocked but delighted "to find that I'd dropped six pounds."

In the fall of that same year, the program's executive producer recommended to Joan that she travel down to Miami, Florida and do a health segment for their television audience from The Spa at Doral. She readily accepted this assignment, looking forward to the bright prospect of shedding more weight. "I came home," she wrote in her book, "down another six or seven pounds—and totally motivated to stay on track."

Soon after this she met Barbara Brandt through her middle daughter, and discovered that this woman was a personalized fitness trainer. "Up to this point, I had only really been concerned with losing weight," she stated. But Ms. Brandt endowed her with something special that most people on weightlosing binges seldom ever have: a fitness *consciousness*.

In her own words, here is how she described this health *psyche* of mind and heart. "My skin was clearer, my eyes were brighter—I felt stronger, healthier, and had more energy. I was no longer in fear of living my life as an overweight, unhappy, unhealthy woman." Just *that* realization alone, she claimed "was like losing 50 pounds." It truly was a defining moment in Ms. Lunden's life.

🌱 Good Nutrition Critical to Successful Weight Loss

Because her knowledge of nutrition was extremely weak, *Good Morning America's* lovely hostess turned to board-certified nutritionist Hermiene Lee, R.D., M.S. One of the first recommendations made was for her to keep a daily food diary for up to several weeks. "I was told to write not only everything I ate on a particular day," she observed, but other things as well normally not connected with a food diary.

These items are worth mentioning here for those willing to discipline themselves enough to keep food journals of their own for a week or more. I've arranged them here just as Ms. Lunden listed them in her own book, but have put them in my own words.

1. Record all periods of hunger.
2. Describe the place you were and activity when cravings came.
3. Mention your thoughts and emotions when stomach growling began.
4. Compare your eating options with your frustration levels.
5. Honestly admit what you really ended up chowing down.
6. Specify time and location of what you consumed (i.e., sitting by TV).
7. Explain your emotional state after eating (i.e., angry, unhappy?).

Joan claimed she "learned a lot" by keeping this food diary for a few weeks. With a record in hand, she discovered, for instance, that she ate more food than she realized. She explained how this came about with her hectic work and home schedules. And once she began tracking her eating patterns from this food diary, she was better able to plan her meals and come to grips with her in-between snacking desires.

It used to be that after finishing a live in-studio shoot of *Good Morning America*, Ms. Lunden would feel a dramatic drop in her energy levels and so resort to munching on doughnuts and danish rolls provided by show personnel. But her qualified nutritionist recommended she purchase a small camper-size fridge for her dressing room and keep it stocked with healthy foods like "fresh fruit, nonfat milk, yogurt, and nonfat cheese." Additionally, she was told to keep nearby crunchy snacks that would allay most of her hunger pangs. "I chose Shredded Wheat," she revealed, because "it has almost no fat, and no added sugar or salt." This is also one of the very same foods that I incorporate into my daily diet, believing it to be one of the healthiest things around because it is such a simple food to begin with.

Ms. Lee reminded her, too, of consuming things she liked, "not just foods you think you're supposed to eat." Many weightloss diets, for example, call for eating water-packed tuna fish, But, by Lunden's own admission, she hated it with a passion. So, why eat it, came the response. The lady nutritionist pointed out that "deprivation will only lead to cheating." She thought it was much better for a dieter "to eat foods you want, but in moderation, and if possible, in lower-fat versions."

It took some time and effort to carefully shop around for the foods she wanted, but that were still good for her to eat. "I now have . . . unfried potato chips, potato skins—things I love, but with the fat taken out," she wrote. "I adore Mexican food and still eat quesadillas; I just use nonfat cheese and nonfat sour cream." In other words, Ms. Lunden became an expert in wise food substitution.

Having two teenagers and a young child in the house didn't make things any easier for her either. She had to *slowly* educate them on the reasons for mommy's different food choices, emphasizing that it wasn't just for dieting only but also for a *healthier lifestyle* for the whole family. The kids reaped nutritional rewards from this, since her kitchen cupboards were no longer "stocked with sodium-filled, fat-filled, sugar-filled junk."

Joan also taught herself and her youngsters—she divorced her husband awhile back—that occasional "food trade-offs" were okay and nothing to feel guilty about. "They eat a low-sugar cereal during the week, but on weekends can have any cereal they choose," she said. "They can still eat mashed potatoes; I just don't make them with cream, salt, and butter."

One very unique feature to Ms. Lunden's remarkable diet and exercise programs are the elements of positive thinking, relaxation, and, most of all, *meditation*. What do these things have to do with cooking anyway, she asked rhetorically in her new cook book. "They're all ingredients in my new healthy lifestyle. And like any good recipe, there are several ingredients that go into making that recipe work. Her ideas on these things can best be summarized this way:

A. Work to build more confidence within yourself.

B. "It's just as important to learn how to slow down," she wrote.

C. Choose those activities that have a quieting effect on your system.

D. Put your thoughts on hold and give your mind a rest with meditation.

❦ Find Cans, Lose Weight; If You Think You Can, Then You Can

One of the most singular weight loss stories I've ever heard in my life came from a man by the name of Clyde Arnold, whom I interviewed in person, while in the city of Spokane, Washington, attending a naturopathic health conference. I met this chap on the street of all places; he was pushing along a large green cart piled high with a dozen gunny sacks crammed full of aluminum cans.

Clyde was then 85 years of age, smoked a pipe, wore glasses, and was outfitted in a khaki shirt, tattered overalls, white socks, and an old pair of gym shoes. He appeared so singular, this cart-pushing grandpa, that I just had to stop out of curiosity, more than anything else, and introduce myself. He gave a cordial greeting back and we shook hands.

Clyde informed me that he had been on the streets ever since his own house burned down sometime in the early 1980s. "I hang my hat over at Summer Manor (a group home for the elderly) sometimes or when it gets too cold to be out on the streets," he said in an almost carefree manner. He noted that he had been doing this particular activity "going on 10 years or better, I suppose."

But, what really struck me with amazement was the old photo of himself that he produced from his wallet. It was taken sometime in 1984 when he was then 75 years old. "Is that *really* you?" I asked in astonishment.

"Yup," he replied back very matter-of-factly. "All *311 pounds* of me! Big cuss, wasn't I?" I could hardly have agreed more.

"What on earth happened between then and now?" I anxiously inquired, while surveying him at a fit and trim 160 pounds. My mind was eager to know that "miracle" food, beverage, herb, or pill this man had taken to get to the slender size he now was. All of my instincts seems to rush forward at once to embrace whatever new or undiscovered "health secrets" he had to tell me.

But, as is so often the case in life, some of the greatest things come wrapped in plain, little packages of ordinary appearance. "I walk a lot," he said.

That's it? That's all there was to it? Talk about an adrenaline let down! I could feel my excitement fizzling fast, but didn't want to show my disappointment. "Oh really?" I asked somewhat incredulously.

"Yup!" came that same self-assured response. "I reckon I do about 27 miles a day. 'Course that don't include slinging all those sacks of cans around either."

As my brain was trying to cope with the simplicity of his statement and attach some greater meaning and value to it, we continued chatting together. He told me that as "long as I'm moving around my arthritis doesn't get to me in my legs." But in the evening when he retires to bed, "then the stiffness slowly sets in and by morning I'm in a lot of pain." He said that getting up and out "is the worst part of starting every day, but I manage to do it anyhow." After a few hours of walking around though, pushing his cart in front of him, "I'm just fine and don't hurt any more after that."

I deliberately shifted our discussion into the area of obesity. "A lot of people spend a small fortune trying a wide variety of diet programs," I observed, "as well as engage themselves in fancy workout exercises in order to shed weight. There's a real 'battle of the bulge' out there as millions of Americans are trying to get rid of big guts, wide hips, large thighs, and flabby buttocks. And here you are, just a common street person collecting cans for a little money to survive on, and you've managed to accomplish something that many others, better educated and economically advantaged than yourself, haven't been able to do. What an irony!"

"Yeh, ain't it?" he laughed. "But picking up cans just isn't for the money alone. It helps to keep me focused and my mind busy so I don't notice how far I've walked every day. I take it slowly and in measured steps. I pace myself every day and make sure I don't wear myself out. This is something I think people need to do more if they expect to walk a lot like I do to get rid of their weight."

Before we parted, I wanted to offer him some money for his time and wisdom, but he casually waved it aside. "Keep your bucks, doc. You'll probably need them for tipping the baggage guys at the airport. I always can get my hands on cash when I need to."

Oh, did he have a bank account or a little stashed away in a mattress somewhere for a rainy day? "Nope, none of them," he stated with emphasis. "In a special place no one knows about, I got me 212 burlap sacks stacked ten feet high and filled with cans just like these here in my cart. Whenever I get broke, I just go to this place and take a load down to Clark's Recycling, where they give me 35¢ a pound for them."

Not bad, I thought, as we parted. Sure beats the heck out of Medicare and a lot healthier for him, too.

THE FASTEST WAY TO BURN FAT

Exercise instructors around the country just love to tout "fat burning" exercises, in which participants go *slower* to get their bodies to run more on fat. Now if that somehow seemed to run against your own intuition, then congratulate yourself. Scientists have now discovered that fast-paced exercise melts away blubber just as easily.

It is true, of course, that during a low-intensity workout the body burns off a little more fat and a tad less carbohydrate than it does during intense activity. But when Georgia State University exercise psychologist Jeffrey Rupp had one group of out-of-shape, somewhat obese women walk on a treadmill while a similar group walked much faster, he learned that the body's different reactions to easy and hard exercise just didn't add up to different results.

Four times a week, the two groups each toiled until they burned exactly 300 calories. And after three months the two groups had lost the same amount of body fat: 3%. So what was his explanation for this? Despite instructors' claims otherwise, the type of calories that a person burns *during* a workout isn't really the issue. "What's important here," he noticed, "is that you've used up calories and created a deficit. Your body then makes up that deficit *later on* by removing fat from your stomach and hips."

So if time is important to you, Rupp claims, then go at it in hard fashion; the faster walkers burned their 300 calories in 30 minutes or less. On the other hand, the slowpokes took almost an hour. Otherwise, walk at the pace you prefer. Rupp's two groups not only lost the same amount of fat, they both ended up equally fit.

🌺 GET MOVING—START WALKING

James M. Rippe, M.D., an associate professor of medicine at Tufts University School of Medicine and director of the Center for Clinical and Lifestyle Medicines in Shrewsbury, Massachusetts, shared the following information in 1995. I am grateful to him for it and feel that it will benefit readers of this book.

"For the last ten years or so," he began, "my research laboratory, first at the University of Massachusetts Medical Center and now affiliated with Tufts University School of Medicine, has studied the multiple health benefits of moderate-intensity walking. Our work, along with the findings of many other researchers, has pointed out some surprising and important positive outcomes from regular walking." He then listed what some of them were:

This exercise lowers the risk of coronary heart disease.

The activity definitely helps control weight.

Walking improves HDL or "good" cholesterol.

It tends to slow down the progress of osteoporosis.

This kind of motion improves a person's mood.

"Combine these benefits with the low risk of injury and the pure sensation of walking," he continued, "and you have the ingredients for a great form of physical activity!

"In my laboratory we have become so interested in the benefits of outdoor walking that we have begun to study it seriously, develop programs and tests for it. We've even coined a new name for the activity: *'Rugged Walking.'*

"By *Rugged Walking* we specifically mean: outdoor, offtrail walking on a variety of surfaces including such terrains as those you'd find in an urban park, campground, state forest or national park, for example.

"*Rugged Walking* carries all of the benefits of regular fitness walking as well as some important additional advantages. Like fitness walking, *Rugged Walking* is also a low-impact activity— with only one to one-and-a-half times body weight impact with each stride compared to three to four times body weight with running or high impact aerobics. *Rugged Walking* on hilly terrains or rough surfaces also provides excellent aerobic benefits, builds strength, and allows you, the walker, to burn an enormous number of calories!

"One of the great virtues of walking is its simplicity. All you really need is a good pair of walking shoes and the proper clothing. Look for light-weight, sturdy construction and good biomechanical design that will help control excessive motion and support the foot during the walking stride. And if you will be doing any *Rugged Walking,* look for shoes that are waterproof and mud resistant and will give you good traction.

"Wear layers to counteract the different conditions you will encounter. You can take layers off as you warm up. Waterproof, breathable fabrics are a must for inclement weather. A hat for warmth and sun protection is important, as are gloves if you'll be walking outdoors in cold weather.

"An important part of any walking program is to start at the right level. This will prevent you from getting injured or discouraged or, if you start at too low a level of activity, from achieving optimal results."

Dr. Rippe was kind enough to tally up the number of calories expended in a three-quarter-hour workout. The results appear in the following table. It shows that *Rugged Walking* can exceed jogging for number of calories burned off.

CALORIES BURNED IN A **45-MINUTE** WORKOUT

Fitness Walking	248
Step Aerobics (6" step)	301
Tennis (vigorous singles)	311
Rugged Walking (mild hills: 5% incline)	338
Jogging (5.5 mph)	455
Rugged Walking (moderate hills: 10% incline)	541
On a rough surface	541

Dr. Rippe finished his short essay on the importance of walking, with these additional comments. "Whether you choose to walk indoors, *Rugged Walking* outdoors or pursue another type of regular physical activity, the point is to become more active. Each of us can find the time in our daily lives to fit in 30 minutes or more of accumulated, pleasant physical activity. By being more active, we're making a commitment to be more healthy. So let's get moving!"

(For additional data on walking, see ALLERGIES/ASTHMA/BRONCHITIS.)

Smooth Skin Sensations

"NUCLEAR SUBMARINE NAVIGATOR FOUND RELIEF FOR RASH WITH TOMATO JUICE"

BEAUTY SECRETS FROM GUATEMALA AND THE PHILIPPINES

A number of years ago while working at an archaeological site near the Honduran-Guatemalan border, I noticed that all of the

Chorti women, who were descendants of the ancient Maya, often rubbed their hair and bodies with an oil to keep them soft and resilient.

Through our interpreter, I learned that they were using avocado oil to keep their skin from getting burned by the hot, glaring sun and the rough elements of wind and rain. They even rubbed some on their lips to keep them nice and moist.

Now some of these Chorti women seemed to be in their late twenties or early thirties. Imagine my utter astonishment when my interpreter informed me that most of them were in their mid to late *fifties!* Now I'm a pretty good judge of age because of my training in anthropology, but their constant use of avocado oil caught me off guard about how old I *imagined* they were.

You too can experience a near smooth skin sensation again by using avocado oil in place of other lotions and creams. Avocado oil is readily available in finer health food stores and nutrition centers. Also, frequently consuming ripe avocados will do the same thing for you, only it will take a little longer to achieve.

Not too long ago I traveled to the Philippines on a fact-finding expedition for more health-giving secrets from common folks. I was introduced to a number of different women in Manila through mutual friends and contacts I had there. Now most of these ladies whom I interviewed with the assistance of interpreters, I *assumed* to be somewhere in their forties.

Oh boy! Was I ever wrong. Each of them giggled in amusement as I guessed 40, 42, 44, 46, or 48. Then they took turns telling me their *true* ages: 55, 57, 59, 61, and 66! Not only was I astonished by what my interpreters told me, but I felt somewhat stupid as well. These women certainly *didn't* look that old from the appearance of their skin tones and textures. I was determined to find out just what they did to stay so young-looking.

When I put forth the question to each and every one of them as to what they ate for keeping their skin surfaces so smooth and soft, they unanimously declared *bananas!* That's right, dear reader—*bananas!* Not only did they eat at least one *ripe* banana a day, but they also mashed one-half a banana and covered their faces at night with this fruit mask, removing it the next morning with a cold water rinse.

Later, after returning home, I mentioned this to a noted cosmetologist, who said it didn't surprise her at all. She pointed out that bananas are rich in various oils, which help to keep the skin from drying out. She thought the banana oils helped to keep the skin more smooth and resilient.

✤ MEDITERRANEAN BEAUTY TIP

I used to wonder for years in my travels around the Mediterranean, how so many *older* women in places like Greece, Sicily, and Corsica, kept their skin so smooth and nice. It finally dawned on me one time in a trip through Italy, that it was the huge consumption of *olive oil* that did the trick for so many of these women.

Ever since that time I have been using olive oil myself on a fairly regular basis, taking at least one amount every few days. I have had a number of women tell me over the years at various conventions, speaking engagements and book signings around the country, that my skin really looks great for a man. They've said that most men (including their own husbands or boyfriends) tend to have rough, dry skin as a rule, but that my skin isn't that way at all. When they've asked me for my secret, I tell them it's the olive oil that has been working so well all this time.

As an afterthought, I probably also should mention that I *don't* use shaving lotion or men's cologne on my skin as I discovered years ago that such things tend to dry the skin out in a big hurry. I'm also a strong advocate of dry brushing the skin, which immediately brings a rush of blood to the surface. This not only feels good, but tends to make the skin tone healthier and give it a more ruddy complexion. I recommend using a natural bristle brush for this and to avoid plastic synthetic kinds as they're not good for the body and can prove to be an irritation instead of a help.

🦎 MISSION SO SECRET HE COULDN'T TELL ME MUCH ABOUT IT

Mitchell Wilkie, age 33, called me on Monday, February 12, 1996 from his home in Lincoln, Nebraska. He had a skin problem that started clearing up after he read about the benefits of drinking tomato juice in one of my books and started following the advice given. But more about that later.

For four years, Mitch served his country faithfully in the United States Navy. He did duty on the U.S.S. Spadefish, one of the military's newest and most powerful nuclear submarines that docks in the naval shipyards at Norfolk, Virginia when it isn't out cruising thousands of feet below the sea. His crew consisted of about 130 men, ten of them being officers. About two dozen of the crew, himself included, were involved in the diving and navigational operations of the sub. When he wasn't doing this, he pulled duty as the supply storekeeper.

Sometime in the early part of 1993, his submarine stayed out for 2¹/₂ months at one time. They went far to the North Pole and broke beneath many feet of frozen ice. He was one of the lucky ones to come up on deck for a few hours. The sky was blue, the sun was shining, there was a gentle wind of 10 to 15 mph., and the temperature was *–30° F. below zero!*

Some military scientists, along for the ride, carried out "a lot of sophisticated radar equipment" and took it some distance away to set up. Mitch told me, "Our mission was so secret, that none of us could ever tell exactly why we were up there at the time. But I can say this—it was equipment designed for 'listening' purposes." He and several other crewmen, heavily clad in snug fur parkas, stood nearby on what he described as "polar bear watch." "If any bears would have wandered by out of curiosity that day," he mentioned, "they would have been very *dead* bears in no time at all."

YOUR JUICE BOOK HELPED MY RASH CLEAR UP

When Mitch got out of the Navy, he returned home to Lincoln and enrolled in college on a Veteran's Education Package, courtesy of Uncle Sam and the American taxpayer. At the time we spoke he was studying to be a travel agent.

Mitch said that a while back, he started breaking out in an "acne-like rash" on parts of his face, neck, and back. He said it wasn't exactly like acne, but close to it. "My mom, who is in her fifties, had broken out with it while I was still in the Navy, but could find no relief for it," he said. "When I came back home, the same thing happened to me eventually. We couldn't figure out what was causing it. No dermatologists could explain the source of the problem. Medicated creams and prescription drugs didn't help one bit either," he admitted.

Then, he received in the mail a piece of printed advertisement promoting my book, *Heinerman's Encyclopedia of Healing Juices*. "I decided to order it and found it to be one of the best juicing books that I've read," he stated. "You mentioned that tomato juice is good for the liver" (see page 258). "I suspected that much of my problem could have something to do with this organ, so I decided to give your recommendation a try."

"At the time I wrote my buddy what to tell his commanding officer, who had a similar skin rash problem," Mitch continued. "I honestly didn't think the other guy would really go through with any of it. I figured he'd think it was all a bunch of nonsense and let it go at that. But, can you believe this, that old fool really gave it a try after my buddy passed the advice on to him. 'Course, there was no way for him to make fresh tomato juice on board a nuclear submarine. But the next time they set out for another month-long excursion beneath the ocean, he ordered and brought along with him from Navy Commissary 4 cases of 'Snappy Tom' (a tomato-based juice for mixing with Bloody Mary or Margarita drinks).

"I don't know how many small cans of this stuff were in each case, but my buddy said in another letter later on, that old Beer-Gut really went through the stuff. And get this—he not only drank it but also actually *bathed his skin* every night in his private quarters with some of it. About the time they surfaced at a port in Norway somewhere, the commander was back to wearing short-sleeved shirts as usual and no cap. Everybody who knew of his previous medical condition, including my buddy, were astonished to see that the patches of red, raised bumps on his head and elbows were gone. In fact, my buddy claimed that his skin looked almost 'as new as a baby's behind'."

Stress Reducers

"RELAXATION TECHNIQUES OF A MIDDLE-AGED OPERA STAR-TURNED-SKI SHOP OWNER"

🦁 OPERA DROVE HIM BATTY

One of America's great ski resort areas is the renovated historic mining town of Park City, Utah. This place marked the end of a 12,400-mile journey for Gary Cole, 50, and his wife, Jana, who left the Seattle area in search of a Rocky Mountain ski area they would feel comfortable in for a winter.

Before their move, Cole had studied music at Western Washington University and received his master's degree in vocal music. Eventually he became an opera singer and practiced for many hours every day at his profession. But "I finally got burned out," he told me in an international telephone interview from Germany during the week of February 5–10, 1996, while on a buying trip there for next winter's new ski wear. "I got so sick of the stuff it nearly drove me batty. That's when I started thinking about maybe teaching ski classes."

Gary and his wife found Sun Valley, Idaho to their liking. But back in 1972 this particular ski resort had minimal snowmaking facilities and they feared the season would be too short. The one at Aspen, Colorado was going through its "hippie movement" at the time, so it wasn't a conducive place to start a family. And Vail "seemed kind of ritzy and expensive," Gary recalled for me.

In the end, "we settled for Park City, with its small-town atmosphere." It was then just beginning to cut its teeth as a ski town, offering a perfect match for Gary and his wife.

❧ GETTING INTO THE WINTER SKIING BUSINESS

During those early years, Cole worked as a ski instructor at the Park City Ski area. This enabled him to make valuable contacts, not just within the ski and real-estate industries, but also with clients who today are avid Cole Sport customers. They proved invaluable in 1980 when a snow drought led him into the real-estate business. Cole peddled condos and second homes for a while before being hired on by a big San Diego developer to open up a ski shop in the Resort Center at the Park City ski base.

While the developer agreed to finance the operator, Cole agreed to run it and headed to Europe to find soft goods—gloves, hats, jackets, pants—they could carry and to get ideas on designing the shop. "This is what I'm over here doing right now," he said from his hotel room in Munich. But in that first trip abroad, "Jana and I traveled around in a rental car looking at all the swank shops on the Swiss-French border, back over through Switzerland and Austria and into Munich," he recalled. With a small tape recorder in hand, "I walked around and talked to myself" whenever he saw an idea or display he liked. "This drew a number of strange stares from quite a few astonished people," he added. "We were noting the different ski apparel lines that we hadn't seen in America. We were looking at shops, how they were laid out, and how they were mechanized."

❧ FIRST MAJOR STRESS AND HOW HE DEALT WITH IT

With hundreds of thousands of dollars in orders in hand, the Coles returned to Park City. But "upon our return," Gary noted, "we were in for the shock of our lives." He and Jana soon learned that their financial partner had totally abandoned the deal even as the store was being put together. "At first the temptation was to pull out and call it quits," he said. "But we figured that was the easy approach. We talked it over and together decided to take the more difficult one instead."

What they did was to essentially "wing it." They took out a large mortgage on their home and sold some additional property on the side. Divine Providence also seems to have played a major role as well. The two winters of 1982–84 were really snowy ones for the Park City area. The onslaught of thousands of new customers enabled Cole Sport to operate without the need for a bank loan.

But before the unexpected "good" weather with all of its snow actually happened, Gary experienced what he described as "a first class stress out of major proportions." There we were with all this new apparel we'd just brought back from Europe, only to discover that our money backer had pulled out of the deal without even notifying us. It was big-time panic for me then."

Cole figured he might have gone over the edge and "become a victim of my own self-created paranoia and anxiety," if it hadn't been for his music. No, not opera, he reassured me, but "rather some classical stuff," something soothing like Beethoven's "Pastoral Symphony," which he claimed "soothed my agitation and calmed my despair."

Gary also decided to try some nutritional supplements. "I took a high-potency B complex in tablet form (3 with a meal) and some Ginsana capsules (2 with a meal) every day." (The Ginsana is a popular brand of ginseng root available in health food stores.) They both seemed to work quite well for alleviating his first major stress crisis.

✿ OTHER IMPROVEMENTS MADE FOR BETTER STRESS MANAGEMENT

Business prospered and in 1987 Cole bought the Park City building that now serves as his six-store chain's flagship. In only $1^{1}/_{2}$ months he closed on the purchase and transformed the structure, which had previously housed a property management business and a family-planning clinic, into a respectable ski shop.

The store underwent another metamorphosis in 1994 when Gary and Jana expanded it from 6,000 square feet to 15,000 square feet. The result was a handsome, open, two-story shop.

Cole's success—more than $1 million in annual sales—is built around just plain "common horse sense," as Gary aptly stated it by phone. He and his top managers are always traveling around the country or elsewhere in the world looking at things. "We've borrowed innovations from other shops. We try harder to please customers than our competitors do. We strive for higher quality merchandise." These are just some of the things that he attributed to the astonishing sales success of his sporting goods chain.

But even with things going great from a material perspective, "you're still faced with stress, even though it may be of a happy kind," he admitted. To cope with that, Cole changed his diet radically. "No wheat, no dairy, no red meat," he mentioned. "More on the fruit and vegetable side. And rice . . . I really enjoy brown rice. I think it's the one food that the body can handle well enough to prepare your system for stress."

"And what about meat?" I asked. Most red meat was definitely out, he countered. "The emphasis with me has been more on fish and chicken." For some reason, he finds that consumption of red meat, dairy products, and wheat "increases my levels of stress dramatically." But since he reformed his diet some years ago, "I've been able to handle almost any stress thrown my way."

Every morning Cole fixes himself several different tea blends. He finds chamomile "very soothing to the system when it's sipped warm." He likes the cooling effects of the menthol in refrigerated peppermint tea, which "calms my anxieties." And, as for the raspberry-mint combination, "it comes to terms with my driving energies in a responsible way," he said with a modest laugh to his voice.

Making any of these teas is quite simple. Pour $1^{1}/_{2}$ cups boiling water over 2 tea bags of chamomile or peppermint; if making the combination, use one tea bag each of the raspberry and peppermint leaves. Let them soak for about 7 minutes in a ceramic mug. They are ready to sip when slightly cooled, but still quite warm. The peppermint works best, he insisted, when it is chilled in the refrigerator for 20 minutes or so.

Another way is to boil two cups of water, then add 1 level teaspoon of any of these coarsely cut herbs. Cover the pot with a lid, set aside, and steep for 20 minutes. Then strain and drink. The peppermint should be cooled in the icebox first before drinking. And when making the combo, add only one-half teaspoon of raspberry and mint.

Music also plays an important part in helping this highly successful businessman to relax. "Some years ago when we still lived in Seattle," he remembered, "I used to sometimes attend the old cathedral on top of Capitol Hill. It was there that I heard one time a Gregorian chant being sung. I fell in love with its hypnotic influence and have since become a strong fan of this type of music. I find that it 'massages' my nerves—if that's an accurate way to describe it—better than anything else I could listen to." Apparently such sounds do for Gary what the constant monotone chanting of Navajo medicine-men does for their feverish-minded and excited patients: it calms both mental and emotional agitations amazingly well.

And, finally, Gary admitted something else that helps him a lot. "Whenever I'm by myself, I love to sing. My wife and I belong to the Community Church in Park City. Often when I need to unwind after a hard day at the store or just after having come off a long trip, like the one I'm on now, I will go to church and sing solos or blend in with the rest of the choir. Singing is for me, one of the most satisfying releases for all of the stresses that can build up in us because of the busy lives we lead."

Stroke Prevention

"HOW THE DISCOVERER OF PLANET PLUTO KEPT
HIMSELF FROM HAVING A STROKE"

 ## "PLANET X" FOUND

Way back in 1930, a young astronomer by the name of Clyde
Tombaugh made an incredible discovery. For some time scientists had felt that there was a mysterious something on the
fringes of our galaxy, but didn't know exactly what to look for.
But Tombaugh found the planet the old-fashioned way by eye-
balling thousands of black-and-white photos of tiny specks in
space with a magnifying glass.

"I was 24 at the time," this crusty curmudgeon told me from
his home near Las Cruces, New Mexico, in a long-distance telephone interview conducted on my brother's birthday of Friday,
March 8, 1996. He was then working at the Lowell Observatory
in Flagstaff, Arizona.

 ## STILL ACTIVE AT 90

Tombaugh is far from rocking chair status. He still keeps up on
his science, reading the latest journals and devouring academ-
ic reports as a blazing fire in a fireplace might do with a cord
of wood. "Don't write me off yet, *sonny!*" he said with characteristic sarcasm. "As long as I'm a kickin', there's still some life
in these old skin and bones. And I don't let *no one* forget it
either."

 ## STROKE-FREE LIFESTYLE

Tombaugh admitted that "other old codgers my age have either
kicked the bucket by now or are so damned paralyzed from stroke

that they can't even wipe their runny noses with a good hand any-more." He attributed his good health to a number of things.

First was his attitude. "Astronomers don't think like other folks do. We tend to keep our sights quite high and our per-spectives very large. We don't deal in narrowmindedness or let our potentials be limited in some way. I also think a lot of that good night air while we're out surveying the heavens with our instruments has something to do with why we live longer than the rest."

Second was his diet. "I *despise* salads with a passion. Were I a rabbit then I might like them. But I'm a guy and just plain hate them." So what does Clyde eat instead? "Well, I'm a sucker for potatoes—just can't seem to get my fill of them. The wife fixes them mashed, baked, and creamed, and I still eat them. I think they're good for you. I have her leave the skins on. I believe you get more potassium that way, which keeps the heart in good health. I also enjoy cooked cereal, usually a small bowl of shred-ded wheat with milk. No fruit in it, just plain old cereal and cow juice. My wife keeps me away from fried things; she thinks they're not good for my health and I'm inclined to agree with her on this point."

Next in line would be his humor. "I try to keep a keen sense of fun about me at all times. I figure that if you don't, your insides will rust up. Humor is the stuff that oils the machinery of the heart and the gears of the mind. It keeps me feeling young, whenever I think of telling something funny.

"When I was a kid I exercised a lot. I was a pole vaulter in high school and did some track. When I grew to manhood I retained my agility for many years. Although I'm now getting a little slower in my step, I still manage to get around pretty good. I think that walking every day has something to do with keeping the heart in good shape."

The final thing he mentioned in avoiding a stroke "is not to worry about the damned thing in the first place. Worrying over it or something else is bound to get you in trouble with yourself. Think well, act well, and you'll be well! That's my motto and I live by it. Well, thanks for your call, and don't go printing any-thing bad about me."

And thus ended my vibrant conversation with one lively astronomer. He may be old, but he sure wasn't dull. What a chat! What a fellow! What a planet that Pluto must be!

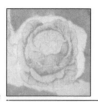

Ulcers Whipped

"63-YEAR-OLD ASSISTANT TO A VETERINARIAN FINDS THE PERFECT SOLUTION"

🌿 ULCERS ARE NOT CAUSED BY STRESS

If there is one thing you need to know about ulcers, then it is this: they are not—repeat *not*—induced by stress! Nor do coffee, spicy food or too much stomach acid produce many ulcers. The real culprit is a spiral-shaped bacterium called *H. pylori* that burrows into the lining of the stomach and duodenum.

Ulcers are an infectious disease, just like pneumonia or strep throat. It turns out that about half of all adults in America are infected with *H. pylori*. Most don't get ulcers. But when ulcers do occur, the bug is usually responsible for 87% of them. The only major exception is ulcers triggered by aspirin and some other types of pain killers.

ACID BLOCKERS ARE ONLY A BAND-AID APPROACH

For millions of Americans afflicted with ulcers, it seems that the front-line treatment of taking acid-blocking drugs such as Tagamet, Zantac and Pepcid AC has been the tried and true one. These medicines will heal an ulcer, but only temporarily. In time, better than 96% of the ulcers eventually recur, and usually with a stronger vengeance than before.

In 1992, articles started appearing in the medical literature about *H. pylori*. Since then there have been over 2,000 published reports about it. This discovery that bacteria can cause stomach ulcers has been labeled by the news media as one of the most amazing medical breakthroughs of this generation. Yet it is only slowly, grudgingly working its way into routine medical practice.

The reason is very simple and will, perhaps, even startle you a little. Most gastroenterologists who treat stomach disorders, get much of their new medical information from drug sales people, instead of journals as one might expect them to. These "detail men" (as they're widely known in the pharmaceutical industry) make numerous office calls on doctors all over the country. And because the aforementioned acid-blocking drugs they were touting had been selling so well, they had no real incentives for calling doctors' attention to an amazing new discovery.

MAKING MEDICAL HISTORY WITH KOALAS AND KANGAROOS

This revolutionary medical discovery happened in, of all places, the "Land Down Under." While working as a pathologist at the Royal Perth Hospital in Australia in the early 1980s, Dr. Barry Marshall (currently with the University of Virginia) and Dr. Robin Warren first observed an odd-looking bacterium in the lining of the digestive system.

To this day, some scientists still marvel at Marshall's talk given at a bacteria conference in Brussels, Belgium in 1983. This then virtually unknown medical researcher got up, described isolating a new bug and then made the incredible announcement that he had discovered the real cause of ulcers.

At first, very few in the medical community bothered to look into his evidence further. And big and small drug companies had little or no incentive to rush into the research themselves to prove his find. But by the early 1990s, the connection between bacteria and ulcers had been indisputably proven.

❧ VETERINARY ASSISTANT PERMANENTLY CURED OF HER OWN ULCERS

Mildred Hodges, aged 63, works as an assistant to a professor of veterinary medicine at a large university in the western United States. About three years ago she began experiencing a gnawing pain in the upper stomach area several hours after eating a meal. Sometimes it would come on as a dull, aching pain instead.

She went to a Health Management Operation (HMO) and was told by the doctor on duty there that her problem was probably caused by her slight overweight or else maybe some stress. "He put me on Tagamet," she related, "saying that it was the standard acid blocker preferred by many doctors. He guaranteed that it would soon clear up."

When that didn't work, she was put on several other brands of common acid-blocking medicines. Each time, she experienced temporary relief "for maybe a couple of months or so" before the pain would come back with even greater intensity. One day another professor at the university where she worked, called her attention to an article in a major medical journal concerning the germ called *Helicobacter pylori*.

She knew then that what she needed wasn't more histamine-2 receptor antagonists such as Tagamet, but something that could cope with the problem directly. Being somewhat disillusioned with doctors by now, she sought my advice in a letter.

I counseled Mildred to use some herbs known for their natural antibiotic effects. These, I said, would help her more than anything else in getting rid of the bacteria for good.

Once a determination had been made through inquiry that she wasn't hypoglycemic or suffering from low blood sugar, I recommended goldenseal root and garlic to her. "You can obtain both of these from your local health food store," I added. It was suggested that she take one capsule of goldenseal root with her noonday or evening meal. I told her that the Japanese made the world's most reputable garlic known as Kyolic. She was to use Kyolic's Formula 105 with vitamins A, C, and E and selenium included with the aged garlic extract—two capsules twice daily with meals. This therapy was to continue for two months, if necessary.

Within $5^1/_2$ weeks, all of her painful symptoms ceased. She went to a different gastroenterologist, who gave her a thorough checkup and pronounced her "completely free" of this nasty stomach bug. She proclaimed the herbs as "a total success" for her recovery and thanked me, accordingly.

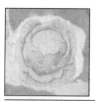

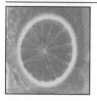

Vision Impairments Improved

"GOSHIUTE INDIAN REMEDY FOR BETTER EYESIGHT"

 PRESERVING NATIVE AMERICAN WISDOM

Some time ago I met Chrissandra Reed, a member of the Ibapah Goshiute tribe. We chatted amicably on the plants her grandmother used to heal people with. But with the exception of one formula written down many years ago, she didn't remember what the rest were.

There was a time, she said, when every tribe member knew how to use the desert as a grocery store, a lumberyard and a pharmacy. Unfortunately, much of that knowledge hasn't been passed on to younger generations. Reed, 38 at the time I spoke with her in 1995, used sage and other plants found on the Ibapah reservation in western Utah for cold remedies and teas.

But she regretted that only a handful of elderly Goshiutes still retain an exhaustive mental catalog of which plants are good for what purposes.

Many people in the 413-member band have been worried for a long time about keeping their 1,000-year-old culture alive. Todd Capson and Elaine Barton were also concerned. The pair of University of Utah scientists wanted to record the diversity of a botanical island in the sea of desert and the way the people who live on that enclave use plants for food, medicine, and spirituality.

But getting on to the reservation was a tough sell. Some tribal members were skeptical when the scientists came to them in 1995 requesting permission to collect plants. "My first impression was that they had run out of resources and so they were coming to us," tribal secretary Genevieve Fields told me.

What persuaded the five-member governing business council was the chance to use the plant collection as a tribal teaching tool. "It's mainly for the benefit of the young people," Fields noted.

Barton and Capson, co-directors of the Sego Ethnobotany Project hoped that someday the collection of 90 specimens would be housed in a cultural center on the reservation somewhere. They have received some funding from the Utah Humanities Council for the project. But most of their work has been on their own time and at their own expense. Their plan is to develop a CD-ROM tutorial that describes how the Goshiutes utilized plants and the role of herbs and flowers in tribal legends.

During the summer of 1995, Capson, a medicinal chemist, and Barton, who has a master's degree in biology education, spent two or three weekends a month on the reservation. Before they began collecting, they talked to older women in the tribe. "We asked them, 'Where do you think a good place would be to pick up plants?' And they pointed us in the direction of 15-Mile Creek," Capson later said.

The pair collected samples and took photographs in the reservation's swath of green at the edge of the western desert in the shadow of the rugged Deep Creek Mountains. When they returned from the hills, they asked the seniors about the plants. Some of the herbs, they were told, have been used in basket-making, some for medicine, and others for spiritual ceremonies. They learned from their native informants that most plants are used in multiple ways.

EYE-SAVING INDIAN FORMULA

Ms. Reed showed me a piece of old paper that had been considerably yellowed with age. "My grandmother had an uncle who wrote down this formula before she died. I don't know if she left any more written records of other formulas. But this one certainly has seen a lot of use over the years."

She noted that all of the herbs in her grandmother's formula were scattered across the Ibapah Reservation. They were collected in the latter part of August to the latter part of September, dried, mixed together, and eventually made into a tea. The eyes were frequently bathed with a strained solution of it; some of the tea was also consumed internally. Judging from the list of ingredients I would venture to say 1 to 2 cups a day would be adequate.

Goshiute Eye Formula

angelica root	1 teaspoon
bluebottle flower or cornflower	1 tablespoon
eyebright herb	1 tablespoon
mule's ear flower (optional)	1 teaspoon
plantain herb	1 tablespoon
wild Oregon grape rootstock	1 teaspoon
yucca root	1 teaspoon

Chrissandra remembered her grandmother putting everything into a coffeepot of water (which she judged to be about a quart, more or less), putting the lid on top, and boiling the contents on a low fire for 20 minutes. After the brew had cooled awhile, she strained it several times before bottling and refrigerating.

She used it to treat a variety of eye problems, ranging from cataracts, conjunctivitis, and diabetic retinopathy to glaucoma, macular degeneration, and weak vision. She recommended that the eyes be washed a couple of times each day and that two cups of the tea be taken internally as well.

Knowing how well ginkgo biloba works in promoting circulation to the eyes and how well it has worked for retinopathy and macular degeneration in Europe, I suggest that some be taken every day in conjunction with the Indian formula. Take 3 capsules of Ginkgo Biloba Plus from Wakunaga of America (see Product Appendix).

When I mentioned one of these ingredients to Barton the biologist later on, he noted that a couple of the alkaloids [nitrogen-based chemical compounds] in the wild Oregon grape rootstock are the same found in over-the-counter eyedrops. Now how's that for Native American plant influence on modern pharmacy?

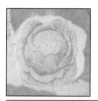

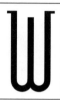

Warts Worn Away

"BRITAIN'S OLDEST HERBALIST (106) HAS 'SURE CURES' FOR WARTS"

🌿 ENGLAND'S OLDEST COLLEGE STUDENT

A friend of mine, who works for the *London Daily Mirror*, recently sent an interesting item to me which came from the Reuters News Service. He enclosed it with his annual Christmas card wishing this American Yankee "Royal Holidays."

Reuters reported at the end of December, 1994 that a British woman named Tabitha Barker had set out to prove that you are never too old to learn. At the incredible age of 106, she had just enrolled at her local college.

Reuters said that this retired herbalist would be taking a course in Reminiscence at Farnborough College of Technology

335

in southern England. The course encouraged students to think of themselves as a living part of history. Senior college lecturer Jennie Espiner remarked, "We couldn't have asked for a more appropriate student."

The feisty and witty Mrs. Barker was asked by Reuters what had been her most popular remedy over the many long decades of her folk medicine practice. She promptly retorted, "Me milkweed salve for warts, of course!" She explained how to squeeze the juice from any broken milkweed stem on to a wart—any wart—and then lightly rub the milky latex into the skin using a circular clockwise motion. Old dandelions picked in the summer and their stems broken for the latex inside, also worked just as well. She said the application should be repeated morning and evening for up to 2 weeks, if necessary.

She claimed 100% success with this. "Had a wart on me nose once, and dabbed some of this on, and it was gone," she said with certainty.

🦟 Banana Cure Works Well

Hector Morales is 62. Several years ago he bought a copy of my national best-seller, *Heinerman's Encyclopedia of Fruits, Vegetables and Herbs* (Prentice Hall, 1988). He read in my book under "banana " how a West Virginia plastic surgeon had cured over 200 cases of warts.

He followed the same procedures outlined in my book. Cut a square half-inch piece of *ripe* or dark banana peel and tape it skin side *down* to the wart. Leave in place for 24 hours, then repeat the same procedure with another piece of *dark* banana peel. Do this for up to a week. An enzymatic action within the near-rotten peel itself will kill the human papillomavirus causing the wart.

He wrote me a letter telling how a wart on the web of skin between his thumb and forefinger disappeared by doing this.

🦟 Additional Remedies

Nutritional therapy has been used by some alternative minded doctors to successfully remove and even prevent the recurrence of warts. A good vitamin B complex (50 mg.) taken 3 times daily is helpful. Also 5,000 mg. vitamin C exerts potent antiviral activity. Vitamin A normalizes the skin and epithelial membranes (i.e., vagina) where warts sometimes occur. Start out with 50,000 I.U. daily for two weeks, then decrease to 25,000 I.U. for the remainder of time.

An especially helpful product is vitamin E. In some of my health books, I've always recommended Rex's Wheat Germ Oil. This is only obtained from a local veterinarian or animal supply house. Internally, between 400-800 I.U. daily can be taken. But some can also be applied externally as well. Hold a cotton ball to the metal rim of the opening and tip the container gently. Don't soak it too much or else you will have a runny mess. Just get it moist enough to apply directly to the wart and hold in place with tape. Repeat same process 24 hours later.

Remember: As one ages, warts and similar skin growths run a *greater* risk of becoming carcinomas. Therefore, it is *imperative* that any suspicious looking wart be immediately examined by a qualified oncologist or dermatologist to determine if it may be malignant or not.

Women's Health Wisdom

"INGENIOUS SOLUTIONS FOR SOME COMMON PROBLEMS"

🌿 HELP FOR HOT FLASHES

In my many years of stomping around the world in search of health secrets for the American public, I've been amazed by one thing. In fact, it would have probably crept by me on little cat's feet almost without notice, had a lady nutritionist not brought it to my attention.

In a discussion once with Jeanie English, Registered Dietitian, on the advantages of the Mediterranean Diet, she commented on how well it seemed to have worked for women periodically experiencing hot flashes. It then set me to thinking about the obvious *lack* of hot flashes among younger women in Greece, Sicily, Corsica, and Italy, where the diet persists the most.

The Mediterranean Diet, as such, is rich in carbohydrates and fiber, low in saturated fats, and high in monounsaturated fat. In food terms, this implies lots of olive oil, wholegrain bread, soups, beans, vegetables, and fruits. In some places, this may also include the regular consumption of cheese and yogurt, and moderate amounts of wine with nearly every meal.

The Harvard Heart Letter (April 1996, pp. 7–8) and the *British Medical Journal* (December 2, 1995, pp. 1457–60) have both reported how the Mediterranean Diet contributes to longevity even among those who've already hit 75. Their implications are plain enough: eat that kind of food more often and you'll add at least 10 to 12 or more years to your life without any health problems to go with them.

 ## VAGINAL DRYNESS ALLEVIATED

I recently came across the following piece of health wisdom for resolving this physical aggravation in a neat and efficient manner. Start consuming more nuts and seeds, eat more avocados, and swallow one teaspoon of extra virgin olive in the morning. Also, it may not be a bad idea to lubricate the vagina with a little bit of the same oil. Simply pour on or dip your finger in a small amount of olive oil before rubbing either side of the vagina with it. Repeat this procedure both in the morning as well as in the evening.

When these things have occasionally been mentioned in health lectures by myself, invariably someone (always a female) will ask in an insistent tone of voice: "How do *you* know if they work? You're not a woman, so how would you know?"

And my classic response has always been to this effect. "It is true that not being a woman does put a man like myself at some obvious disadvantage when discussing strictly female matters like this. But rest assured that I have consulted with the best *female* minds around who are experts in their particular fields of women's health, and have also observed in the field among different native cultures, what women do for this particular condition. Consequently, I've been able to distill the best of all this *female*-derived wisdom down into essential kernels of fact that will be of definite assistance to women everywhere who suffer from vaginal dryness (or anything else particular to a woman's anatomy)."

🌿 VARICOSE VEIN DISAPPEARANCE

The following true story was shared with me by Donn Hecht, age 67, of Miami Beach, Florida. He included it with his lengthy letter to me, dated November 20, 1995. Before getting into the story itself, however, I need to mention that the anecdote has absolutely nothing whatsoever to do with varicose veins. It intrigued Donn to think that a common vegetable like ordinary leaf lettuce could be so wonderful.

He started juicing it up in a Vita-Mix Total Nutrition Center with some other vegetables such as tomato or carrot or a fruit like pineapple or pear. He claimed that after being on this regimen for awhile, he noticed that most of the varicose veins in his legs had simply cleared up. He was baffled but obviously quite pleased with the results. "I drank an average of one small [6 oz.] glass every afternoon," he insisted. The ratio was usually one-third lettuce juice and two-thirds juice of something else. "It really worked for me," he stated.

🌿 A SOLDIER'S STORY

Here is what Mr. Hecht concluded his three-page correspondence with:

" . . . A mysterious experience reported from the Korean War.

"A squad of soldiers were in bad trouble, seperated [sic] from their fellows, with survival seriously in question due to their need to carry a badly wounded soldier. [He] implored them to leave him behind and thereby stand a better chance of saving themselves. In addition to a leg and chest wound, the poor fellow suffered, as is usually the case, from general shock and anxiety, which have been known to be more lethal than bullet wounds.

"As the prospect of escape grew dimmer, as did the wounded soldier's condition, which worsened with each step, they decided on a compromise. Coming upon a lettuce field (rare for that area), it was decided that they would dig a trench-like foxhole, about two feet deep. [They placed] the lad with rations and water in [the] same [hole] over a bed of lettuce leaves. And [covered] him with a blanket of the same [lettuce leaves], in hopes of hiding him from view until proper help might be sent for his rescue.

"As they left, they stopped and looked back, with somber thoughts of guilt, as they feared that lettuce field would surely mark their comrad's [sic] grave.

"Unincumbered [sic], they finally reached a friendly unit five days later, pinpointed the location of the lettuce field, and a rescue team was dispatched.

"To their amazement, what they found was their comrad [sic], not only very much alive, but in such a relaxed state of near euphoria that he appeared to be under sedation—with no apparent fever, or major infection in spite of his wounds.

"In his later accounting, the soldier told of laying still throughout the day, quietly chewing lettuce leaves throughout the night when running out of rations and water, and lining his field jacket with more lettuce leaves to help insulate him from the cold . . . [Also] . . . that soldier's cough, which invited certain detection, [had] subsided completely."

Wrinkle Wrappers

"WHAT WOMEN AROUND THE WORLD HAVE DONE TO MAINTAIN YOUTHFUL-LOOKING SKIN"

❧ SOPHIA'S SECRETS

Sophia Loren is an international star, who at the age of 61 (as of 1996) still looked quite beautiful, rather youthful—and even *sexy!* Believe me, I know, because I went to see her film *Grumpier Old Men,* in which she starred opposite movie veterans Jack Lemmon and Walter Matthau.

So, how does she manage to keep herself looking so great, when you consider that she is a "sun worshipper" every chance she gets. "I adore the sun," she told a reporter, "but have the kind of skin that tans easily. I don't have a tendency to burn, and my skin doesn't get dried out. If you want to have a tan but not ruin your skin with wrinkles, make sure you never allow yourself to get burned."

Sophia also watches her diet very carefully. She eats a lot of cottage cheese and yogurt. "I love melons, grapes, berries, cucumbers—anything with lots of water in it." She thought that this probably had a lot to do with why her skin has stayed so wrinkle-free through the years. "While other women put moisturizers on their skin, I *eat* mine," she said with a mischievous laugh, while at the same time pressing another succulent grape between her lips with a teasing, flirting motion.

Her intake of oils must also have something to do with it as well. "I grew up in the land where olive oil is famously used," she said, making an obvious reference to her native Italy. "I use olive oil a lot. I think it's good for you. And that it keeps the skin young and resilient." She also likes avocados and bananas, both rich in natural fats that are safe for the body. "I think getting your fats that way is better for you."

Then there are the enzymes in her diet. No, she *doesn't* take them in supplement form. Rather she *eats* them in food form often. "I'm crazy about papaya, mangos, and guavas. When they're ripe, they're perfectly delicious. I've discovered that they've kept my skin blemish-free, besides wrinkle-free."

SHUT UP AND TRANCE

Ms. Loren's last and "best kept secret" is her sleep. "I create an aura of tranquillity about me by meditating on things I enjoy," she said. "I tend to get a lot of sleep. I sleep very soundly and without nightmares. I stay away from TV and avoid that temptation as much as possible. I usually go to bed very early, sometimes in the late afternoon, and I sleep till 6:30 the next morning. I believe that an abundance of rest creates for you not only a healthy attitude and emotions, but also a very fine complexion. And, as for sex," she purred in her diminutive and alluring way—"I like to seduce and be seduced in return."

A professor friend of mine in India sent me an article by syndicated columnist Tara Patel which appeared in *The Daily*, a large Bombay newspaper sometime in January 1995. The writer, a woman of some noted literary talent, was writing about the many virtues to be had from meditation.

Now I've read lots of articles on the subject over the years and have amassed a sizable collection of them. But none struck my fancy so much as this did. Ms. Patel was writing about meditation and how it related to the *skin*. She stated that *vipassana* or insight meditation was the best form to practice for this.

"Envision the sky without clouds. Then picture a clear lake. After this look at the outward self from within. Imagine your face—not a blemish, not a mark anywhere to be found. Tell yourself that it is as clear as the moon and fair as the sun. Then if you do this each day for 20 minutes, you will have radiantly healthy skin that belongs on a young maiden instead of a middle-aged matron."

BEAUTY SECRETS FROM MANILA

In the summer of 1994 I went to the Philippines for several weeks for some more health research. While there, I looked up a friend named Gloria Cruz.

But it is not Gloria that I wish to write about. Rather, it has to do with her mom, a woman aged 59, who looked as if she were only 25. I sincerely mean this and am not joking one bit. Here was a lady old enough to be my older sister, who didn't manifest so much as one crease or line on her exceptionally smooth and shiny face. The skin was the most supple and soft I believe I had ever seen.

I was deeply intrigued by her stunning beauty at such a mature age. What was she doing right that so many other women in America, Canada, Europe, Australia, and New Zealand were doing wrong? What were *this* woman's secrets for terrific skin? I *just had* to know and intended not to leave until I found out what they were.

❧ IT'S IN THE LOOFAH AND THE FRUIT

My friend Gloria acted as our translator and the older Mrs. Cruz and I sat down to discuss business. Being somewhat of a shy person by nature, it took her awhile to warm to the idea of a face-to-face chat. Perhaps my over-eagerness to learn her beauty secrets may have had something to do with her feeling uncomfortable. But she handled everything like a trooper and the interview came off without too many glitches.

One of the things which the mother routinely did every morning was to give her skin a *dry* brush rub with a loofah brush. She did it slowly and carefully all over her forehead, face, throat, neck, shoulders, arms, and hands. It took her about half an hour to do this. She told Gloria for me that this removed old, dead skin and brought a healthy pink to the surface as blood circulation inside dramatically increased. She stated that she always felt a tingling exuberance after massaging her skin in this manner.

The next thing out of her mouth took me by total surprise. The woman *never* used any bar soap on her body. She thought it was much too harsh for her skin. Instead, she used a mild—are you ready for this one, dear reader?—*dish detergent*, which was diluted with a little water. Talk about your very own bubble bath! Palmolive and liquid Joy will never be seen in the same light again. And she only used *cold* running water to rinse with. And instead of gently patting her skin dry with a towel as so many women are apt to do, the older Mrs. Cruz rubbed hers vigorously.

The other part to this curious equation lay in the foods she preferred consuming. She ate very little meat, maybe having a small piece of roasted *dog* or boiled *monkey* heart every now and again. But her chief staples centered around rice cooked in different ways and fruit—*lots* of it as a matter of fact! She always ate them fresh and especially *in the morning*. I compiled a short list of what was given to me, but in my haste to scribble it all down—where was my pocket recorder when I needed it?—I may have missed a couple of items.

Fruit Diet For Wrinkle-Free Skin

Avocado	Nectarine
Banana	Nuts
Fig	Orange
Date	Papaya
Grapefruit	Pineapple
Guava	Squash
Mango	Tangerine
Melon	Watermelon

🦁 Hungarian Grandmother's Wrinkle Prevention

I've mentioned my dad's mother Barbara Leibhardt Heinerman in several of my other health encyclopedias. She was born in Temesvar, Hungary, but emigrated with her husband Jacob Heinerman, Sr. and young son George to America in the early part of the 20th century.

She lived well into her 80s and raised me to about the age of six before she passed on. Yet the thing that still sticks in my mind about her after all of these years is the *total lack* of wrinkles on her face. My dad was fond of saying, "Your grandma's face is as smooth as your little behind." Grandmother's approach to this success was entirely different from anything I'd ever encountered.

Every evening I would sit down on the floor in her bedroom to quietly watch her regular preparations. "Oh, you like to see your grandma make herself pretty, do you?" she would often tease me with in her accented English. Grandmother Barbara had a "secret" formula that she used throughout her entire life. It was marked by its naturalness and its extreme simplicity. *She mixed 2 to 4 tablespoons of heavy cream with 1 teaspoon of lemon juice* together in a small dish. Afterwards, she would dip her forefingers into the liquid and then begin applying it to her skin. She would start from her forehead and gradually move downward until all of her neck and throat had been done. She always rubbed in a circular, clockwise motion and made sure to spend extra time around her eyes, nose, and mouth. Whatever was left over, she would rub over her forearms in long strokes and finished the procedure off by a vigorous rub between her hands. Then she'd clap them together and announce, 'Your grandma's done; now you can give her a kiss." At which time I'd get up, go over and put my arms around her neck. She smelled good and her skin always tasted quite flavorful when I gave her a peck on the cheek somewhere. It reminded me of citrusy cream.

❧ QUEEN CLEOPATRA'S HONEY-BASED SKIN CONDITIONERS

One thing that hasn't been lost on federal government numbers counters is the fact that at the turn of the century, *some 76 million baby boomers will start aging.* That's a lot more seniors and a bigger burden to an already overtaxed Social Security system. And it also means there will be a great many more wrinkled women, too.

No wonder Johnson & Johnson was betting the house when the baby-products giant unveiled the first wrinkle cream to be approved by the Food and Drug Administration in mid-February, 1996. According to *The Wall Street Journal* Tuesday, February 13, 1996; p. B–1) this R_x cream "offers J&J rich potential."

Heather Hay, an analyst at J.P. Morgan & Co. in Manhattan said, "Demographically, everything is working in favor of something that diminishes wrinkles. The population is aging, and people need something to make them look young again." The product is called Renova and sells at $60 for a four-to-six month supply.

Maybe someone should tell the top executives at J&J that almost 3,000 years ago, Queen Cleopatra—heralded as "the most beautiful woman in Egypt" at the time—knew what to do for wrinkles and it didn't cost her a fortune either. Her servants-in-waiting bathed her skin every day in ass's milk and honey to keep it luxuriantly soft and smooth.

While you don't need an ass to duplicate this recipe, you will need some honey. I'm giving you two of her famous beauty formulas that kept her looking young enough to entice every man from lofty pharoahs to lusty Roman generals to her side. Regular daily use of both will make your own skin feel and look a lot younger and help to bring out your true, full beauty.

Cleopatra's Honey Mask

Mix one tablespoon of honey with one tablespoon of fine white flour. Add a few drops of rose water, just enough to make a smooth paste that's easy to spread. Cleanse your face thoroughly. Apply the honey mask generously over your entire face except around your eyes. Let the pack remain on your face for half an hour, then remove it with tepid water and a soft cloth. This mask will leave your skin soft as silk and smooth as crushed velvet.

Cleopatra's Honey Hand Cream

Rub together one pound of honey with the yolks of eight farm-fresh eggs. Gradually add one pound of sweet almond oil. Work in a half pound of bitter almonds, powdered. Perfume the mixture with two drams each of Attar of Bergamot and Attar of Cloves. This cream makes a very fine softener for the hands.

Hide the Years and the Wrinkles

One other thing I might add here in closing, but which appears in the final entry following this one, is the use of a very similar mixture by modern women in Sicily, Corsica, and Greece for keeping their skin fairly smooth and supple with the advancing years. Only in those countries, *unrefined* grape juice or white wine is substituted and a 50:50 mixture of both employed.

And the oils themselves can vary from common olive to sesame or sunflower seed. Equal parts of oil and wine are considered to be a better blend for the skin. I've watched older women dip their forefingers into such mixtures and liberally rub them across their foreheads, down the sides of their faces and throats in long strokes or rotating fashion. I'm amazed at how so many of them have stayed youthful looking even into their fifties and sixties with so few wrinkles that you need a magnifying glass to notice them up close.

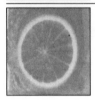

Young Lifestyle

"THINKING YOUNG, STAYING YOUNG"

TEN WAYS TO PUT A SPRING IN YOUR STEP AND A SONG IN YOUR SOUL

Nineteenth-century researchers helped formulate today's basic biomedical approach to disease as they tracked the links between germs and illnesses. People like Louis Pasteur basically had no concepts of the influence of the human psyche upon the well-being of the body itself. Instead, with marvelous ingenuity, they doggedly kept testing for the germ that "made" the disease and then for the vaccine that would thwart the germ.

But lately, medical research has shifted gears and pointed itself in an entirely different direction. An entirely new field has opened up called psychoneuroimmunology, which stresses that there is a definite link between states of mind (the psycho part), the brain (the neuro aspect), and the immune system (the immuno link). In short, the mind can affect the body for better or worse, younger or older.

The medical publication entitled *Advances: The Journal of Mind-Body Health* (Subscription Dept. AVN, POB 3000, Denville, NJ 07834; published quarterly at $49 a year), is a good place to start. Two issues in particular (Fall 1994 and Winter 1996) were both devoted almost exclusively to "New Directions in Psychoneuroimmunology." It is from these and several other related journal articles that the following data have been extrapolated.

In a telephone conversation sometime ago with Dr. Robert N. Butler, chairman of geriatrics at Mt. Sinai Medical School in New York City, he noted that a number of studies have demonstrated that "people have a lot of control over aging and better health when their attitudes and behavior are right." He thought that if people could change the way they think, "it is entirely possible to actually *slow* down the biological aging process."

With his assistance and the two issues of the foregoing mentioned medical journal, I've compiled ten ways to help you, the reader, get back on the correct track to *thinking* young again.

1. ADOPT NEW BELIEFS. People who have "tunnel vision" and refuse to recognize new things, will invariably turn old, get sick, and die in misery. Mental and emotional stagnation set in, and they eventually "wither on the vine" and soon pass away. Open yourself up to new concepts. Not only will it stimulate your mental energy, but will also provide you with a sense of renewal throughout the rest of your life.

2. ACT HAPPY. According to David Myers, Ph.D., a professor of psychology at Hope College in Holland, Michigan, *acting* happy could ultimately help you to *become* happier. In his book, *The Pursuit of Happiness* (New York: Avon, 1993), he wrote: "You can't just sit around waiting for the inspiration to become happier to strike you. Rather, you need to get up and start acting more like happy people act, talking like happy people talk."

3. TAKE CONTROL OF YOUR OWN DESTINY. Studies have revealed that people who have control over their own environments live twice as long and have happier lives than those who are controlled by the circumstances around them. But, realistically, you need to know and accept just what can actually be controlled and what can't.

4. ALWAYS EXPECT THE BEST. Negative thinking can get you sick more often and even decreases longevity. For instance, a group of 99 Harvard University graduates were followed for 35 years. Those who explained their misfortunes and disappointments in an optimistic way tended to have better health later in life than did their pessimistic classmates. Don't ever ignore the positive. Try to hone in on your negative thoughts and feelings and bring them into perspective. Ask yourself this question: "Is this or that *really* so bad that it can't ever be rectified somehow? Isn't it possible to look for hope at the end of this dark (situation) tunnel?" Invariably you will find that *nothing*, and I *do* mean *n-o-t-h-i-n-g*, is ever that bad that it can't, with a little time and patience, become brighter and better for you in the long run.

5. DON'T SWEAT THE SMALL STUFF. Those of us who suffer from chronic anxiety, long periods of pessimism and unremitting tension and anger are more apt to get sick. Many people have learned, usually the hard way, that life is just too short to sweat over the endless minutiae in life with which we're constantly confronted: long lines at the supermarket checkout, traffic gridlock or rude people. Take a reality check next time on yourself. Adopt a policy I've lived with for years: Let most things *slide*. They'll eventually become resolved, one way or another, without you developing anxiety attacks in the meantime.

6. BE OPEN TO NEW OPPORTUNITIES. Trying out new things can be unsettling, if not downright scary. I recall my very *first* public speaking appearance at the tender age of 12. I was asked to give the opening prayer in a Mormon Sunday School meeting in the old Fourth Ward in Provo, Utah (nearby Sears department store). I had written it out ahead of time on a small slip of paper, which I then read from as my head was bowed. Everyone thought it was nice and many even congratulated me afterwards with a pat on the head or verbal praise. That is, all but my ward bishop, who saw what I had done from his seat directly behind me. He took me aside and whispered, "Your prayer was very good, John, but

next time let's try to have it come from the heart instead of a piece of paper, shall we?" He then smiled and walked away, leaving me to my own chagrin for awhile. But I vowed from that hour on that I would *never* again have anything written or prepared whenever called up to speak or pray in public; and so it has been ever since in my lengthy speaking career!

7. CULTIVATE INTIMATE RELATIONSHIPS. Those people I've found to be the most endearing, exciting, and interesting, are the ones who remain open to new relationships. They manifest a positiveness in their lives and, above anything else, *like* to meet new people. As an anthropologist who has studied the cohesiveness of many cultures, I can tell you that one reason today's generation is growing older a lot faster, is because they've lost a sense of their community spirit. They are no longer connected with the tribe they belong to or the village they live in. But those who develop a sincere interest in others, usually experience heightened confidence in themselves and a vibrant attitude.

8. GET HELP. Everyone needs some assistance at one time or another in their lives. But it's difficult to admit it, and even harder to want to seek professional counseling. Still, clearing the air, solving or letting go of a problem is another key to getting and keeping a youthful mindset. One of the main reasons people seldom reach out for help is that they're afraid they can't be helped. Or else they think there is some shame attached to seeking for assistance. People who can't quite cope with life's many frustrations, shouldn't fret or stew. Instead, they should practice a philosophy I incorporated into my own life many years ago: Let slide what you can for the time being and work out the rest, piece by piece and step by step. Confer with someone you can trust—a minister, friend, relative, or psychologist. Seeking a sympathetic ear always seems to help in the tightest of moments.

9. DON'T TAKE LIFE TOO SERIOUSLY. Humor can help to alleviate stress, make us think more creatively, and avoid narrow-mindedness. Often life presents us with the absurd, the silly, or the ridiculous. Look for life's "little ironies," because there are plenty of them around. Or watch nature programs on educational television that show the antics of animals in the wild—otters sliding into the water, bear cubs at play, and chipmunks racing up and down trees always cracks me up when I'm down. The same goes for real live animals: cats and dogs are fun to watch and can be very amusing sometimes.

10. SET A GOAL OR FIND A PURPOSE. People who seem to always live the longest have distinct purposes outside of themselves. They feel an inner sense of self-worth, that is not to be confused with pride or self-esteem. Those who have a passion for life forever see themselves as young (even though their bodies may sometimes act otherwise). Ask yourself these soul-searching questions: What are my values? How can I share them? Who may benefit from them? When you become useful to others, then there is an evident spring in your step and a noticeable song in your soul.

ARE YOU YOUNG AT HEART?

Want to know if you're young or old at heart? Well, the following ten traits of people who think young, and ten traits of those who think old, will tell you which category you fit in the best. Go ahead and answer "yes" or "no" for each one listed. Then, tally up your "yes" answers. The side that has the most affirmative responses will indicate if you're thinking young or old. (I'm indebted to Cal Orey of San Francisco, California, for this arrangement, and thank her most graciously for its inclusion here.)

YOUNG THINKERS	OLD THINKERS
Do you look forward to events and seeing people?	Do you anticipate a negative result?
Are you proactive and initiate actions?	Do you take yourself too seriously?
Do you give others the benefit of the doubt?	Do you lack a sense of humor?
Do you laugh at yourself?	Do you stay stuck in a bad mood?
Do you enjoy a sense of humor?	Are you reclusive and withdrawn socially?
Are you easygoing?	Are you close-minded?
Do you trust other people?	Are you set in your ways?
Are you upbeat?	Are you resistant to change?

YOUNG THINKERS	OLD THINKERS
Are you open to new relationships?	Do you have a sense of bitterness?
Do you engage in new ideas?	Are you closed to new friendships?

❧ HELPFUL HINTS ON HOW TO PUT YOUR AGE ON INDEFINITE HOLD

Believe it or not, you can almost put your age on an indefinite hold for just about as long as you like (assuming, however, you have no current lingering health problem). Here are some hints on how to accomplish the nearly impossible.

A. MUSCLE MASS: Americans tend to lose 6.6 pounds of lean body mass each year, with the rate accelerating after age 50. *Control factor: moderate activity everyday.*

B. STRENGTH: The average person loses 30% of his or her muscles and nerves between age 20 and 70. Strength and size of remaining cells can be increased. *Control factor: intensified exercise everyday.*

C. CALORIES: At age 70 a person needs 500 fewer calories per day to maintain body weight. *Control factor: reduce caloric intake.*

D. BODY FAT: The average 65-year-old sedentary woman's body is 43% fat compared to 25% at age 25. *Control factor: convert fat into muscle by exercising periodically.*

E. BLOOD PRESSURE: Most Americans show an increase of blood pressure with age. *Control factor: Walk more, ride less.*

F. BLOOD-SUGAR TOLERANCE: Some diabetes cases are caused by an increase in body fat and loss of muscle mass. *Control factors: Exercise frequently; avoid sweet things; lose weight, if necessary.*

G. CHOLESTEROL: Bad cholesterol leads to heart disease, good cholesterol helps protect against it. *Control factors: Low fat diet; moderate exercise; daily walking.*

H. TEMPERATURE: The body's ability to regulate temperature declines with age. *Control factors: routine exercise; moderation in eating habits; consumption of more high-fiber foods.*

I. BONE DENSITY: Bones lose mineral content and become weaker with age. *Control factors: Consumption of these health food supplements everyday: Mighty Greens drink mix from Pines; ConcenTrace Trace Mineral Drops from Trace Minerals Research; Badmaev 28 from America's Finest; and Kyo-Ginseng from Wakunaga of America.* (See Product Appendix for further information. Also see under HEALTHY BONES for additional data.)

J. AEROBIC CAPACITY: The body's efficient use of oxygen declines by 30–40% by age 66. *Control factor: Engage in frequent aerobic exercises such as rope-jumping, mini-trampoline bouncing, swimming, jogging, tennis playing, or horseback riding.* (Some of the foregoing material was adapted from *Biomarkers* by William Evans, Ph.D., Irwin H. Rosenberg, M.D., with their permission.)

SCIENTISTS DISCOVER THE "AGING GENE"

In the April, 1996 issue of *Science* journal there appeared an intriguing report prepared by scientists in Seattle, Washington. It told how they had managed to capture and analyze the first human gene thought to be actually involved in aging. The gene, which in mutant form causes a rare premature aging disorder called Werner's syndrome, is "a kind of Holy Grail of aging research," said molecular biologist Gerard Schellenburg, leader of the research effort.

This discovery, the report noted, opens a door toward fundamental understanding of why and how the human body ages. It also is expected to assist scientists to understand the panoply of diseases that typically accompanies old age.

Other scientists have hailed this event as "a very good discovery." They hope it will now permit them to "make rapid progress toward determining if this gene is a factor in normal aging." The discovery of the gene now gives real weight to the belief that aging is caused by DNA damage. However, because aging is a very complex issue, scientists prefer the plural—aging process*es*—instead of the more common single variety—aging process.

Although the Washington researchers aren't quite ready yet to call it a Methuselah gene, they think it plays a pivotal role by resisting the accumulation of genetic errors that are part of aging. The gene has to be working properly, or DNA damage is allowed to build up, making aging accelerate.

🦎 How to Keep the "Aging Gene" Functioning Properly

So now that we know about this one presumed "aging gene," just how does each one of us go about keeping it in a state of good health and from ever turning mutant? The answer is so simple, it's going to surprise you.

Eat less! But be sure to have sufficient protein (preferably soybean, fish, lamb, or veal); adequate amounts of fat (derived most from nuts, seeds, seed oils, avocados, and some dairy cheese/butter); and ample vitamins and minerals (check out the Pines Mighty Greens drink mix or the ConcenTrace Trace Mineral Drops from Trace Minerals Research listed in the Product Appendix). This prescription has always done wonders for the health and longevity of rodents. Might it not work the same for humans?

Way back in 1936 scientists at Cornell University made a star-tling discovery. By placing rats on a very low-calorie diet, they were able to extend the outer limit of the animals' life span by 33%, from three years to four. Clive M. McCay and his research associates subsequently found that rats on low-calorie diets stayed youthful longer and suffered fewer late-life diseases than did their normally fed counterparts. Since the 1930s, caloric restriction has been the *only* intervention definitely shown to have slowed aging in rodents (which are mammals, like us) and in creatures ranging from single-celled protozoans to round worms, fruit flies, and fish.

Obviously, the terrific power of the method begs the question of whether or not it can extend survival and good health in peo-ple. The issue is very much open to discussion at the moment. But the fact remains the approach *does* work in an array of organisms. Also, some intriguing clues from monkeys and humans support this idea quite well. So the answer appears to be "yes."

Below are three separate categories for man, rat, and fish. Each one displays the estimated length of life on a normal diet and a greatly enhanced life span with restricted caloric consumption in place.

HUMAN

Normal Diet

Average life span:	75 years
Maximum life span:	110 years (with a few longlivers beyond this figure)

Caloric Restriction

Average life span:	95 years
Maximum life span:	135 years

WHITE RAT

Normal Diet

Average life span:	23 months
Maximum life span:	33 months

Caloric Restriction

Average life span:	33 months
Maximum life span:	47 months

GUPPY

Normal Diet

Average life span:	33 months
Maximum life span:	54 months

Caloric Restriction

Average life span:	46 months
Maximum life span:	59 months

Studies have been conducted with rhesus and squirrel monkeys and Wistar mice (a common species raised exclusively for laboratory testing), in which comparisons were made between normally fed animals and those reared entirely on low-calorie diets. The latter ones on caloric restricted diets invariably *looked young, were more animated, and seemed healthier all around.* The conclusion to be drawn from these experiments is that by cutting your daily intake of calories, you are also preventing that Methuselah gene in each of us from turning mutant and, thereby, possibly damaging the integrity of your body's DNA structure. And when this preventive step is taken, *you won't age so fast!*

Below are two very different meals: one is a typical supper and the other is a calorie-restricted meal. See which one you would prefer if you intend to be around a long time.

Typical Meal

Beef sirloin (before broiling), 6 oz.

Peas, $1/2$ cup

Carrots, $1/2$ cup

French bread, 2 slices

Butter, $1 1/2$ tablespoons

Lettuce, $1/4$ head

Tomatoes, $1/2$ cup

Salad dressing, 2 tablespoons

Baked potato, 7 oz.

Sour cream, 1 tablespoon

Apple strudel, 1 piece

Sparkling water

Calorie-Restricted Meal

Salmon (before broiling), 3 oz.

Summer squash, 1 cup

Broccoli, 1 stalk

Brown rice, ½ cup

Sweet potato, 4 ounces

Spinach, 1 cup

Soybeans, ¼ cup

Plain yogurt, 3 oz.

Brewer's yeast, 2 tablespoons

Fruit salad, ½ cup

Skim milk, 8 oz.

It will probably take another decade or two before scientists have a clear concept of whether caloric restriction can be as beneficial for humans as it definitely is for rats, mice, and a variety of other creatures. In the meantime researchers studying this intervention are sure to learn much about the nature of aging and to gain ideas about how to slow it. This is according to the conclusion reached by Richard Weindruch in an article he wrote on the very subject of "Caloric Restriction and Aging" for the January, 1996 issue of *Scientific American* (p. 52).

For further reading on the subject, I recommend:

The Retardation of Aging and Disease by Dietary Restriction. Richard Weindruch and Roy L. Walford. (Springfield, IL: Charles C. Thomas, 1988).

Free Radicals in Aging. Edited by Byung P. Yu. (Boca Raton, FL: CRC Press, 1993).

Modulation of Aging Processes by Dietary Restriction. Edited by Byung P. Yu. (Boca Raton, FL: CRC Press, 1994).

❧ CURIOSITY MAKES YOU SUPER YOUNG

Ah, the awe and wonderment of our childhoods, when everything seemed so special and interesting to us at once. When the simple spider's web or caterpillar's silk cocoon held an amazement all to themselves. Those were the years we were intrigued the most with whatever we encountered. Did the tiny snail *really* slide along on a path of slime? Or, why weren't there any gentlemen among all those hungry ladybugs greedily devouring the aphids on the tomato plant leaves?

It was in those precious years of growing up that we were at our best. And at our *youngest*! The curiouser we became, the more we used our imaginations. And the more we imagined, the greater our brain muscles expanded. And with each expansion came a flood of *new* brain cells.

But when we grew up and had learned everything we needed to know, then we ceased to be as easily amazed. Our childhood wonderment slipped away with the encroaching years. The so called "gray (brain) matter" of human intelligence became a little thinner. Brain muscles started to slightly atrophy and fewer new brain cells were produced. *We became old*, but not necessarily wiser.

Truth of the matter is, if you want to stay *super young* and stay as smart as your little grandkids are, then you've got to revive that insatiable curiosity you once had long ago as a child yourself. The *key* to becoming *super young* is to get back *the awe of wonderment* you knew as a kid. It's that plain and simple, and doesn't take a college degree to figure out either.

❧ "DON'T EVER THINK HOW OLD YOU ARE"

Sometime in 1979 I met artist Harry Lieberman at the Akrum, a prestigious gallery in Los Angeles. It was the opening day and there he stood, ramrod straight, shaking hands with about 400 collectors, viewers, reporters, art critics, and one lone anthropologist. Above the goateed gentlemen was a sign which simply read: "Harry Lieberman at age 102: New Works."

He had sometimes been referred to as the American version of Chagall. Lieberman was heralded as a master of the primitive art form. Not bad, I thought to myself, for someone who only started painting at the age of 80.

Mister Lieberman blinked his eyes incredulously when several reporters asked him about his age. "I don't ever call myself 102 years old. I prefer to think of myself as 102 years *mature*. At my years, you tend to age very gracefully, like a good vintage wine."

I elbowed my way through the mob of reporters and posed my own question. He shot back with obvious wit and rugged charm: "Special diet? Hell, I eat any damn thing I can chew. Just so long as it doesn't wiggle on my plate."

"What's that?" he asked another reporter. "Speak up son, you're making yourself look like a jackass mumbling so low that even the flies can't hear you." The poor guy tried again, only this time considerably louder in tone.

"Hmmm," the senior artist sounded as he stroked his gray goatee in contemplative fashion. "I'd like to show the people who *think* they are elderly, that 70, 80, 90 years is *not* old by any means. So, sonny, you want to know the secret to my long life? Well, let me tell everyone this: *'Don't think how old you are.'* Think only of what you would accomplish. In plain words, a person's mind can make him live or make him die."

He then informed us that at age 74, he "retired" from his regular line of work and ended up playing chess every day at the Golden Age Club with "an old codger sicker and unhappier than I was." "Those six years of retirement," he snorted in disgust, "were *the* most miserable six years of my entire life. I didn't know what to do with my time. Hell, I was *bored stiff!* And I came to discover that boredom just about finished me off." (Also see the entry for BOREDOM elsewhere in this text.)

So, he started experimenting with painting. "First it was all by the numbers game," he emphasized. "Then, as I got better, I started becoming more inventive. Finally, I got to master the brush strokes and techniques enough to become rich and famous at 98. But, if anybody intends living for a long time, they'd better not think of how old they are. 'Cause the minute they do is when their bodies begin slowly shutting down. It's like telling all of your internal organs, 'Wow! I'm old . . . guess I'd better quit while I'm ahead.' That's when they start pushing daisies instead of lawn mowers."

Product Appendix

The following companies offer outstanding products designed for the health of consumers everywhere. I recommend them because they are good, because I believe in them, and because I know that *they work*!

PINES INTERNATIONAL, INC.
P.O. Box 1107, Lawrence, KS 66044
1-800-MY-PINES / 913-841-6016 / Fax 913-841-1252

Pines International are makers of the finest vegetable nutrition your body needs—in an instant! Their delicious Mighty Greens drink blend is a nutritious mix of 27 different vegetable powders for quick energy and a younger appearance. They also manufacture an organic Beet Root Juice Powder, Rhubarb Juice Powder, and a Peppermint Powder. They also market the best vitamin C product around—Super C from Native American Nutrition. A portion of the proceeds from this subsidiary goes towards funding of Native American education programs. Pines also sells wheat grass and barley grass juice concentrates in powders or convenient tablets. The company is owned and operated by American farmers in the Midwest.

SABINSA CORPORATION
121 Ethel Road West, Unit 6, Piscataway, NJ 08854
1-800-248-7464 / 908-777-1111 / Fax 908-777-1443

Sabinsa Corporation specializes in natural pharmaceuticals, phytochemicals, and herbal extracts. Right now it's curcuminoid Complex C-3 product from turmeric root that is the world's proven, leading antioxidant. This is based on numerous research studies. It is marketed exclusively through **America's Finest, Inc., 1-800-350-3305.** AFI also markets an herbally enhanced aspirin called Tri-Prin, which delivers fast pain relief and reduces inflammation almost instantly but without causing any stomach upset. AFI also carries the exclusive marketing rights for Badmaev 28, a particular formula developed by the Badmaev family, who were physicians to the old Russian Czars from 1851 to 1918. Badmaev 28 is especially designed to enhance the immune system. AFI also distributes a Male Formula, which is intended primarily for men.

TRACE MINERALS RESEARCH
1990 West 3300 South, Ogden, UT 84401
1-800-624-7145 / 801-731-6051 / Fax 801-731-7985

Trace Minerals Research does something no one else in the entire health food industry has ever managed to achieve—they manufacture nutritional supplements derived exclusively from the health-giving waters of the Great Salt Lake (the largest inland body of sea water in the world). Their top-selling products include ARTH-X Plus for relieving joint and muscle aches and pains; Circu-Ease I & II for improved circulation; ConcenTrace, a complete nutritional supplement; Transcend for women passing through the change of life; Stress-X for coping with life's many challenges; and Inland Sea Water.

VITA-MIX Corporation
8615 Usher Road
Cleveland, OH 44138
1-800-VITAMIX / 216-235-4840 / Fax 216-235-3726

The Vita-Mix Corporation manufactures the world's best whole food machine and juicer under the name of Vita-Mix Total Nutrition Center. Not only is it the simplest machine to operate and the easiest one to clean up afterwards, but it also is the *only* one of its kind in existence to *juice even the fiber.* There is *no* waste of produce at all—*everything,* including very tiny seeds is shredded to microscopic size particles. This way a person can obtain the *whole* benefits of fruits and vegetables the way Nature intended, without losing any of the precious nutrients. More Vita-Mix machines are sold throughout the world than any other commercial juicer around. You won't find a more reputable product of this kind around.

WAKUNAGA OF AMERICA CO., LTD.
23501 Madero
Mission Viejo, CA 92691
1-800-421-2998 / 714-855-2776 / Fax 714-458-2764

When the owners and operators of other present-day garlic companies were still in diapers and just learning to walk, Wakunaga Pharmaceutical Company of Hiroshima, Japan, was also entering its research adolescence with the world's premier selling, *odorless* garlic called Kyolic. I've personally used and have recommended this particular garlic product now for a number of years to more than a million people through my many published books (50 to date), hundreds of published magazine articles, numerous lectures and countless talk radio shows. Wakunaga has Kyolic Garlic available in a number of different formulas—I prefer their liquid Kyolic and Kyolic EPA. They also make a superior garlic-ginseng product called Kyo-Ginseng and an outstanding ginkgo biloba-garlic extract called Gingko Biloba Plus. As far as I'm concerned the Japanese wrote *the* book on the *perfect* garlic product—Kyolic Garlic! All other brands are just cheap imitations of the real thing!

Index